PSYCHOLOGY FOR NURSES AND THE CARING PROFESSIONS

3rd edition

Jan Walker, Sheila Payne, Paula Smith and Nikki Jarrett

Open University Press

Open University Press
McGraw-Hill Education
McGraw-Hill House
Shoppenhangers Road
Maidenhead
Berkshire
SL6 2QL

email: enquiries@openup.co.uk
world wide web: www.openup.co.uk

and Two Penn Plaza, New York, NY 10121-2289, USA

First Published 1996. Reprinted 1997, 1998, 1999, 2000, 2001 (twice), 2002
Second edition published 2004

First published in this third edition 2007 © Jan Walker, Sheila Payne, Paula Smith
and Nikki Jarrett 2007

A catalogue record of this book is available from the British Library

ISBN10: 0 335 22386 9 (pb)   0 335 22385 0 (hb)
ISBN13: 978 0335 22386 2 (pb)   978 0335 22385 5 (hb)

Library of Congress Cataloging-in-Publication Data
CIP data has been applied for

Typeset by RefineCatch Ltd, Bungay, Suffolk
Printed in Finland by WS Bookwell

The *McGraw·Hill* Companies

£24·99

PSYCHOLOGY FOR NURSES AND THE CARING PROFESSIONS

SOCIAL SCIENCE FOR NURSES AND THE CARING PROFESSIONS

Series Editor: Professor Pamela Abbott
Pro-Vice-Chancellor, Glasgow Caledonian University,
Glasgow, Scotland

Current and forthcoming titles

Community Care for Nurses and the Caring Professions
Nigel Malin *et al.*

Epidemiology: An Introduction
Graham Moon, Myles Gould *et al.*

Nursing People in Psychiatric Systems
Chris Stevenson

Research Methods for Nurses and the Caring Professions (2nd edn)
Pamela Abbott and Roger Sapsford

Research into Practice (2nd edn)
Edited by Pamela Abbott and Roger Sapsford

Social Perspectives on Pregnancy and Childbirth for Midwives, Nurses and the Caring Professions
Julie Kent

Social Policy for Nurses and the Caring Professions
Louise Ackers and Pamela Abbott

CONTENTS

Preface ix
Acknowledgements xi

Chapter 1   Psychology in the context of health and social care   1
Key questions   1
Introduction   1
What is psychology?   1
Why is psychology important in health and social care?   2
The importance of working together   3
Current schools of thought in psychology   4
Psychological facts versus psychological theory   9
Research methods in psychology   10
Professionals involved in the prevention, management and
   treatment of psychological problems   15
Psychology in practice: introduction to the scenario   16
Summary of key points   17

Chapter 2   The perception of self and others   19
Key questions   19
Introduction   19
The self-concept   19
Self-esteem   23
Body image   23
Social roles   27
Attitudes   29
Stereotyping, prejudice, stigmatization and discrimination   30
Attribution theory   33
Personality and health   35
Summary of key points   39

Chapter 3   Development and change across the lifespan   41
Key questions   41
Introduction   41
The development of thinking and understanding   42
Social development   49
Development in adolescence   55
Development in adult life   57
Development in later life   59
Approaching life's end   61
Summary of key points   63

Chapter 4	Memory, understanding and information-giving	65
	Key questions	65
	Introduction	65
	Memory	65
	Short-term memory	67
	Long-term memory	70
	Understanding	71
	Mental schemas and scripts	71
	Recall and false memories	73
	Context-specific memories	74
	Forgetting	74
	Memory loss	75
	Communicating effectively with patients	78
	Breaking bad news	80
	Summary of key points	82
Chapter 5	Learning and social learning	84
	Key questions	84
	Introduction	84
	Types of learning	84
	Background to the development of learning theory	85
	Conditioning theories	86
	The importance of fear-reduction in hospital settings	89
	Fear, avoidance and phobias	90
	Operant conditioning	91
	Lifestyle and behaviour	95
	Behaviour modification	96
	Self-modification	98
	Reinforcement or control	100
	Learned helplessness, uncontrollability and depression	100
	Social learning theory	102
	Self-efficacy	103
	Locus of control	104
	Applying behavioural principles to designing a health education programme	106
	Summary of key points	108
Chapter 6	Understanding anxiety, depression and loss	109
	Key questions	109
	Introduction	109
	What is an emotion?	109
	What do we mean by anxiety and how can it be managed?	111
	Comparing different approaches to anxiety and its management	113
	What do we mean by depression and how can it be managed?	116
	Theories of depression and approaches to management	117
	Cognitive Behaviour Therapy (CBT)	121
	Post-traumatic stress disorder (PTSD)	122
	Dealing with loss	124
	Hope	131
	Summary of key points	133

Chapter 7	Social influence and interaction	134
	Key questions	134
	Introduction	134
	Persuasion	134
	Audience influences and effects	140
	Obedience	141
	Conformity	143
	Social desirability	145
	Helping others	146
	Non-verbal communication	148
	Interpersonal skills	149
	Group interaction	153
	Leadership styles	155
	Summary of key points	155
Chapter 8	Stress and coping	157
	Key questions	157
	Introduction	157
	Definitions of stress	158
	The transactional model of stress and coping	159
	Cognitive appraisal	159
	Coping	162
	Review of the transactional model of stress	163
	Stress and stress-related illness (psychoneuroimmunology)	164
	Mediators and moderators of stress and stress-related illness	167
	Social support	171
	Other mediators of appraisal and coping	175
	Stress in different contexts	179
	The reduction and management of stress	182
	Summary of key points	184
Chapter 9	Psychology applied to health and illness	185
	Key questions	185
	Introduction	185
	Defining health, illness and disease	186
	Promoting health and preventing ill health	187
	Social cognition	189
	The health belief model (HBM)	189
	The theory of planned behaviour (TPB)	191
	Stages of change (transtheoretical) model	195
	Self-regulatory theory: the importance of having a goal	198
	The motivational interview	200
	Medical help-seeking	200
	Tertiary prevention: managing illness	201
	Understanding chronic illness	204
	Self-management in chronic illness	207
	Summary of key points	211

Chapter 10   Psychology of pain   213
Key questions   213
Introduction   213
Perceiving and expressing pain   213
Gate control theory of pain   214
Learning to perceive and express pain   216
Psychological principles of pain assessment   219
The aim of pain management   225
Types of pain   226
Psychological issues in acute pain   227
Psychological issues in terminal illness   229
Psychological issues in chronic or persistent benign pain 231
Evidence-based therapies for acute and chronic pain   235
Case Study: Pam   237
Summary of key points   242

Exercises   244
Glossary   246
References   251
Index   269

PREFACE

This book aims to encourage those working in the fields of health and social care to use psychological knowledge to enhance their practice. Topics have been selected to reflect priorities in the delivery of person-centred care, drawing on classical psychological theory and research as well as contemporary developments and applications in health psychology. Our aim throughout is to illustrate how practitioners can apply this knowledge in their everyday work.

The text for this third edition has been comprehensively updated to include new theoretical concepts and contemporary research. We have very carefully selected psychological theory and research that, in our opinion, will enhance practice in health and social care. In preparing this text, we have attempted to retain the strengths of the previous editions while addressing issues raised by students and reviewers. These include reinserting a chapter on pain and including a separate chapter on emotions, where we have relocated loss. In so doing, we have retained the emphasis on normal psychology. We have added some exercises to assist the learning process.

The sequence of chapters has been changed to allow us to build on previous material when presenting complex issues like stress, health and pain. But since each chapter stands alone, readers are free to select chapters or topics in any order and follow suggested links as appropriate. We have included many references to classic works and all have been carefully chosen to illustrate a point. Readers will observe that some topics are more fully referenced than others. This is primarily an introductory text and for ease of reading we have not referenced much of the basic psychological theory and research that can to be found in other introductory psychology textbooks. It is inappropriate to offer a critical review of all aspects of psychology, but we have done so when introducing contentious aspects, and when applying it to more complex issues in health and social care, as in Chapters 8, 9 and 10.

Throughout the text, you will find the following symbols:

⚲ refers to original research

👪 refers to applications of psychological principles to characters who are drawn mainly from the scenario presented in Chapter 1

- A suggested exercise to support each chapter is given after Chapter 10.
- The glossary includes most terms that are unlikely to be familiar to a basic learner or non-psychologist.
- Words given in bold in the text are explained in the glossary.

How you might choose to use this book

Students studying at different academic levels might find the following guide helpful:

First level (UK HE levels 0 and 1)

- Select a relevant chapter.
- Read the questions at the beginning of the chapter.
- Read through the chapter in its entirety, or read at least a whole section, so you don't take statements out of context.
- Follow up links to other chapters and further reading.
- Go back and see if you can answer the questions at the beginning of the chapter. What have you learned that will help you to function more effectively in practice?

Diploma level (UK HE level 2): analysis

- Select a specific issue, topic or question.
- Use chapter headings and index to locate relevant material.
- Read relevant sections, making a note of key references.
- Follow up further reading and referenced articles. Seek help from tutors if these are not available or are difficult to understand.

Degree (UK HE level 3): critical analysis

- Focus on a specific aspect of practice.
- Use the index to identify relevant issues, refresh your memory, identify possible lines of argument, identify key words and seek out relevant references.
- Follow up relevant references and use these as ideas to help develop and conduct your own literature search to find more recent sources of evidence.

Postgraduate level

- If you have not previously studied psychology, use this text to gain an overview of what psychology has to offer in practice.
- If you have some knowledge of psychology, use this text to refresh your memory and gain ideas to assist with your own literature search.

ACKNOWLEDGEMENTS

We would like to thank the nursing students at the University of Southampton who provided constructive feedback on the previous edition. We would also like to thank the reviewers, most notably Tim Ley of the University of Plymouth, whose detailed and helpful comments have made an important contribution to the development of this edition.

PSYCHOLOGY IN THE CONTEXT OF HEALTH AND SOCIAL CARE

- **What is 'psychology' and why is it so important in the context of health and social care?**
- **What do we mean by 'health' and why is psychology central to the effective delivery of health and social care?**
- **What are the main approaches to psychological thinking and research?**
- **Who are psychologists and what do they contribute to the promotion of health and well-being?**

Introduction

This chapter emphasizes the importance of psychology in the context of health and social care. For many years, psychology and the other social sciences were viewed by the medical profession as 'soft sciences', interesting but unimportant. With the advent of research into the links between physical and mental states in the late twentieth and early twenty-first centuries it is now possible to demonstrate that psychology can make a fundamental difference to physical as well as mental health.

In this chapter, we explore the nature of psychology and its relevance to health and social care. We outline the different schools of thought and methods of inquiry in psychology. We seek to distinguish between psychology as an academic discipline and popular notions of psychology, and identify professionals whose practice is mainly concerned with the application of psychology. In order to show how psychology can be applied to health and social care, we introduce a family scenario whose characters appear in examples throughout the book.

What is psychology?

Psychology is the study of human behaviour, thought processes and emotions. It can contribute to our understanding of ourselves and our relationships with other people, if it is applied in an informed way. Health psychology refers to the application of psychological theory and research to promote evidence-based personal and public health. To do this, psychology must take account of the context of people's lives. Certain sets of beliefs and behaviours are risk factors for illness; therefore some knowledge of public health and the public health agenda for change is essential. Those we care for come from a variety of different social and cultural backgrounds that value certain beliefs and behaviours above others. These may place some people at greater or lesser risk of illness than others; therefore some knowledge of sociology is essential. In order to understand the link between psychological and physiological processes, some knowledge of the biomedical sciences is also essential. Therefore psychology sits alongside these other disciplines to make an important contribution to the health and well-being of the population. But it is important to note that the psychology we draw on has evolved entirely from western philosophy, science and research, and may therefore be viewed as specific to western cultures.

Why is psychology important in health and social care?

Those working in the caring professions spend most, if not all, of their working lives interacting with other people. A key part of their job is to promote health and well-being. Most people are familiar with the following definition of health: 'a state of complete physical, mental and social well-being and not merely the absence of disease or infirmity' (WHO 1946). If this is seen as an important goal, those working in health and social care need the knowledge and skills to help people work towards achieving it. There are many ways in which psychological theory and research can contribute to improvements in health and social care including:

- appreciate how people's understandings and needs vary, so that we can try to ensure that the individualized care we provide is both appropriate and optimal;
- gain a better understanding of communication processes so that we can identify ways of improving the therapeutic relationship and work more effectively in interprofessional and inter-agency contexts;
- identify factors that affect how people cope with such situations as acute and chronic illness, pain and **loss**, and the demands of everyday life, so that we can help them, and ourselves, to cope better and reduce the risks of stress-related illness;
- inform us about factors that influence people's lifestyles and what motivates certain **health-related behaviours** such as smoking, dietary change and exercise;
- apply evidence-based **interventions** to enhance health and well-being, and help people to change or modify their lifestyles.

Western medicine emphasizes the importance of evidence-based health care. Whereas much of twentieth-century health psychology was characterized by models and theories, the twenty-first century demands research-based evidence to support these. An important recent contribution to the psychology of health has emerged through a field of study called **psychoneuroimmunology** (pronounced psycho-neuro-immun(e)-ology). Studies now show that our emotions play a key role in the link between the world we inhabit and our immune responses (Chapter 8). This is conceptualized within the '**biopsychosocial**' model of health which emphasizes the complex interaction between biological factors and physiological systems (life sciences), psychological processes (thoughts, feelings, behaviours) and the social and cultural context in which people live and children grow up (see sociology and social policy). This field of study provides strong evidence to support the need for holistic care.

The main purpose of this book is to enable practitioners to apply evidence-based psychology to enhance their therapeutic work, work more effectively with members of the multiprofessional team to promote the health and well-being of patients (or clients) and their caregivers, and preserve their own health and well-being.

The importance of working together

John is aged 9 years. He lives with his unemployed father and alcoholic stepmother. He has diabetes that is well controlled in hospital but poorly controlled at home. His school attendance is poor. He was admitted to hospital in a diabetic coma and found to have an MRSA (methicillin-resistant staphylococcus aureus) infection at his main injection site. He is quiet and compliant.

John's type of problem is not uncommon and serves to highlight the importance of interprofessional and inter-agency working. A few days in hospital treating his infection and controlling his diabetes will save his life but will not promote John's long-term health. Establishing links between school and home and supporting John and his parents under the joint guidance of the doctor, school nurse, psychologist or mental health nurse, and social worker could make a real difference to his future health.

Understanding barriers to integrated care

Holistic care and service provision for someone like John and his family requires an integrated approach. But there are many barriers to overcome and it is helpful to understand why and how these have arisen. The problems go back to the seventeenth century when Descartes, a French philosopher, proposed that body and mind could be understood independently of each other. This is referred to as mind–body '**dualism**'. In medical science, this has legitimized the study of diseases and body systems without focusing on the whole person and is termed '**reductionism**'. This would lead doctors to focus on John's diabetes, rather than the circumstances that lead to poor control over his diabetes. In the human sciences, dualism has led to the separation of the life sciences from the social sciences.

The various health and social care professions have also developed independently, each with their own sets of assumptions and theoretical perspectives. These include medicine, physiotherapy, occupational therapy, midwifery and social work, while nursing has been subdivided into adult, child, mental health and learning disability. Each of these disciplines seeks to explain human responses, predict human needs and/or treat human problems. But they often draw on different bodies of knowledge, including different aspects of psychology. Such differences in knowledge and values can lead to interprofessional conflict. There have been economic separations between health and social services, and hospital and community services in the UK and other countries. These have reinforced the divide between physical treatment and **social supports** with potentially disastrous effects for those with complex physical and mental health and social care needs, such as John and his family.

Within education, divisions have been brought about by the development of a series of unrelated academic disciplines including physiology, psychology and sociology. Each discipline has its own sets of theories, terminology and research methods with which to study the human condition. Within psychology itself, reductionist approaches to the study of the mind meant that people were often studied in isolation from their social context and social groupings. Prior to the twentieth century, the study of the mind was primarily the preserve of philosophers. This changed at the end of the nineteenth century with the emergence of psychology as a scientific discipline, dominated by positivist philosophy. According to **positivism**, human beings are objects of nature, sharing common functions or attributes that can be studied in an objective, scientific way.

Since the early twentieth century, psychological theory and research has developed into different schools of thought, each with its own theorists and researchers, some of whom (humanistic and narrative psychologists) reject positivism and reductionism. Academic psychologists tend to focus on a discrete field of psychology which has its own specialist network of communication via specialist journals and conferences. Thus a psychologist who specializes in one field of study, such as memory, may have little exposure to serious dialogue with those working in other areas of psychology. This makes it very difficult for those wishing to understand and apply psychological theory and research to their work in health or social care in an integrated way. It also means that many psychology textbooks can seem quite fragmented and confusing.

Current schools of thought in psychology

There are five main schools of thought in psychology in which academic psychologists normally work and on which health psychology is based. They are:

1 *Cognitive science* (including cognitive psychology): the study of **cognition** (mental processes) including memory, perception, information processing, psychophysiology, psychoneuroimmunology and **social cognition**.

2 *Behavioural psychology* (based on **behaviourism**): the study of learning by observing the direct effects of external environmental stimuli on behaviour and behaviour change.

3 ***Psychodynamic*** *psychology* (developed from **psychoanalysis**): the study of the influence of childhood experiences on current psychological and emotional states.

4 *Humanistic psychology*: the subjective study of human experience.

5 *Social psychology*: the study of the influence of social settings and social interactions on human behaviour.

Psychology is continuously developing new concepts, theories and methods. A recent addition is the field of '***narrative psychology***', which we have added to this edition. It studies people subjectively through the stories they tell about their lives. Figure 1.1 shows how each of these fields of study relates to different aspects of human experience.

Psychologists working in these different fields of psychology usually agree that people tend to respond in predictable ways in certain clearly defined situations. What they usually disagree about is the theoretical explanation and interpretation of these observations. People working in health or social care may draw on any or all of these approaches, but it is

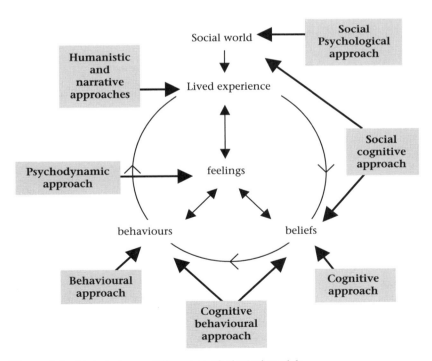

Figure 1.1 Links between different psychological models

helpful to understand the assumptions and principles that underpin them. Therefore we have provided a brief introduction to each one, highlighting where in the book applications are to be found.

Cognitive science

Cognitive psychology is concerned with thought processes. It was originally based on experimental studies of memory, perception and information processing. Until the 1990s, cognitive theories were largely based on assumptions about how information might be transmitted and stored in the brain. More recently, the introduction of brain imaging techniques has enabled psychologists and neuroscientists to map this against brain function. As a result, cognitive psychology has been incorporated into 'cognitive science', which is now the dominant field of academic psychology and closely linked to the biomedical sciences.

Psychologists working in the field of psychoneuroimmunology are increasingly able to make direct links between **psychosocial** processes, immune function, and health and illness (Chapter 8). Social cognition refers to the study of beliefs and attitudes in a social context and currently dominates the psychology of stress and **coping** (Chapter 8) and health behaviour (Chapter 9). In the field of mental health, Aaron Beck is best known for his theory of **depression** (Chapter 6) and the development of cognitive therapy as a treatment for depression. Cognitive behaviour therapy (CBT) currently leads the way in helping people change the way they respond to problems (Chapters 6, 8, 9 and 10).

Behavioural psychology (behaviourism)

Behavioural psychology refers to the study of behaviour change. It is based on the assumption that behaviour change signifies that learning has taken place. Behaviourists did not concern themselves with mental processes since these could not be directly observed. From its beginnings with the work of Pavlov in the early twentieth century, behaviourism grew to prominence during the 1940s to 1970s under the influence of B.F. Skinner, whose theories predicted a direct relationship between behaviour and its consequences in given situations.

Behavioural psychology declined in popularity during the latter part of the twentieth century. Research with animals became unacceptable and some psychologists argued that human mental processes are qualitatively different from those of animals. Most disliked its **'deterministic'** principles, which contradicted the notion of free will. But by then, behavioural research had become more sophisticated and enabled psychologists to draw inferences about the thought processes involved in behaviour change, most notably perceptions of control. These aspects were incorporated into cognitive science and remain influential. Behaviourism's greatest impact has been the development of therapies for fears and phobias (Chapter 5), **anxiety** disorders (Chapter 6), the management of unwanted or challenging behaviours (Chapter 5), and its contribution to CBT (Chapters 8, 9 and 10).

Psychodynamic psychology

Psychoanalysis was founded by Sigmund Freud as a method of inquiry, a theory of mind, and a mode of treatment for complex psychological problems. Freud was a medical doctor who studied neurological problems, moving on to treat physical illnesses that were believed at the time to be manifestations of psychological problems. The correct term for this is **psychogenic** illness (physical illness that has a psychological cause), as distinct from a **psychosomatic** disorder, which refers to a physical illness that has a psychological influence, or vice versa.

Central to Freud's theory was the proposition that certain experiences during childhood are too uncomfortable to remember and are unconsciously 'repressed'. According to Freud, these repressed thoughts, which he proposed were commonly of a sexual nature, eventually give rise to a state of anxiety or depression which may be expressed in terms of physical symptoms. Repressed thoughts may be revealed through dreams, word associations and slips of the tongue. Their release (termed **catharsis**) is an aim of the psychoanalyst.

The terms '**denial**, **repression** and **ego**' entered everyday conversation, but are actually theoretical concepts and not verified facts. Freud's ideas have been influential in psychiatry, clinical psychology and counselling. But many aspects of psychoanalytic theory have been difficult to prove or disprove using scientific methods. Psychoanalytic explanations are usually offered '**post hoc**' (after the event) and some would argue that psychoanalytic theory is therefore unable to fulfil the primary purpose of a theory, which is to *predict* outcomes. This has led to attack from members of the scientific community who regard psychoanalysis as a '**pseudoscience**'. Following Freud's death, psychoanalysis largely gave way to what was termed 'ego' psychology. This gave rise to a number of important developmental and cognitive theories, including theories of lifespan development and **attachment** (Chapter 3), loss (Chapter 6) and coping (Chapter 8).

Psychodynamic psychotherapy evolved from psychoanalysis under the influence of Melanie Klein and others. It retains the notion that many emotional problems are caused by unresolved difficulties in attachment relationships formed in childhood (Chapter 3), and clients are helped to retrieve and resolve difficult or traumatic memories. This approach to therapy has given rise to some concerns about the possibility of introducing false memories (see Chapter 4). Psychodynamic counselling is currently one of the most popular approaches, in western societies, for the treatment of anxiety and depression (Chapter 6).

Humanistic psychology

Humanistic psychology has its origins in existential phenomenology in which causal explanations are of relatively little interest. Humanistic psychologists do not deny the existence of an objective external reality, but are concerned with individual perceptions and interpretations, which are influenced by social and cultural meanings and past experiences. Therefore, individual perceptions may change over time and vary in different social and cultural settings. Psychologists who accept this philosophical view reject the scientific method as an appropriate method of investigation, preferring **qualitative research** methods such as phenomenology. They would argue that there is no single truth, no single 'right way' of doing things, and no 'one size fits all' treatment for emotional problems.

The main focus of humanistic psychology is on the individual's sense of **self** (Chapter 2). An important theoretical contribution to humanistic psychology came from Abraham Maslow in the 1950s. Maslow observed human needs in different settings and used these observations to construct a 'hierarchy of needs' (see Figure 1.2). He predicted that for all people, lower order needs (such as basic needs for food, drink, warmth etc.) must be satisfied before higher order (intellectual) needs can be fulfilled. The pinnacle of achievement is described as **self-actualization**, which means accepting self and others for what they are; the ability to tolerate uncertainty; creativity; the use of problem-centred rather than self-centred approaches to dealing with issues (see Chapter 8); and strong moral and ethical standards. Maslow's hierarchy has provided an important foundation for human services including nursing where it forms the basis of most nursing models. However, it is not popular with academic psychologists because it lacks scientific evidence.

Carl Rogers is best known for the development of humanistic counselling. He trained as a psychoanalyst but eventually rejected that approach. He observed that people who came to him with psychological problems exhibited a natural tendency towards growth and maturity (self-actualization) that enabled them to overcome many of their own problems. He developed non-directive counselling as a therapeutic technique which encouraged people to explore their self-understanding. Humanistic counselling is quite

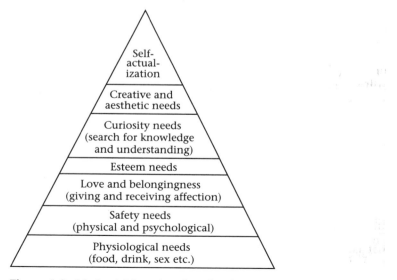

Figure 1.2 Maslow's hierarchy of needs, adapted from Maslow (1970)

different from psychodynamic counselling in that the therapist makes no attempt to interpret the client's problems or direct a course of action. Rogerian counsellors act in a non-judgemental, non-directive way, displaying warmth, empathy and 'unconditional personal regard' towards their clients. These humanistic principles are central to the development of the therapeutic or caring relationship and define the qualities needed by those who seek to work in a holistic and person-centred way.

Social psychology

Much of social psychology lies in a grey area between psychology, sociology and anthropology. It owes much to the work of Erving Goffman, a sociologist and social anthropologist, and his field studies of human interaction. Social psychologists seek to explain how humans behave in certain social contexts and predict social influences on human thought and behaviour. Research in social psychology includes games and experiments that manipulate 'real world' type situations to see how people respond. This often involves some degree of deception because people tend to change their behaviour if they think they are being observed. Social psychologists also use participant observation to study people's responses in naturalistic settings. In the field of health and social care, social psychology has done much to enhance our understanding of the interactions between professionals and patients or clients (Chapters 2 and 7). It has also contributed much to our understanding of the ways in which individuals make sense of illness and disability (Chapters 9 and 10), and how those with altered minds or bodies are perceived by others (Chapter 2).

Narrative psychology

In the late 1980s, Mary and Kenneth Gergen, both social psychologists, became interested in the ways people naturally construct stories to make sense of their lives. Personal stories normally have a narrative thread that links our past with our present, and contain a trajectory towards a desired goal. This provides an aim or purpose in life and an overall sense of meaning and coherence. Research methods and therapeutic interventions based on eliciting personal accounts or stories have since been developed. Narrative therapies provide psychological ways of achieving 'closure', by which is meant bringing an emotional conclusion to traumatic or difficult **life events**. The increasing range of applications are illustrated in Chapters 2, 3, 6 and 9.

Psychological facts versus psychological theory

In spite of recent advances in brain technology, it is rarely possible to study the human mind directly. We can never 'know' what someone is really thinking. We can only find out by studying what people say, how people behave and, more recently, how the electrical activity in their brains varies in different situations. Therefore, psychology, as with all social sciences, is not a body of 'facts', but a body of theories that change over time in the light of new information, new research methods, new technologies and new ways of thinking about (conceptualizing) things.

The purpose of scientific theory is not merely to explain what has happened in the past, but to predict and control what will happen in the future. For example, while it is helpful to be able to explain why people get ill, the main use of health-related theory should be to help prevent them from becoming ill in the first place. Similarly, the main purpose of psychology is to be able to predict and control certain aspects of human beliefs and behaviour.

The test of a good scientific theory, according to Karl Popper, a famous twentieth century philosopher of science, is that it must be clear and concise. This is known as the principle of parsimony, or 'Occam's Razor'. A good theory generates a logical statement or **hypothesis** that is falsifiable. Popper argued that no theory can ever be proved, but it can be disproved. He used the example of white swans: it is possible to observe thousands of swans over many years and record that they are all white. The logical deduction is that all swans are white. But it takes only one black swan to overturn the theory that all swans are white. Therefore, even the best available theory should not be treated as fact.

Psychological theory, as with all scientific theory, should be treated with caution. Theories predict what is likely to happen, not what will happen to an individual. People vary in their genetic make-up, experiences and circumstances, so no theory or research evidence can ever tell us precisely what will apply to a particular patient or client. When applying theory to practice, it is important to apply IF–THEN logic, and then to use cautious language such as 'may be' or 'is likely to'. For example 'If X theory is applied, then the best course of action is likely to be . . .' or 'If X theory is applied, then this person may be at risk of . . .'.

Research methods in psychology

Research methods are systematic methods of inquiry by which theories are tested and new knowledge gained. The main methods used in psychology are set out below. These are divided, for convenience, into:

- *quantitative methods* which involve the collection of objective measurements to test ideas and theories;
- *qualitative methods* by which researchers collect and analyse subjective reports and observations to develop new ideas and theories.

Quantitative methods

Quantitative methods are usually designed to test a hypothesis or prediction, based on a theory. They are therefore termed deductive (or hypothetico-deductive). For example, a theory might predict that a particular set of beliefs predict a certain type of behaviour; or a particular psychological intervention will lead to a certain outcome. Quantitative methods require that psychological concepts can be measured.

The development of psychological measures

Psychological instruments have been constructed to measure each concept such as anxiety or **self-efficacy**. They consist of a series of statements or questions (items) that represent different aspects of the concept. A fixed range of responses is offered, such as in a '**Likert scale**':

1 Strongly agree   2 agree   3 neutral   4 disagree   5 strongly disagree

Having developed the measure, researchers test its **validity** (to ensure it measures what it is intended to measure) and **reliability** (it does so consistently). It can then be used to measure **variables** in experiments, or in questionnaire surveys. We give information about a range of health outcome measures in Chapter 9.

Experimental methods

The scientific method most commonly used to test theory is the experiment. This involves measuring a set of responses before and after the introduction of a new intervention or change. The intervention might be a new treatment, method of disease management, health promotion programme or care package. The experimental design recommended as the 'gold standard' within the biomedical sciences is the **randomized controlled trial** (RCT), illustrated in Figure 1.3. Here the new 'experimental' intervention is compared to a dummy treatment (**placebo**) or standard care. These are termed the control intervention because it controls for changes that are not attributable to the new intervention, such as the natural propensity to get well or sort out problems. Recruits are randomized to receive either the experimental or control intervention using **random** numbers to ensure that there is no bias in the selection process. Ideally, neither the researcher nor the patient should know which treatment option (experimental or control) the patient is receiving. This is called 'blinding' and is used to ensure that patients' expectations do not lead to a **placebo response** that favours a particular intervention. Experimental designs work well for testing new drugs, but are problematic when applied to interventions that depend on therapeutic interactions. It is often difficult for ethical or practical reasons to randomize people to groups, and it is impossible for the therapist or client not to be aware which treatment is being used. These issues are often seen to damage the scientific credibility of the research.

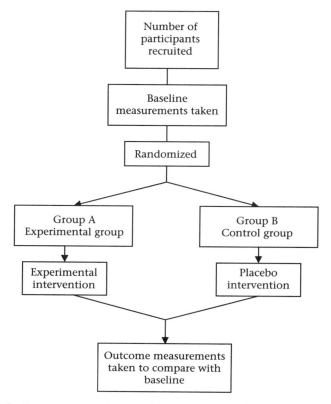

Figure 1.3   Randomized controlled trial (experimental) design

Survey methods

Survey methods use structured interviews or questionnaires as instruments
to collect self-report data about such issues as health-related beliefs and
behaviours (see Chapter 9). They allow the researcher to identify patterns
of response within a population, differences in response between groups
(e.g. men and women), and relationships between variables, such as the
relationship between beliefs and behaviours. These methods are very popular in health psychology to test models and theories. For example, it is
possible to test if the belief that 'exercise is important for health' is related
to the age of the respondent. The findings might then be used to investigate
if different approaches to intervention are needed for different age groups.
Although surveys are used to test psychological theory, it is difficult to
distinguish between cause and effect. Longitudinal surveys, in which data
are collected from the same people at different points in time, can be used
to help establish these relationships, but are less common because of the
extra time and expense involved.

Qualitative methods

Qualitative methods seek to describe or explain psychological events from the point of view of people involved. They can be used to generate new theory, in which case they are termed **inductive** methods. It is difficult to produce explanations that are not based on preconceived thoughts or ideas. Therefore the researcher must be aware of this and try to approach data collection and analysis with an open mind. Data collection normally involves semi-structured or unstructured interviews, conducted individually or in **focus groups**, participant or non-participant observations in care settings, diaries and/or other documentary analysis. The data presented in qualitative research reports is usually in the form of direct quotations or rich description, rather than statistics, which makes it easier to read and understand. The findings can strengthen or challenge existing assumptions. Qualitative methods are particularly helpful for understanding psychological or care processes, including patients' needs and the nature of patient and staff interactions. As such, they offer a real contribution to improving care. There are a range of different qualitative methods used by psychologists to explore different types of issues:

- *Phenomenology* is a philosophy and a method of inquiry well suited to psychology. Loosely structured or narrative interviews are collected and analysed to understand the 'lived experience' of various aspects of life including health and illness. Within health psychology, interpretive phenomenological analysis (IPA) has become a popular method for identifying common aspects of the patient experience of disease, illness or social problems.
- *Narrative analysis* is used to investigate the structure as well as the content of the stories people tell about important events in their lives. It contributes to our understanding about the ways people construct meaning in their lives.
- *Ethnography* is derived from anthropology and is traditionally associated with participant observation. It provides an insider understanding of behaviours and interactions within specific social and cultural contexts.
- *Grounded theory* was designed for use in sociology. It tends to be based mainly on interview data, but can include observation and documentary sources to construct new theoretical accounts of social situations and interactions. It offers a clearly defined approach to data analysis.

Some pieces of research draw on a mix of these approaches and are referred to quite simply as qualitative research. The choice of research method must suit the needs of the topic and client group. The following example is used to illustrate how qualitative research has relevance for those working in health and social care.

Garley *et al.* (1997) wanted to understand what it was like for children to have a parent with a mental health problem, so that better support might be made available and subsequent problems avoided. Children are reluctant to be interviewed on their own, so children aged 11 to 15 years who all faced this problem were invited to join one of four focus groups. A number of important themes emerged, including the struggle to gain information and understand what was happening, and what it was like to act as a caregiver. The researchers observed that being part of a group with a shared experience seemed beneficial. This type of information enables practitioners to develop a suitable programme of support.

A piece of work such as Garley's allows professionals to identify transferable issues and solutions that are relevant to their own practice. They might identify changes to improve their own care, or it might prompt them to conduct their own research. Researchers might use the findings to construct a questionnaire to survey the needs of others in similar situations or develop and test a new care package.

Qualitative and quantitative methods are complementary because they answer different types of research question, as illustrated in the following examples:

- *Experimental design*
  - What is the effect of a particular intervention?
  - Which is the best intervention for a particular condition?
- *Questionnaire survey*
  - What factors influence beliefs about a particular issue?
  - Which beliefs are most likely to predict behaviour?
- *Phenomenology*
  - What is it like to experience a particular illness?
  - What do people understand by 'good quality' care?
- *Ethnography/grounded theory*
  - How is a particular intervention (or care) currently delivered in a particular context and how does this affect all concerned?

Pop psychology and pseudoscience

It is important to discriminate between psychology as a serious academic discipline and 'pop psychology'. It is often said that psychology is just common sense. But there are many examples where common sense is contradicted by good psychological research. For instance, some professionals still believe that the reduction in a symptom as a consequence of administering a placebo indicates that the symptom was 'all in the mind' (see Chapter 10 for correct interpretation). Much of what we think of as psychology has no scientific foundation and is therefore myth. A body of knowledge or theory that cannot be tested or has never been tested is called a pseudoscience. Some psychologists might regard psychoanalysis as a pseudoscience because it offers persuasive explanations for an event after it has already occurred (a post-hoc explanation), but does not predict what will happen in the future (an **a priori** prediction). In an age of 'evidence-based' health and social care it is important to be cautious about applying any aspect of psychology unless there is reasonable evidence to support it.

Professionals involved in the prevention, management and treatment of psychological problems

The number of psychologists working in health and social care and other fields has increased considerably over the last few decades. Their tasks focus on preventing, assessing, treating and/or helping individuals to manage emotional, behavioural and cognitive problems using psychological theory and research. They also work alongside, or provide consultancy to, other health professionals. It is helpful to be able to distinguish between the skills available to different types of therapists who use psychology. Definitions of psychologists given below are based on those provided by British Psychological Society (BPS): www.bps.org.uk from where further details of their work and training requirements can be obtained. All chartered psychologists have a first degree in psychology and further training to masters or doctoral level that includes practice placements. All undergraduate and postgraduate education must be approved by the BPS.

- *Clinical psychologists* aim to reduce psychological distress and enhance and promote psychological well-being. They work with people with mental or physical health problems, including anxiety and depression, serious and enduring mental illness, adjustment to physical illness, neurological disorders, addictive behaviours, childhood behaviour disorders, personal and family relationships. They work with people throughout the life span, sometimes specializing in fields such as learning difficulties.
- *Health psychologists* apply psychological research and methods to the strategic prevention and management of disease, the promotion and maintenance of health, the identification of psychological factors that contribute to physical illness, and the formulation of health policy. As examples, they study why and when people seek professional advice about their health, why they do or do not take preventative measures, how patients and health care professionals interact, how patients adapt to illness, and the links between perception, health behaviour and physical functioning.
- *Counselling psychologists* apply psychology to working collaboratively with people across a diverse range of human problems. This includes helping people manage difficult life events such as **bereavement**, past and present relationships and mental health problems such as depression. Counselling psychologists accept subjective experience as valid for each person, explore underlying issues and use an active collaborative relationship to empower people to consider change. Counselling psychologists adopt a holistic stance, which involves examining issues within the wider context of what has given rise to them.

The roles of psychologists overlap with the roles of other health care professionals who have similar aims, including:

- *Counsellor*. Similar to a counselling psychologist, except that anyone can describe themselves as a counsellor. Training courses vary from a few days to several years. There are short courses that provide a certificate of attendance, longer courses that provide a 'certificate' or 'diploma' (though the academic level may be unspecified), and MSc programmes that include a period of supervised training. Some training programmes offer an **eclectic** mix of psychological approaches, though most follow a particular psychological model such as Rogerian or psychodynamic counselling.

- *Psychoanalyst.* Someone who has trained in psychoanalysis under the supervision of an approved psychoanalyst. All approved psychoanalysts can trace the provenance of their trainers back to those who were trained by Freud himself. All analysts undergo psychoanalysis themselves as part of a lengthy period of training.
- *Psychodynamic psychotherapist.* A therapist who has undergone a period of intensive training, including personal analysis and supervised practice, and who bases their approach on a psychodynamic model.
- *Psychiatrist.* A medical doctor who, since qualifying, has specialized in the diagnosis and treatment of people with mental health disorders. They may use a range of psychological therapies, but these usually include drug treatments which they have the right to prescribe. They sometimes use physical interventions such as electroconvulsive therapy (ECT). They are in charge of psychiatric beds and have the authority to admit people to hospital for treatment on a voluntary or compulsory basis. They usually assume the clinical lead of a multiprofessional mental health team that includes clinical psychologists, mental health nurses and social workers.
- *Cognitive behaviour therapist.* A qualified health or social care professional, such as a mental health nurse, who has completed undergraduate or postgraduate specialist training in CBT for the treatment for such disorders as depression, psychosis or obsessive-compulsive disorders. All clinical psychologists are trained to offer CBT.

Psychology in practice: introduction to the scenario

In order to understand psychology, it is important to appreciate how it can be applied in different contexts. We have devised a family scenario that will be used throughout the book to provide examples, as in a soap opera. Figure 1.4 contains a family tree for the 'psychosoap' family. We have included a thumbnail sketch of each family member to help you make sense of the examples.

Anna is currently on a diploma programme at university, training to be a nurse.

Anna has a brother, Jo, who drifted after leaving school at the age of 16. He is currently unemployed and living with his girlfriend, Sasha, and her son, Lee. Sasha is pregnant with Jo's baby.

Janice and Mark are parents to Anna and Jo. Mark recently retired early from his job as a groundsman because of the onset of Type 2 diabetes, hypertension and angina. Janice works as a health care assistant in a local nursing home.

Janice's mother, Margaret, was divorced 25 years ago and lives on her own in a town not far from Janice and Mark. She was born in the West Indies and came to this country in the 1950s, where she married Fred who was then a postman. They separated nearly 30 years ago and he died in 1989.

Mark's father Ted is a former factory worker. He is a widower whose wife died three years ago. He has chronic heart disease and has recently given up his home to live with Janice and Mark.

Mark's sister Lillian is unmarried and lives alone close by. She has been unwell and has recently been undergoing medical tests.

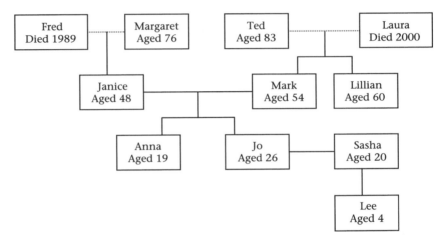

Figure 1.4 'Psychosoap' family tree

The characters from this scenario are used throughout the book to illustrate the application of psychological theories to health and social care and exemplify good practice.

Summary of key points

- Psychology is the study of human behaviour, thought processes and emotions.
- The study of psychology is essential to the achievement of good outcomes in health and social care.
- We have discussed six different approaches to psychology:
  - behaviourism
  - cognitive science and cognitive psychology
  - psychodynamic approaches

- humanistic psychology
- social psychology
- narrative psychology
- Different approaches to psychology are based on different sets of assumptions about the nature of human beings, have different ways of explaining human thought and behaviour, and use different methods of research.
- Each approach to psychology offers a unique contribution to our understanding of health, illness and human interaction in health and social care.
- Psychology is used by a range of psychologists and other professionals working in fields related to mental and physical health care, social care, and health promotion.
- A scenario (psychosoap) is introduced as an aid to understanding and applying psychology.

Exercise

See after Chapter 10.

Further reading

Background information about the nature of psychology and the schools of thought in psychology are to be found in any introductory undergraduate textbook on psychology. We have selected the following texts because they support the approaches to psychology introduced in this book. We recommended you look for the most recent edition.

Introductory psychology texts include:
Gross, R. (2005) *Psychology: The Science of Mind and Behaviour*, 5th edn. London: Hodder & Stoughton.
Smith, E., Nolen-Hoeksema, S. and Frederickson, B. (2003) *Atkinson & Hilgard's Introduction to Psychology*, 14th edn. London: Wadworth/Thomson.

Health psychology texts include:
Marks, D.F., Murray, M., Evans, B.E., Willig, C., Woodall, C. and Sykes, C.M. (2006) *Health Psychology: Theory, Research and Practice*, 2nd edn. London: Sage.
Taylor, S.E. (2006) *Health Psychology*, 6th edn. Boston, MA: McGraw-Hill.

Social psychology texts include:
Brehm, S.S., Kassin, S.M. and Fein, S. (2005) *Social Psychology*, 6th edn. Boston, MA: Houghton Mifflin.
Taylor, S.E., Peplau, L.A. and Sears, D.O. (2006) *Social Psychology*, 12th edn. London: Pearson.

THE PERCEPTION OF SELF AND OTHERS

- **What is the 'self'?**
- **How do we learn about and understand our 'self'?**
- **What are the social influences on the way we behave and present ourselves?**
- **What do we mean by 'attitudes'?**
- **What influences stigmatization and prejudice?**
- **Why do we justify our own behaviour differently from the way we explain other people's behaviour?**
- **Do personality traits provide a useful way of categorizing people?**
- **Why is individualized care important?**

Introduction

In this chapter, we explore perhaps one of the most intriguing concepts in psychology, the sense of 'self'. This is particularly important in health and social care because we are often dealing with people whose sense of self and self-worth has been changed or damaged in some way by illness, disease, disability or social deprivation. In the context of working in health and social care, we need to be aware of the ways in which other people perceive us and what influences how we perceive them. The demands caring makes upon us can also lead us to review our own sense of self. We start by considering what self means and how we come to acquire our sense of who we are.

The self-concept

Everyone holds some kind of mental representation of themselves which is referred to as the self-concept or self-schema. It seems to be part of human nature to wonder exactly who or what we are. There are so many ways to describe ourselves: what we look like, how we feel in different types of situation, how we behave towards others, what we do at work, the roles we have in the family or society. At the beginning of the twenty-first century, people seem to be obsessed with the need to feel good about themselves to the extent that people spend years 'in therapy' or seeking to change their bodies through cosmetic surgery. Present-day western societies place great emphasis on the body: its size, shape, complexion, hairstyle and adornments including clothing, jewellery, piercings and tattoos. But what do these really tell us about ourselves and others? How do we gain our sense of self?

Psychological theories are dominated by western cultural beliefs that view the 'self' as a discrete and personal entity. In western cultures, the worth of an individual is commonly defined in terms of having a good job, earning a lot of money and owning a nice house or smart car. In contrast, certain other cultures emphasize the collective nature of human beings in which an individual's worth is evaluated according to their contribution to their family and community. In some cultures, individuals are more likely to be respected for their position of seniority within their family and local community. But in this chapter, we focus on western psychological theories that seek to explain how we come to understand ourselves. We then review some of the social influences on our perceptions of ourselves and others, and ways in which the construction of the self influences health and well-being.

The looking-glass self

We all have theories about our own self and probably most of us assume that our self-understanding is gained through a process of **introspection** or inward reflection. But an early explanation of the development of the self-concept and one that is still widely respected was offered by Cooley in 1902. He proposed the notion of 'the looking-glass self'. According to Cooley, the concept of self develops through social interaction; it is a reflection of how we are regarded and responded to by other people. For example, other people confer labels on us such as good-looking or hard-working. We internalize these labels and use them to define ourselves in relation to others. Positive labels make us feel good about ourselves and can motivate us to do well. Negative labels make us feel bad about ourselves and can reduce our belief in ourselves. Similarly the labels we attach to others can affect their self-concept.

Most of us remember labels placed on us by our parents and others during childhood. These are often used to distinguish between siblings. In the scenario family (Chapter 1), Anna was labelled as the one who worked hard while her younger brother, Jo, was labelled as lazy. Such labels may or may not reflect the 'truth', but can become self-fulfilling prophecies. This may help to explain why Anna is anxious to work hard and achieve success in her training as a nurse, while Jo failed to achieve at school and is currently unemployed. This type of explanation suggests that what is commonly referred to as 'personality' is not just a consequence of inherited disposition but is substantially created and modified by our interactions with those around us. You may care to reflect on the labels placed on you as you were growing up and consider the impact these might have had on your own life.

Self defined by social comparison

Leon Festinger, a social psychologist, introduced social comparison theory which proposes that we construct our sense of self by making comparisons with important others (Festinger 1954). That someone is 5 feet 8 inches tall is a statement of fact, but whether they consider themselves tall or short depends on who they compare themselves with. For example, they might consider themselves tall if a women and short if a man. Downward social comparisons (seeing one's self as better than others) tends to boost **self-esteem** (feeling of self-worth) and maintains a sense of well-being. For example, people who are older or disabled are often heard to comment that there are others worse off. This seems to help them feel better about their own situation.

When we are young, we tend to accept the labels others confer on us. But as we get older, we make our own comparisons with those who are important to us. Much of our self-concept and self-esteem depends on the choice of **reference group** (the group the individual aspires to be part of). Thus those who gain a place at the University of Poppleton might consider themselves very successful if they are from a family with no history of going to university, but a failure if they are from a family where there is a strong tradition of winning Oxbridge scholarships.

George Kelly, a psychologist and psychotherapist, proposed that as we grow up we learn about ourselves and the world around us in much the same way that scientists produce and test theories. According to Kelly (1955), we organize this knowledge into a series of dimensions (personal constructs) that define our sense of self. Examples might include 'intelligent', 'attractive', 'outgoing', if these are important to us. We identify ourselves somewhere between positive and negative in relation to each one. Distorted beliefs about the self can contribute to anxiety and other mental health problems, as can distorted body image (see later).

When Anna was a teenager, she was desperate to be interesting, attractive and outgoing, but rated herself negatively when compared to her selected significant others, as in Figure 2.1. This made her feel quite depressed. Based on Kelly's approach, a therapist would work with her to focus on her positive characteristics and encourage her to try out new roles that facilitate positive comparisons with others.

The creation of identities

According to social identity theory (Tajfel 1982), one's identity must balance the need to be similar to one's reference group with the need to be a unique individual. Children become very aware of the need for a group identity and are often afraid of dressing or acting differently from their peers for fear of victimization. As they approach their teens, they often seem torn between the need to assert their own individual identity and the

	Myself as I am (actual self)	Myself as I would like to be (ideal self)	Brother	Best friend
Interesting (✓) Dull (✗)	✗	✓	✓	✓
Attractive (✓) Plain (✗)	✗	✓	✓	✓
Outgoing (✓) Shy (✗)	✗	✓	✓	✓

Figure 2.1   Anna's **repertory grid**

need to conform to their reference group. Distinctive or rebellious group identities seem to emerge at this time, associated with particular styles of dress and behaviour. Later, new identities are forged in relation to work, parenthood, economic status and ageing, and during their lives most people develop several different identities.

Anna has recently acquired a new identity as a nurse. With this comes a uniform, bedside manner, code of conduct and set of public expectations. But when she goes off duty and out with her friends, she will assume a quite different identity.

The identities we confer on others, based on our assumptions about them, are often rejected by them. For example, one 80-year-old might refer to another 80-year-old as 'that poor old soul' because they mentally distance themselves from being old. As a result, many older people decline to join seniors clubs. It becomes clear that, in many circumstances, people just don't see themselves the same way that others see them. It is a mistake to assume that individuals share common attributes or have anything in common with each other just because they happen to belong to a particular age or social group, or any other group.

Identity as narrative

A recent focus in psychology has been on what is termed 'the narrative self'. According to this, our identities are the stories we tell. We each have our own unique life story that encompasses the past, present and future. Our story represents our map, our destination and our purpose. It defines us as someone who is unique and distinguishes us from others. Our story may not be entirely factual because, as Murray (2003) explains, we construct a narrative that makes sense of our life experiences. Narrative provides a sense of continuity over time and we use it to justify our actions and our existence. Major life-changing events, including chronic illness, disability or loss, cause biographical disruption and thereby challenge the existing sense of self (Radley 1994; see also Chapter 3). Frank (1995) argued that a story demands a listener; therefore the narrative self is one to be heard, rather than measured. Listening to someone's account of their illness tells us a lot about the way they see themselves in the context of their illness and their life and helps us to see them as individuals. It gives them a unique identity with which others, including professionals, can readily identify (see also Chapter 3).

Self-esteem

Self-esteem reflects a critical personal evaluation of self-worth and is a central component of psychological well-being. There is no single theory of self-esteem. Accounts depend very much on the field of psychology they are drawn from, though different explanations are not mutually exclusive. For example, according to personal construct theory, self-esteem reflects the degree of discrepancy between the ideal and actual self (the greater the discrepancy, the lower is self-esteem). A psychodynamic psychologist may view self-esteem as resulting from the type and strength of attachment relationships formed in early life. Research evidence supports the view that there are stable elements to self-esteem which are formed early in life, though life experiences may serve to raise or lower self-esteem (Rubin and Hewstone 1998).

According to Bandura's social learning theory (Bandura 1997a, Chapter 5), self-esteem comes from the confidence in one's ability to be able to achieve important goals. This is usually the result of one's own endeavours, but may also be a consequence of collective effort, depending on cultural norms (Abrams and Hogg 2004). Personal efficacy may be a more important determinant of self-esteem in western societies that value individual effort and personal achievement. Drawing on social comparison theory (Festinger 1954), self-esteem is influenced by the extent to which we feel our beliefs and behaviour are valued by others who matter to us. This is often referred to as the '**social norm**' (Chapter 9).

Feedback on self-worth commences at birth and is particularly important during the formative years. Therefore childhood experiences in the family and in peer groups are very important (Chapter 3). Changes in adult life, particularly those involving change of work or family role, are important influences on self-esteem. Injuries or alterations to the body can also have important positive or negative effects on self-esteem, as evidenced by the enthusiasm for cosmetic change.

Body image

Our bodies are important determinants of our identity and self-esteem. Bodies have certain unique features that remain relatively stable over time and by which other people recognize us. Other body features change with age and life experiences. Work as health or social care professionals brings us into contact with many people who have to deal not only with life changes but with changes to their actual bodies. Some of these are abrupt results of trauma, disease processes or surgery. Other changes are insidious, as in disease processes such as rheumatoid arthritis or chronic heart disease, those caused by exposure to toxic environments, or ageing processes including menarche and menopause. All types of bodily change can result in the need to change the self-concept and may seriously challenge an individual's sense of identity.

Body image is described as having three components: body reality, body ideal and body presentation.

Body reality

Body reality refers to the physical structure of the individual body, whether an individual is tall or short, fat or slim, fair or dark. Basic aspects of our body reality, such as eye and hair colour, height and body shape, are determined by genetic factors. Certain aspects of body structure change over time from infancy to old age although most people retain a sense of continuity about their own bodies. Sudden disruptions may be deliberately engineered, or may result from trauma or disease.

Body ideal

Body ideal is part of an individual's ideal sense of self. This is likely to be gender- and age-specific and is also influenced by social norms that define appropriate size, shape and contours. Magazines and other media provide a lot of information about appropriate body shape, size and colour, for example urging women to be slim, suntanned or have large breasts. A brief look at the history of fashion will show how women's, and to a lesser extent men's, ideal body shapes have varied over time. There are also cultural variations in what is considered desirable at any time. Discrepancies between body reality and body ideal lead to dissatisfaction and distortions have been blamed for serious health problems, such as anorexia.

Anna's friend, Clare, judges herself to be fat in relation to her ideal self when she is in fact of normal weight in relation to population norms. This leads her to continue to diet in order to lose even more weight. She eats quite a lot, but has started making herself sick and taking laxatives to try to keep her weight under control. Anna suspects that she might be developing bulimia and has encouraged her to seek help from the college counsellor.

The effect of body image on self-esteem is influenced by the roles that are important to the individual. For example, a mastectomy scar may damage self-esteem in the role of lover, but be of little importance in the role of, say, accountant.

Al-Ghazal *et al.* (2000) compared the impact of different types of breast surgery (local excision, mastectomy and mastectomy plus breast reconstruction) on measures that included body image and self-esteem for women aged between 20 and 70. Perhaps not surprisingly, they found that cosmetic outcome was closely associated with psychological outcome. In all age groups, mastectomy was associated with poorer body image and lower self-esteem. As a result of this and previous findings, the team of researchers concluded that breast reconstruction should automatically be offered to all women undergoing mastectomy. However, this was a retrospective study and the findings may have been influenced by treatment preference. An earlier prospective study by Morris and Ingham (1988) indicated that providing choice, rather than the type of operation performed, led to improved physical and psychological functioning.

Body presentation

Body presentation includes the characteristic ways in which the body moves or functions in social situations, including gestures and physical actions. Some 'innate' responses, such as smiling or laughing when we are happy, are shared by all people. Other 'acquired' responses, such as hand-waving, nodding or winking, mean different things to different cultural groups. People acquire many of these behaviours during childhood, through the process of socialization and use them in a largely unconscious way. In fact, we may feel very awkward if we try to suppress innate or acquired behaviours.

Each culture has its own norms of body presentation. What is acceptable in some cultures is totally unacceptable in others. Some are quite subtle and difficult to learn. It is very noticeable if people behave differently from what is normally expected, or act out of character, and can make others feel quite uneasy. In multi-ethnic societies which have high levels of immigration, this can cause particular misunderstandings.

Some people are unable to control their movements. If interpreted as socially inappropriate, this may cause offence, intimidation, ridicule or misunderstanding. For example, someone who has Parkinson's disease may show very little facial movement and, to others, this can make them seem quite disinterested in what is going on around them. People with cerebral palsy used to be ridiculed because they are unable to control body movements. Having a body that does not conform to the norms of a society or reference group can cause psychological harm.

Stigma

Goffman (1963) introduced the concept of stigma to refer to visible or distinguishing features in an individual or group. The concept is important in psychology because stigmas lead to negative perceptions and behaviours by others, a process referred to as stigmatization. Goffman described three types of stigma, linked closely to the three types of body image:

1 Physical deviations that may be interpreted as deformity or disfigurement.
2 Appearance, attributes or behaviour that violate cultural or social values, which Goffman referred to as 'moral' stigma.
3 The adoption of badges, dress and other adornments used to signify group membership, which he described as 'tribal' stigma.

Physical stigma refers to alterations in the body or in bodily functions. Facial disfigurement is a particularly important stigma. Parents are often very distressed by the appearance of a baby with a cleft lip and/or palate and may, as a result, find it difficult to form a close attachment to the baby. Seeing another baby who has been successfully treated can be very reassuring to the parents at an early stage. Research suggests that fears about the social consequences of facial disfigurement are well founded.

Houston and Bull (1994) conducted a series of studies that involved marking the face of a normal individual with a port wine type stain. The 'stigmatized individual' then took up a seat in a railway carriage while an observer recorded the behaviour of the other passengers. They found that when the subject sat with the marked side or the face towards an adjacent empty seat, people tended to avoid sitting there until the other seats were occupied.

More recent work by Coull (2003) highlighted even worse personal experiences reported by burns patients. It appears that people with physical differences, whether congenital or acquired, are probably quite right to fear being stared at, ignored or avoided. Therefore, professionals need to know how best to help them to deal with such situations. Useful reviews of these issues, together with advice for professionals on how to help adolescents and adults with disfigurements are provided by Newell (2002a, 2002b) and Rumsey and Harcourt (2004). Social skills training to help people deal with the social anxiety of facial disfigurement appears to offer benefits. Face transplant might appear to offer hope for those with the most severe facial disfigurements. But the recipients most likely to benefit cosmetically are likely to be among those most psychologically vulnerable and may be the least well equipped to deal with the uncertainties of surgery (Rumsey 2004).

Some aspects of appearance are regarded as morally reprehensible in a particular culture at a particular time. Certain body characteristics may be seen to confer a moral stigma. For example, children who are obese are often taunted as lazy or clumsy by their classmates. Certain behaviours may be regarded as moral stigma. For example, smoking has come to be regarded by many as unacceptable. The debate about whether smokers should be offered heart surgery could be said to illustrate stigmatizing attitudes on the part of health professionals.

The wearing of certain garments, such as the head covering or veil worn by Muslim women are forms of stigma in non-Islamic societies. It is important to respect and accommodate the wishes of the individual so far as possible. For example, we do not normally expect married women to remove their wedding rings before surgery.

Social roles

According to Goffman (1959), an important part of the self-concept is determined by the social roles people play. Everyone plays a large number of social roles at the same, as well as different, points in their lives.

Anna has various roles as friend, daughter, aunt, nurse, part-time barmaid and girlfriend. Some of these are a familiar, taken-for-granted part of her life, though recently she has returned home and found that her role as daughter has changed because of her increased independence and confidence. However, she is still learning her role as nurse and frequently faces feelings of uncertainty and self-consciousness.

Goffman likened the experience of living to a drama that takes place in the theatre of everyday life (the 'dramaturgical model'). Thus our social roles may be seen as the roles in a play and the social environment as the stage set. He suggested that any one person will have available to them a number of different social roles according to the setting they are in at the time.

Goffman outlined how we use various props to help sustain our roles and present the image we wish to portray. He termed this 'impression management'. Clothes, hairstyle, make-up, perfume and mobile phone are all examples of the props we use to portray the public image we wish to present. The doctor's stethoscope and white coat are part of the props used to create the image of the doctor. In fact, the performance of some 'bogus' doctors has been so convincing that it has taken a long time before their lack of medical knowledge or expertise has exposed them. Each profession has its own set of props and behaviour into which newcomers are initiated and socialized. These are often learned by **modelling** (copying) rather than formal instruction (social learning, Chapter 5). However, we eventually learn to regulate and modify our own behaviour as necessary.

We often meet patients or clients in situations where they are deprived of their normal props or set. For example, the individual dressed in a hospital gown lying in a hospital bed could have almost any role in 'real life'.

Knowledge of their other roles and identities can significantly influence the attitudes of those caring for them. For example, in order to ensure that she was given greater respect, a colleague reminded staff that her elderly mother had until recently worked as a magistrate.

Social rules

Goffman observed that the performance of a particular role is appropriate only in certain social situations. For example, we may be kind and gentle with patients, but noisy or comical with friends. Each role has its own set of behaviours, expectations and rules of engagement which may be suited only to certain situations. It is possible to cause serious offence if we mis-judge others' social roles. For example, care staff risk offending an older gentleman if they refer to him as 'grandpa' when he feels that this is inappropriate to his present situation. Failure to understand the rules of social engagement leads to social isolation.

When Jo was young, he knew a boy called Matt who was eventually diagnosed as having Asperger syndrome (APA 2000). Matt was unable to read social cues or understand accepted rules of social interaction (see Chapter 6). He interrupted other children's conversations and games and failed to recognize why they got annoyed with him. This meant that most other children did not want him for a friend and he became socially excluded.

The rules of social engagement are culturally determined and normally learned automatically, as part of normal development. Where this fails, it is important to teach these skills from an early age in much the same way that a child can learn to play the piano (Stewart 2002). Difficulties can also arise as a result of mental health problems and may be amenable to social skills training (Chapter 6).

Adapting to changing roles and self-concept

Some people find it more difficult than others to make a transition between the roles they are expected to play at different points in the lifespan. Many transitions are enforced as a result of illness or social change. Some find it easier to adapt to these than others (see also Chapter 8).

During Janice's lifetime, she has had to adjust from being single to being married and becoming a parent. She adapted from being the mother of young children to having adolescent offspring to being alone with her husband again. She was a caregiver to her mother-in-law, Laura, and may

> have to care for Ted. Her role has changed to chief wage-earner since Mark retired. Her role as wife and lover has changed over the years, particularly since Mark's health has deteriorated.

Illness and disability interfere unexpectedly with the ability of the individual to continue with their previous social roles. People who have lived independent lives or cared for others suddenly become dependent. With new social roles comes **adaptation** to a new set of social rules and a new sense of self. The loss of previous identity and roles can lead to psychological harm, as Walker *et al.* (2006) found from listening to the stories of people who had developed chronic back pain.

The self-concept or self-schema is normally relatively stable, but can vary in its ability to adapt to change. In an early study, Linville (1987) found that people vary in their ability to perceive themselves differently in different situations. Linville showed that having a complex self-schema that varies in different situations appears to make people more adaptive and resilient to stress-related illness and depression. Flexibility and resilience is influenced by genetic make-up, socialization and exposure to different life experiences. However, many of the difficulties people have in adjusting their roles following illness are caused not by personal strengths or weaknesses, but by the attitudes of others.

Attitudes

Attitudes are subjective evaluations that predispose people to behave towards an object or person in a positive or negative way. The object in question may be a health-related topic such as HIV or teenage pregnancy (Chapter 9). But it is commonly a person or group of people, for example immigrants or antisocial teenagers. Attitudes are generally conceptualized as consisting of three classes of response:

- *cognitive:*   beliefs about the object;
- *affective:*   a feeling about the object, based on a positive or negative evaluation;
- *behavioural:* actions directed at the object.

Attitudes are formed through feedback from a range of different experiences. They are culturally shaped through formal socialization processes, including childrearing, schooling and professional training. They may also be the product of identification with social groupings such as religious, kinship or friendship groups. These groups exert strong influence or 'peer pressure' on the behaviour of group members. **Conformity** to 'social norms' laid down by the group is very strong and attitudes towards 'others' may be hostile (Chapter 7).

Negative attitudes are an important part of stigmatization, prejudice and discrimination. First impressions are very important in generating positive or negative attitudes, therefore subjective and judgemental statements in letters of referral, handover or case conferences can have a profound effect on subsequent care. When recording or reporting personal information, it is a good idea to imagine that the patient or client is reading over your shoulder, or listening to what you say.

Stereotyping, prejudice, stigmatization and discrimination

Stereotyping refers to the attaching of attributes to an individual on the basis of group membership. Sociologists refer to this process as labelling. It is a convenient form of shared **schema** for describing and categorizing people and draws on certain salient characteristics that usually have some foundation in fact or experience. Some categories, such as personality types or diagnostic categories, are determined by objective assessment using scientifically valid and reliable instruments. They are intended to assist with psychological or medical treatment, but even these can lead to stereotyping if the group label takes precedence over individualized care planning.

Most stereotypes are based on selective attention to limited characteristics which emphasize differences rather than similarities in others. These often involve characteristics that are exaggerated and generalized at the expense of individual attributes. Stereotypes are often based upon features such as age or gender, ethnic, national or regional characteristics, personal appearance or ethnic origin. Some stereotypes are positive, but many are negative. For example, it is often said that people with red hair have fiery tempers, Scots people are mean and fat people are lazy. These assumptions are usually untrue when applied to individuals and can be very damaging.

The negative effects of stereotyping are to be found in prejudice, stigmatization and discrimination. Prejudice refers to the combination of negative beliefs and attitudes towards an individual or group, and discrimination to the negative behaviour associated with prejudice. Many beliefs about others are based on limited knowledge about their social group. Religious affiliation has become a recent target for stereotyping and prejudice. Negative stereotypes usually ignore the fact that each religion has many different subgroups, ranging from a few extremists to those who are very liberal in their beliefs, attitudes and behaviours.

Stigmatization

Having any sort of distinguishing feature or stigma can lead others to assign a negative stereotype. Once such a label has been attached to an individual, it is difficult to remove.

A classic study by Rosenhan (1973) 'On being sane in insane places', illustrated how a diagnosis of mental illness, once established, can be difficult to shake off. In Rosenhan's study, several 'normal' people, including a psychologist, paediatrician and psychiatrist, worker and housewife presented themselves at a psychiatric clinic complaining of hearing voices. During their assessment, all details of their stories were correct apart from their claims to hear voices. All were diagnosed as having major mental illness, in most cases schizophrenia, and were admitted to hospital. Following admission, they stopped complaining about the voices, but in most cases it took several weeks to convince staff that they were in remission and well enough to be discharged. Only fellow inmates were suspicious about their true identities. This study was later the subject of the film *One Flew over the Cuckoo's Nest*.

Those with mental health problems are probably the most stigmatized group. Even those who have suffered an episode of depression or other less serious mental illness are perceived by others to be less trustworthy and intelligent, more incompetent and dangerous, with the result that they suffer serious socioeconomic disadvantage, social exclusion and higher levels of stress (see review by Link and Phedan 2006). Many physical illnesses, such as epilepsy and HIV, are similarly stigmatized. Cancer was until recently a stigmatized disease, to be talked about in hushed tones. Other stigmatized conditions are more visible.

Ann worked on a medical ward where there was a 40-year-old male patient who weighed nearly 40 stone and was described as 'bariatric'. Staff attitudes towards him were very negative because he was difficult to move and even routine observations were difficult. One day, Anna found him crying. She learned that he had suffered from bullying as a child and recently lost both his parents, with whom he had lived. He was well aware of the way staff and other patients felt about him and he wanted to die.

Where possible, people often choose to conceal the source of stigma. For example someone who had had an episode of depression might not admit to this on a job application. Some may choose to mix only with other people who share similar attributes. For example, some deaf people who use sign language may feel more comfortable in social situations where signing is the dominant communication system. They do not need to explain to others that they are deaf nor are they stared at and made to feel abnormal when they are signing. It is often difficult for parents of deaf children to know how much to encourage their children to form relationships with other deaf people or how much they should be helped to integrate into the hearing world. Other problem-solving ways of dealing with an obvious stigma include preparing explanations to share with others and using humour to avoid embarrassment.

The self-fulfilling prophecy

Stereotypical labels lead to positive or negative expectations. The effects of these were well illustrated in a series of social psychology experiments conducted by Rosenthal and colleagues in the 1960s.

Rosenthal and Jacobson (1968) examined the effect of expectation on children in a classic experiment on teacher expectations in the classroom. The result became known as the 'Pygmalion effect'. At the beginning of the school year, students took an IQ test and were then randomly (regardless of the actual results) labelled as either clever or ordinary. The teacher was told to expect that the clever ones would make rapid progress. Students took a further IQ test at the end of the year and the students labelled 'clever' were found to have made greater gains in IQ, compared to the others. This clearly demonstrates that students who are expected to do well, do better, but why? Observations suggested that students labelled as clever received more attention, more encouragement and more positive feedback from the teacher than the other pupils.

In the field of health care, the self-fulfilling prophecy may be an important predictor of patients' behaviour. The expectations of health professionals are often influenced by personal observations or value judgements recorded in, or implicit from, patients' records.

Lillian had previously had little contact with doctors when she was referred to the hospital for investigation. Her general practitioner was sympathetic and wrote in the referral letter, 'This pleasant lady . . .'. She found the staff very sympathetic and helpful. But the lady she sat next to in the waiting room had quite a different experience. She had a thick set of notes that catalogued a series of health problems that had not responded to treatment. She felt that none of the staff seemed interested in her any more and tried to avoid her, even though her health needs were much more complex than Lillian's.

Factors that influence our expectations include 'stigma' such as age or gender, appearance, the way in which an individual dresses, their accent, the questions they ask and their **illness behaviours** (Chapter 5).

In the early 1970s, Stockwell (1984) first reported the findings of a classic nursing study which sought to identify the characteristics of 'unpopular' patients. She found factors that accounted for lack of popularity with nursing staff included physical features, physical defects, nationality, length of stay, complaints and the need for time-consuming care. Other factors include perceptions of low social worth or value (Johnson and Webb 1995). Shelley Taylor (1979) observed that 'good patient' behaviour involves being quiet, passive and undemanding. But these characteristics may also be indicative of dependence and depression, rather than confidence and **self-management**. Being passive is not conducive to the achievement of an effective 'patient-professional partnership' or to self-management of their health problems. Yet those who are most vocal about expressing their needs may become unpopular with care staff.

It is not just patients who are expected to conform to certain stereotypes. Each profession appears to hold a stereotypical set of expectations about members of other professions (Chapter 6). This can interfere with interprofessional working, to the detriment of patient care.

Attribution theory

Attribution theory is a dominant theory in social psychology. It refers to processes by which people understand relationships between cause and effect, and how they make judgements about responsibility and blame. Based on the work of Kurt Lewin in the 1930s, attribution theory was proposed by Fritz Heider in the 1940s and developed further by Harold Kelley in the 1970s. It is based on the premise that people have an intrinsic need to understand cause–effect relationships. This is reflected in a most fundamental question most people ask when they get ill – why?

Unlike other theories of decision-making, attribution theory recognizes that most events take place in a social setting where there needs to be some way of deciding who or what was responsible for what occurred. Attribution theory, as applied in health care, proposes that decisions about causality take place on three separate dimensions:

- *locus:* internal–external (myself, or someone else);
- *stability:* stable–unstable (always, or just on this occasion);
- *globality:* global–specific (in all situations, or just in this situation).

The dimension 'internal–external' is usually referred to as '**locus of control**' (Chapter 5). The theory is illustrated in the following example.

Anna failed her first examination. As a result, she may decide that she is just no good at examinations. This involves an internal, stable and global attribution for failure. On the other hand, she may decide that on this occasion the paper was an unfair test of her knowledge (external,

> unstable, specific attributions). Or she may decide that on this occasion, she did not work hard enough (internal, unstable, specific attributions).

The attributions people make are likely to determine their future course of action. If Anna makes internal, stable and global attributions for failure (I am always a stupid person), she will feel that she is a failure and may become depressed. If she makes external, unstable and specific attributions (it is their fault for setting such a silly test on this occasion), she may blame the module leader. This will help her to feel better about her failure, but will not encourage her to work harder for her resit paper. On the other hand, if she makes internal, unstable and specific attributions (it was my own fault on this occasion because I didn't work hard enough), she is well placed to address the reasons for her failure and make sure that she works harder to ensure a pass next time. There is some evidence in health care that internal locus of control is associated with better health outcomes in a variety of situations (Chapters 8, 9 and 10).

Attribution error

Attribution theory helps us understand how we make judgements about the actions of others. If someone is anxious, we may attribute their anxiety to their personality (internal, stable and global attributions). Or we may, if we have taken a little time to find out the reasons for their anxiety, attribute this to specific worries or concerns about their illness or what is happening at home (external, unstable, specific attributions). The attributions we make about responses such as anxiety will have important implications for the way we respond to others. Quite often, we draw on stereotypes (negative stable and global attributions) when making these judgements.

It appears that there is a tendency to systematic bias in the way we draw inferences about the reasons for other people's behaviour. Ross (1977: 183, see Brehm *et al.* 2002) called this the **fundamental attribution error**. He defined it as 'the tendency for attributers [those making a judgement] to underestimate the impact of situational factors and to overestimate the role of dispositional [personality] factors in controlling behaviour'. The explanation for this is not entirely clear, though it may be related to a dominant western cultural expectation that people are personally responsible for their own actions. Another important source of attribution bias, according to Jones and Nisbett (Hewstone 1989), is the 'pervasive tendency' for people to attribute their own actions to the demands of the situation, while those observing are likely to attribute the same actions to stable personal dispositions (personality traits). These attribution errors or biases can have serious implications for patients and clients as well as professionals, as illustrated by the following examples.

- If I make a mistake, I am likely to believe it is because I was given the wrong information or instructions.

- If somebody else makes a similar mistake, I am more likely to believe that it is because they are stupid.
- If I am anxious about an illness symptom, I am likely to believe there must be a physical cause, even if the doctor cannot find one.
- If a patient is worried about an illness symptom for which there is no apparent cause, health professionals may believe that he or she is a hypochondriac.

These potent sources of error are important causes of victim-blaming judgements.

Anna was working alongside a junior doctor who wrote up the wrong dose of drug for a patient. The staff nurse gave the drug before noticing the error. Luckily the patient was unharmed. The junior doctor was disciplined for his mistake, but it probably happened because he was tired and distracted by too many other demands.

In the case of mistakes, it is common for organizations to seek someone to blame, so that they can be disciplined. In reality, it is often a system failure, such as inadequate information or resources, that causes the error. The Department of Health (DoH) has recognized this as an important cause of persistent medical error and has attempted to introduce a 'no blame' culture into the UK National Health Service (NHS). But systematic attribution bias is often institutionalized and difficult to overcome.

Personality and health

We give little space in this book to the topic of personality because the widespread, inappropriate use of personality labels in health and social care can (and does) lead to stereotyping and stigmatization. The identification and use of personality typologies in the absence of a formal training and adequate patient assessment can be dangerous. In the field of mental health, personality traits are often measured as part of a detailed assessment to establish a diagnosis. Even then, practitioners need to be aware of the potential problems that labelling can lead to. But in general health care, personality traits are often assigned in the absence of proper assessment, or even any assessment.

Personality traits

A trait is a relatively stable set of individual characteristics that include patterns of thought, adjustment and behaviour that are partly inherited, strongly influenced by experiences during childhood, and to some extent modified through adult experiences. Personality and intelligence are examples of such traits. The extent to which inheritance (nature) and childrearing practices (nurture) influence intelligence and personality traits remains a matter of considerable debate within the scientific community, where it is commonly referred to as the nature–nurture debate.

> The relative contribution of nature versus nurture has been examined through the study of monozygotic (identical) versus dizygotic (non-identical) twins. Monozytogic (MZ) twins share identical genetic material, whereas dizygotic (DZ) twins do not. Twin studies normally compared similarities between MZ and DZ twins brought up together with those adopted separately. Borkenau *et al.* (2001) confirmed findings of previous studies that about 40 per cent of personality is genetically determined, and the remaining 60 per cent environmentally determined: 25 per cent was due to shared environment (most of which is likely to be in the parental home), and 35 per cent to non-shared environmental influences.

The names most commonly associated with the measurement of personality are Raymond Cattell and Hans Eysenck. Cattell produced a multi-dimensional measure of personality consisting of 16 traits or personality factors, called the 16 PF. Eysenck is particularly well-known for his work on the dimensions of extroversion, neuroticism and psychoticism, which were measured using the Eysenck Personality Inventory (EPI). Perhaps the most important of Eysenck's propositions was that extroversion and neuroticism are biologically determined.

The personality measure currently in most common use in health psychology is the 'Big Five', which measures the following five traits (Costa and McCrae 1992):

1 *Neuroticism*: anxious, tense, worrying, unstable.
2 *Extroversion*: active, assertive, enthusiastic, outgoing, talkative.
3 *Agreeableness*: appreciative, forgiving, generous, kind, trusting.
4 *Conscientiousness*: efficient, organized, reliable, responsible, thorough.
5 *Openness (or creativity)*: artistic, curious, imaginative, insightful.

Each of these traits lies at one end of a **bipolar** dimension and an individual may score anywhere between positive and negative on each of the dimensions. An alternative approach has been to measure positive and negative affectivity, which simply measures the dispositional tendency to view all aspects of self and life as either positive or negative, regardless of stressful demands or negative events. These contrasting world views are commonly referred to in terms of 'cup half full' versus 'cup half empty'. Many psychologists regard negative affectivity and neuroticism as measuring the same thing (Ekman and Davidson 1994).

Personality and change

Evidence from a wide range of studies appears to indicate that we are born with distinctive personalities, but there is still a lot of room for change.

Longitudinal studies suggest a degree of consistency in personality throughout life, due mainly to genetic factors and the enduring nature of parental influence. But there are also maturational changes resulting from life experiences such as leaving home, mothering, middle age and getting older (Chapter 3). Srivastava *et al.* (2003) conducted a cross-sectional internet survey of adults aged 21–60, using the Big Five personality measure and found that conscientiousness and agreeableness increased throughout early and middle adulthood at varying rates. Neuroticism declined among women but did not change among men. Helson *et al.* (2002) found considerable individual variation in personality over time and confirmed personality changes in response to time of life and cultural climate. The wide variations in response suggest that it can be dangerous for health care professionals to believe that an individual's personality tells them anything meaningful about the way that individual is likely to respond in different or difficult circumstances.

Effects of personality on health outcomes

One reason for measuring personality traits is because some psychologists still believe that they predict adjustment to different aspects of life. In the field of mental health, the relationship between neuroticism and anxiety-related disorders is self-evident, since neuroticism indicates a proneness to negative mood states. However, research has also revealed some interesting relationships between neuroticism and health care use.

Goodwin *et al.* (2002) set out to determine the relationship between personality factors and the use of mental health services among adults living in New York. They found that neuroticism was associated with an increased likelihood of service utilization. Conscientiousness and extraversion were associated with decreased likelihood of utilization. This appears to suggest, perhaps not surprisingly, that reserved, passive people who are emotionally unstable and lack a sense of commitment are more likely to require treatment for mental health problems.

There has long been similar interest on the influence of personality variables on health outcomes for people with physical illnesses.

Friedman (2000) reviewed links between personality and physical health, based on a seven-decade longitudinal study. He offered three possible theoretical explanations for links between personality and health:

1 Certain personality types may be associated with physiological mechanisms that lead to certain diseases, for example coronary heart disease and cancer.

2   Personality traits may set a trajectory towards health or disease. For example, those who are more sociable may develop better support networks than others.
3   Personality may be associated with certain motivational forces that draw people towards rebellion or risk, including substance use.

Friedman examined these explanations in relation to three of the Big Five personality types: sociability (extraversion), conscientiousness and neuroticism. Only conscientiousness was found to be a predictor of good health, possibly because conscientious people are likely to smoke less, moderate their alcohol consumption, have greater work and social stability and adhere to medical treatments where necessary.

Vollrath and Torgersen (2000) observed that the effects of extraversion on health are ambiguous. Extraverts tend to be more optimistic and have good support networks, but are also high risk-takers and more likely to engage in unhealthy behaviours such as drinking and smoking. Therefore the negative effects tend to cancel out the positive.

Friedman (2000) concluded from a review of the available literature that there is little evidence to support the notion of a disease-prone personality. Certain people are more likely to take up unhealthy habits, exhibit unbalanced emotional and physiological responses, and experience unsupportive social environments that are conducive to poor health. Friedman argued that these causal processes, rather than personality, need to be taken into account when offering health advice.

In line with this, Cameron *et al.* (2005) found that patients who have negative affectivity may be less likely to benefit from a self-management cardiac rehabilitation intervention because of poorer attendance and **adherence** to diet and exercise. However, no attempt was made in their study to measure current situational influences, such as home circumstances, major life events or hassles. These conditions can bias self-reports of mood and affect the ability to adhere to action plans.

Walker *et al.* (2006) interviewed people with chronic back pain and found that their negative outlook reflected losses and negative experiences resulting from their back problem. These in turn made them pessimistic about the future. Therefore, it is worth considering that negative affectivity is a consequence of illness and social problems, as well as a cause of negative health outcomes.

Certain patterns of thought and behaviour, such as self-efficacy and locus of control (Chapter 5), have been shown to influence health-related ways of coping with difficult life changes or events. But these have been shown to be amenable to change and are not considered to be personality traits. Watson and Pennebaker (1989) studied the relationship between negative affectivity and health and concluded that it is likely to have a negative impact on satisfaction with, and complaints about, health care. This can turn such people into unpopular patients.

Health and social care professionals need to be very careful not to use stereotypical explanations when working with individuals who experience mental or physical illness or other life-changing experiences. If we believe that the way an individual behaves is a consequence of their personality, we will also believe that they are unlikely to change. This is sometimes a convenient way of absolving professionals from their responsibility to help people manage change. If we believe, as do humanistic psychologists (Chapter 1), in the potential for human growth, we will encourage people to talk about their beliefs and their reasons for responding as they do, and then endeavour to facilitate positive change and adaptation for that individual.

Person-centred care

Feeling valued is one of the key determinants of patient trust and satisfaction (Walker *et al.* 1998). The opposite of feeling valued is feeling depersonalized and alienated. 'Depersonalize' in this context means to treat someone as an object, rather than a person. The medical model of care can encourage this by focusing attention on the disease or the injured part, or by emphasizing dispositional factors in accounting for people's responses to illness.

One of the main antidotes to depersonalizing and discrimination, particularly in health care, is individualized, person-centred care, which recognizes individual beliefs, expectations and needs during the assessment, planning and implementation of care strategies. Kleinman (1988), one of the originators of narrative medicine, asserted that the ability to listen to and interpret people's experiences of illness should be seen as core skills for health care professionals. We offer exercises at the end of the book to support this approach.

The rewards of caring for people become apparent once a person-centred approach to care is adopted. In nursing, task-oriented care focuses mainly upon the rituals of toileting, bathing, changing and feeding, which can easily become demoralizing for caregivers and patients. In contrast, individualized care can elicit rich rewards by establishing relationships and revealing anecdotes and personal histories. The tasks become less onerous for the patient and the nurse as they engage in a closer rapport. Some tasks may become less necessary as professionals and patients work together to explore person-centred solutions. The remainder of this book is devoted to psychological theory and evidence that support person-centred solutions.

Summary of key points

- Much of what we think of as our 'self' is actually defined by the ways that other people respond to us.

- Looks are important. Looking or behaving differently, whether through disability or choice, can lead to avoidance or labelling as 'different' or deviant.
- The labels we attach to ourselves and others can become self-fulfilling prophecies.
- If we treat people positively, they are more likely to respond in a positive way. It is never too late to change.
- There is a pervasive tendency within western health care to focus on dispositional (personality) explanations, rather than situational explanations, for the ways people behave.
- The labelling of people according to personality traits or types may lead to attribution error, stereotyping and discrimination.
- Listening to people's stories is informative and can have therapeutic value and is an important part of individualized care.

Exercise

See after Chapter 10.

Further reading

Brewer, M.B. and Hewstone, M. (2004) *Self and Social Identity*. Oxford: Blackwell.

Goffman, E. (1959) *The Presentation of Self in Everyday Life*. London: Penguin.

Goffman, E. (1963) *Stigma: Notes on the Management of Spoiled Identity*. Harmondsworth: Penguin.

Rumsey, N. and Harcourt, D. (2004) *The Psychology of Appearance*. Maidenhead: Open University Press.

Stapel, D.A. and Blanton, H. (2006) *Social Comparison Theories: Key Readings*. New York: Psychology Press.

Stockwell, F. (1984) *The Unpopular Patient*. London: Croom Helm.

DEVELOPMENT AND CHANGE ACROSS THE LIFESPAN

- **How do children of different ages understand complex issues related to health and illness?**
- **Why are attachment relationships so important and what is the impact of separation?**
- **How might parenting influence adolescent behaviours?**
- **How can we explain responses to change throughout the lifespan?**
- **What is special about the psychology of later life?**

Introduction

In order to be able to communicate effectively with people of all ages, it is important to know how their interpretation and ability to relate to others is influenced by their level of cognitive, moral and social development. Cognitive development refers to development of thinking and understanding about the world. Moral development refers to the ways in which children evaluate issues and justify their behaviour. Social development focuses on the development of relationships with others. In this chapter, we start by presenting theoretical perspectives on cognitive, moral and social development in childhood, drawing upon classic as well as contemporary psychological theory and research which we apply to children of different ages. The chapter moves on to consider development across the lifespan, focusing particularly on issues that arise towards the end of life.

Theoretical background

It is important to remember that a theory is simply a system of ideas or principles that are used to explain what is happening and, if possible, predict what is likely to happen. Many traditional theories of child and lifespan development are 'stage' theories, based on an assumption prevalent during the mid-twentieth century that psychological development follows a fixed sequence of separate steps. Freud introduced the idea that children pass through a series of psychosexual stages until they reach puberty. Failure to move successfully from one stage to the next would, Freud claimed, cause 'fixation' and affect later psychological adjustment. Freud's important contribution to psychology was to highlight the influence of childhood experiences on adult psychological adjustment, though there is no evidence to support his stages. Whereas Freud's theory of development stopped at puberty, Erik Erikson proposed an 'epigenetic' stage theory of human development (one in which the stages are determined by an interaction of genetic and environmental influences) that extended across the lifespan. Drawing on psychoanalytic theory, Erikson proposed that an individual is unable to progress from one stage to the next until certain 'crises' have been overcome and psychological adaptations accomplished (Erikson 1980). Many of the challenges faced by adults are, we feel, better addressed under the headings of stress and coping (Chapter 8). Nevertheless, Erikson's ideas continue to inform research into developmental processes, most notably the psychology of later life.

In contrast to Freud and Erikson, Piaget (1952) was interested primarily in the development of intelligence. He rejected biological theories that assumed developmental changes to be entirely 'pre-programmed'. He also dismissed behaviourist theories which proposed that children learn entirely through reward and punishment (Chapter 5). He based his theory of cognitive development on direct observation and developed a unique developmental framework that is still used to inform educational, health and social care practices. Piaget assumed that each child progresses through certain stages of development in a fixed sequence, each building on learning acquired at the previous stage. Like Freud, Piaget stopped short at adolescence, at which point he assumed that the capability for adult reasoning was attained.

Although psychologists no longer subscribe to stage theories, we have included Piaget's theory because it is well established as a framework for understanding child development within health and social care. It is relatively simple to understand and still useful to apply in practice. But we also offer the work of Vygotsky as a flexible and useful addition to our understanding about the ways in which children and adults can be helped to learn and develop throughout the lifespan.

The development of thinking and understanding

Piaget's theory of cognitive development

Piaget's specialization in intelligence testing led him to study in detail the development of learning in his own children, introducing experiments to test their understanding as they grew older. At the centre of Piaget's theory is the concept of mental structures or 'schemas' which form the building blocks of understanding (see also Chapter 4). According to Piaget, the child is born with certain hard-wired reflexes, such as sucking and crying, with which they interact with the world around them. As the child interacts with the physical and social environment, they develop mental structures he called 'schemas' which form the 'building blocks' of cognitive development. Just as in a building, it is not possible to build the second floor before the building blocks for the first floor are in place. Schemas may be behavioural (e.g. learning to tie shoelaces), symbolic (use of representations using symbols, such as language) or operational (e.g. learning to add up or subtract). The development of schemas imposes constraints on the child's level of understanding – hence the division into developmental stages.

According to Piaget, schemas are developed through a process of 'assimilation' and 'accommodation'. New information about the world is assimilated (incorporated) into existing schemas. When these schemas no longer allow adequately for the interpretation of new information, they are altered or modified to 'accommodate' it.

It has been conclusively shown that babies are born with the ability to recognize the human face (Johnson and Morton 1991). This means that newborns can assimilate information about the human face into a pre-existing 'face schema' which enables them to distinguish the human face from other images. Through interaction with the mother or main caregiver, this face schema is modified within as little as four days to enable the baby to distinguish the mother's face from others (Pascalis *et al.* 1995). This modification is an example of accommodation of the face schema. From 5 weeks of age, the face schema has undergone further accommodation to enable the infant to recognize the mother's face in a photograph (Bushnell 2001).

Piaget proposed that the process of assimilation and accommodation underpins cognitive development. His own observations led him to define a series of invariant developmental stages. We have highlighted the main stages below.

- *0–2 years: sensorimotor stage*, so called because infants use sensory information gained through the mouth and hands to learn about the properties of objects around them. During this time, the child quickly learns to recognize and later label familiar objects. They also learn that objects continue to exist when they are not in sight.
- *2–7 years: preoperational stage*, so called because children are influenced by how things look, rather than by logical reasoning. This is the stage at which children learn to use imagination and language (symbolic thought). They become self-aware, but remain egocentric (unable to see how things look from the point of view or perspective of someone else).
- *7–11 years: concrete operational stage*, so called because the child is now capable of using logical reasoning. They can view things from the perspectives of others, understand the notion of relativism (taller, hotter), the concept of reciprocal relationships, and number conservation (e.g. if I start out with two oranges and you have none, when I give you one of my oranges there are still two oranges in total). But as the term 'concrete' indicates, children at this stage have difficulty in dealing with abstract concepts. For example, they would probably view health in terms of not feeling poorly.
- *11+ years: formal operational stage*, so called because the child becomes

capable of engaging in abstract thought. This means that they should be able to manipulate ideas and follow a hypothetical argument, using logic and without reference to a concrete object.

Clearly, much change takes place within these age bands and Piaget sub-divided them into a series of sub-stages. For those who are interested, these are detailed in any specialist text on child development.

> One of the best-known examples of Piaget's experiments is the 'three mountains' experiment (Piaget and Inhelder 1956). The child was sat in front of a table, on which stood a model of three mountains and a doll. The child was shown a selection of photographs and asked to choose the photograph of the view the doll is likely to see. Very young children did not understand the task and until around the age of 7 the child selected their own view, rather than that of the doll. This appeared to demonstrate that children at this stage are unable to see things (literally) from the perspectives of others. Piaget termed this **egocentrism**.

The 'three mountains' experiment subsequently came in for criticism because the task is complex and uses a scene that is not part of most children's normal experience. Donaldson (1978) demonstrated that by using familiar objects, such as teddies and building bricks, children of the same age or younger can accomplish the task. Children in her study were able to hide a 'naughty teddy' behind building bricks so that the doll cannot see it, demonstrating that the child is able to take the dolls perspective (literally). However, a problem with these types of experiment is that they focus only on visual perception, whereas the term 'egocentrism' is normally applied to the inability to understand someone else's feelings. Further experiments using dolls led Donaldson to conclude that young children are often quite good at understanding how other people are feeling and what they might be thinking or planning to do (Donaldson 1990). In other words, many young children have the ability to empathize with others and cannot be truly held to be 'egocentric'. In the field of health and social care, these findings imply that young children's understanding can be disrupted by unfamiliar objects or surroundings and quite young children are likely to be affected by the feelings and emotions of those around them.

> When Sasha first became pregnant, she experienced a lot of morning sickness and became very tired, which made her tearful. At this time, Lee became upset when left at the nursery, telling the staff that mummy was poorly. With encouragement and help from the nursery staff and the health visitor, Sasha tried to reassure Lee and explained things to him using simple examples so that he could understand. She worked out a routine with Jo that enabled them to help Lee feel more secure until this phase of her pregnancy passed and things were back to normal.

When questioned, it is quite difficult to tell if a young child is saying what they really believe, or what they think adults want to hear, particularly if they feel that their knowledge is being put to the test. Professionals who wish to explain things to children in this age range using play must make sure that they use familiar objects. They also need regularly to check out the child's understanding by asking them to describe what is happening, rather than asking direct questions, as happened in Piaget's experiments.

Piaget's theory remains influential in the contexts of education and child care, because the notion of developmental stages provides a simple rule of thumb for children's levels of understanding that is easy to apply.

Vygotsky's sociocultural theory of cognitive development

Vygotsky was a Russian contemporary of Piaget, although his work was little known in the west until more recently. Like Piaget, Vygotsky acknowledged children as active explorers of the world around them and that they learn in incremental steps. But while Piaget seemed to view this as a mainly solitary activity, Vygotsky was interested in the role of social interaction and language in the child's' development. Vygotsky (1978) argued that children are particularly likely to learn from others when there is only a small gap between what children are able to do on their own and what they could do with a little help from someone more skilled. Vygotsky called this gap the 'zone of proximal development'. Essentially, this means that the child learns 'one small step at a time, with help and guidance'.

> Lee was having difficulty opening a box and became very frustrated. Jo observed that the cause of Lee's frustration was his failure to distinguish the top of the box from the bottom. If Jo had assumed that Lee was not old enough to open the box for himself, he might have taken it and opened it for him. Instead, Jo showed Lee where he was going wrong, and then gently guided him while he did it himself. In this way, Lee learned a new skill that would enable him to open the box for himself in future.

The term 'scaffolding' is used to describe the interactive process whereby the amount of help and guidance given is tailored to the individual's responses, so that they can gradually achieve more and more. These concepts have been influential in education by encouraging active, guided participatory learning. They have also led to the introduction of peer teaching, where older children who are more skilled are encouraged to teach those at a slightly lower level of skill development. This has been used in the field of health education (Chapter 9). An important and useful feature of Vygotsky's theory is that, unlike Piaget's theory, it has no upper age or stage limit, and this principle applies equally to adult learning.

Vygotsky's theory predicts greater flexibility in the ways children learn. A child may attain greater understanding about certain issues because they have had more opportunities for learning within their social environment. Therefore, while some children with health problems appear to be very advanced for their age in terms of their knowledge about their body, illness, drugs or procedures, others have little knowledge or understanding. This means that professionals need to take account not just of the child's age and developmental stage (from Piaget), but must take account of the individual child's experience and understanding.

Veldtman *et al.* (2000) sought to evaluate knowledge and understanding of illnesses in children and adolescents, aged between 7 and 18 years, who had congenital and acquired heart disease. They found that less than a third had a good understanding of their illness; 77 per cent did not know the medical name of their condition and 33 per cent had a wrong or poor understanding of their illness. Even some older adolescents had an entirely wrong concept of their disease. Of particular importance is their finding that understanding was not directly related to age.

Rushforth (1999) reviewed the available evidence in order to enhance information-giving and consent-taking for children in hospital. She proposed that children's understanding is often related to the explanations they have been given. For example, in relation to pain, they were more likely to be able to explain why an injection hurts than why they have a headache. She suggested that this is because adults are more likely to spend time explaining an injection. She also pointed out that ambiguity in the English language can lead children to make misinterpretations (e.g. children might hear IV as ivy). Rushforth argued that many childhood fears related to illness may originate from such simple misconceptions. Therefore, it is essential to check the child's existing level of understanding before giving any further information. (Drawing on Vygotsky, the same applies to adults; see also Chapter 4 on memory and information-giving.)

Sasha has been trying to explain to Lee that she is expecting another baby. She has told him that there is a baby growing in mummy's tummy. But when Lee asked how the baby got in there, Sasha was not sure what to say. It is unlikely, at the age of 4, that he will be able to understand an abstract concept such as conception. There are some very good books that help to explain pregnancy and childbirth to young children and Sasha has decided to get one from the library next time she is in town. This will enable her to find out what Lee already knows and help her to provide the 'scaffolding' around which he can develop his learning on this subject.

The development of moral reasoning

As children grow older, the development of moral reasoning is important because it is associated with independence of thought and action, the ability to tell right from wrong and to resist peer pressure where necessary.

Kohlberg was interested in how children learn to tell right from wrong. He studied how boys from the age of 10 dealt with moral dilemmas such as theft and criminal damage (Kohlberg 1969). He found that younger boys conformed to adult rules, but evaluated the goodness or badness of an act by its consequences. They tended to reason that if it is possible to 'get away with it', then it couldn't be that bad. Older children tended to obey the rules of their social group in order to gain praise and avoid censure, but by the age of 16, adolescents tended to demonstrate commitment to a set of principles shared with a reference group. In contrast, the highest level of adult moral reasoning involves the development of a self-chosen moral code and set of ethical principles.

Based on these observations, Kohlberg developed a six-stage theory of moral reasoning. Below are the main three levels of development:

1 Preconventional morality (approximates to Piaget's preoperational stage): consequences are used to distinguish right from wrong. The main aim is to achieve rewards and avoid punishment. The most important value at this stage is obedience to authority.
2 Conventional morality (approximates to Piaget's concrete operational stage): the child's developing concept of self leads them to want to be thought of as a 'nice' person. Behaviour is judged to be 'good' or 'bad' on the basis of social rules set down by the society or subculture in which the child lives.
3 Postconventional morality (approximates to Piaget's formal operational stage): this stage emphasizes the importance of obeying democratically agreed laws and social rules because they are seen to be for the public good. At the highest level of development, people adopt a set of ethical principles based on personal conscience.

Like Piaget, Kohlberg proposed that these stages are fixed in terms of sequence. But unlike Piaget, he claimed that they are not linked directly to chronological age. In fact, he believed that few actually attain a state of postconventional morality. An important criticism of Kohlberg has been that his work is culture-specific, limited to a set of western values that prevailed at a particular point in time. It is possible to argue that since Kohlberg made his observations in the 1960s, punishment for bad behaviour has largely disappeared and younger children are now much more ready to challenge the moral codes of their parents. Similarly, older children are less likely to be influenced by the moral rules of society, and more likely to be influenced by the social code of their peer group. This is particularly noticeable where taking risks or behaving badly is considered 'cool'.

Based on his own observations, Kohlberg argued that with respect to behaviours such as smoking, drug-taking and alcohol consumption, younger boys need careful monitoring to make sure that they don't 'get away with it'. Peer pressure is a strong influence on teenage behaviours and is likely to take priority over 'rational' arguments.

> Sasha had a very strict upbringing but went to a school where she mixed with children from a variety of different social and cultural backgrounds. By the time she was 15 years old, most of her closest friends boasted of having sex and encouraged her to do the same. She knew her parents would be angry and upset, but one evening at a party she gave in to unprotected sex with a boy she was infatuated with and became pregnant.

Kohler only studied boys, and it is possible that moral development in girls might be somewhat different. Nevertheless, appeals to adult reasoning may have little or no effect if the teenager belongs to a social group that rejects them.

Children's understandings of death and dying

According to Piaget's theory, children at the preoperational stage of development may find it impossible to accept the permanence of death.

> Lee has a friend, James, also aged 4, whose father was recently killed in a road accident. James's mother told him that his daddy had died and he was later taken to visit the grave. But a few weeks after that, he said to his mother, 'Now please can we go and dig daddy up?'

Meadows (1993) suggested that most children are unable to accept the permanence of death until they are about 9 years old. Rushforth (1999) suggested that they may be unable to accept death in terms of the impact on the family until adolescence. Viewed from the perspective of Kohlberg's preconventional and conventional stages of moral reasoning, it is possible that a child may see the death or permanent departure of someone they love as a punishment for their own misdeeds. Rushforth has therefore argued that the greatest disservice we do is to try to protect children from the realities of events such as death. In seeking to fill gaps in their knowledge, their imagination may be far worse than reality. It is worth reflecting that even adults have difficulty in accepting death as permanent unless or until they have seen the body or obtained concrete evidence of the death. An abstract concept such as death can be addressed through stories, but may be more easily understood and ultimately less frightening if learned about through the death of a pet, provided family members are themselves willing to confront the reality of death (Chapter 6).

The importance of play

Both Piaget and Vygotsky noted the importance of play in cognitive, motor and social development. During the preconventional and conventional stages of moral reasoning, play also offers opportunities to enact and resolve moral conflicts. Play in the form of experimentation starts at an early age when babies repeat acts that have a direct effect on their environment and those in it, such as hitting a hanging mobile to make it turn, or making a noise to attract the caregiver's attention. Piaget argued that play enables babies to practise motor, cognitive and social competencies and thereby achieve mastery. Both Piaget and Vygotsky noted that children use symbolic or pretend play to act out different roles and situations. This enables them to learn to cope with a variety of possible situations, including emotional crises, interpersonal conflicts and social roles. For example, playing at doctors and nurses, or mothers and fathers, is a good way to learn about different aspects of the social world in which they live.

Sasha has been encouraging Lee to play at mothers and fathers with his friend, in preparation for the birth of his new brother or sister. Boys are often discouraged from playing with dolls, but Sasha has provided him with an old doll of her own that cries and wets its nappy. She hopes that he will be better prepared and less jealous once the baby is born. Meanwhile, Jo has been encouraging Lee to play football and other 'boys' ' games to build up a special type of relationship between stepfather and son and distract from the extra attention required by the new baby.

Play has been promoted as a useful way of preparing children for medical procedures. There appears to be little evidence to support its routine use prior to medical procedures (Kain *et al.* 1996) though it can be effective if tailored to suit an individual child's needs (Watson and Visram 2000). Play therapy is an accepted intervention for use with emotionally or behaviourally disturbed children. A **meta-analysis** by LeBlanc and Ritchie (2001) showed it to be as effective as other therapies, though it may take as many as 30 sessions to achieve optimum improvements in such outcomes as self-concept, anxiety and behavioural problems.

Social development

Social development refers to the development of human relationships. The human infant is dependent on adults for all its needs in the early years. Therefore, there are good reasons why babies need to establish a close relationship with their mother and/or other principal caregiver(s). The early behaviourist operant **conditioning** view was that a bond of attachment to the mother occurred because she provided **reinforcement** (Chapter 5) in the form of food and comfort. This explanation was discounted at an early stage when Harlow (1959) demonstrated through experiments with rhesus monkeys that a baby monkey preferred soft physical contact with an inanimate object, even when it did not deliver milk. Harlow's studies also confirmed that female monkeys who had no experience of mothering subsequently neglected or abused their own children. These experiments identified that a close bond between the child and principal caregiver is an important requirement for normal social development.

Having studied the permanent negative effects of separation at birth on other species, psychologists once believed that there might be a critical sensitive period soon after birth when it was essential for mother and baby to 'bond'. Klaus and Kennell (1976) studied the effect of increased infant-mother contact soon after birth and found that close physical contact just after birth stimulated caring responses in the mother. As a result, maternity units encouraged women to hold and suckle their babies as soon as they had been born. Nevertheless, Rutter (1979) noted the propensity of adoptive parents to develop strong attachments with older babies, casting doubt on the notion of a sensitive period for attachment. Babies undoubtedly benefit from a close relationship with their principal caregiver, but this may take place at any time during the early weeks or months and may involve one or more care providers.

Attachment

Attachment refers to the strong emotional bond which is formed with the principal caregiver(s) in infancy and usually remains life-long. The name most closely associated with early studies of attachment in human infants is John Bowlby. Bowlby (1969) noted that human babies exhibit a number of behaviours that have survival value because they engage the adults who will meet their needs. These include:

- crying, cooing, babbling and smiling – called signalling behaviour;
- clinging, non-nutritional sucking and maintaining eye contact with caregiver – called approach behaviour.

Bowlby's theory of attachment is based on an interactional model. This means that attachment is not dependent solely on the infant's responses or those of the mother. Rather, each influences the other. Therefore, a depressed mother who is unable adequately to respond to the infant's demands for attention may influence the baby's subsequent behaviour. Similarly, a very small pre-term infant may be unable to produce responses like crying or smiling that elicit adult attention. Either of these may affect the relationship between baby and mother. Bowlby suggested that primary attachment in infancy provides a template for subsequent intimate and social relationships. Therefore the failure to develop strong emotional bonds in infancy or childhood may damage the ability to develop close relationships in adult life.

Separation

By the age of between 7 and 12 months, Bowlby noted that babies become very distressed at the absence of their mother or primary caregiver. He termed this 'separation anxiety'. At this age, infants also become very wary of strangers and may protest vigorously if they approach too close. Bowlby emphasized that separation from the primary caregiver before the age of 5 years might damage the mental health of the child. His research was used to argue that women should not go out to work and leave their babies with other caregivers. More recent studies have identified that attachment to multiple caregivers is possible. There is no evidence of adverse effects of other types of child care arrangements on the child, provided stable and good quality sources of care are provided.

Until the 1960s, when a child was admitted to hospital it was common for the mother to be asked to leave the child and only be allowed to visit for limited periods. This was because children were observed to become extremely distressed each time their mothers had to leave. James Robertson worked closely with Bowlby in the late 1940s and, with his wife, made a series of harrowing films that revealed the true nature and extent of distress shown by separated young children (Robertson and Robertson 1967–73). The stages of separation were marked by:

- protest – anger and loud crying;
- despair – withdrawal and less vigorous crying;
- detachment – later, the child outwardly displayed cheerful behaviour but remained emotionally distant.

As a result, children's units reversed their policies and now encourage mothers, or other close caregivers, to stay if possible for the duration of the child's admission. Of course, this can cause separation problems for other children in the family, depending on the availability of alternative trusted caregivers.

Types of attachment

It was observed that not all children respond in the same way when separated from their mothers. This led to a series of experiments into different types of attachment relationships and their effects on separation.

During the 1970s, Mary Ainsworth (Ainsworth *et al.* 1978) conducted a series of classic experiments on the nature of attachment and stranger fear, called the 'strange situation experiment', as in the following scenario. The child and mother are placed in a room full of toys and observed through a one-way mirror. A strange person comes into the room and talks to the mother. Then the mother exits from the room, leaving the child with the stranger. Finally, the mother returns.

Based on the child's responses to these types of event, three main classifications of attachment have been identified (based on Ainsworth *et al.* 1978; Cassidy and Shaver 1999).

Secure attachment
The child uses the parent as a secure base for exploration, plays happily with the toys, reacts positively to strangers and returns to play. Play is reduced during the parent's absence and the child is distressed. On the parent's return, the child seeks contact and then returns to play.

Avoidant attachment
The child avoids physical intimacy with the parent and maintains emotional neutrality. Plays with toys, unaffected by the parent's whereabouts in the room. The child is not distressed on separation and, on the parent's return, ignores her or may move away. If the child is distressed, they are as easily comforted by the stranger as the parent.

Ambivalent
Protests strongly on separation. The child is fussy and wary in the parent's presence and has difficulty leaving her. On reunion, the child seeks contact in a babyish way, but at the same time struggles against the parent and appears angry. The child remains uninvolved in play.

Subsequent research sought to identify features of parenting associated with these styles of response.

- The parents of children who were securely attached appeared more responsive, showed more affection including touching, smiling, and praise, and more social stimulation.
- Those whose children showed avoidant attachment or insecure attachment showed much lower levels of these types of interaction.

These observations indicate that parental (normally maternal) warmth is an important prerequisite for secure attachment. Follow-up studies have indicated that securely attached children are more likely to be initiators of play as well as active participants in play, more curious and eager to learn, and showed more empathy towards other children. Those who have insecure attachment relationships tend to be socially withdrawn and less curious (Maccoby 1980). However, Maccoby noted that (at least until the age of 3) insecure relationships can change if the quality of the parental response improves. This offers important support for parenting classes.

Teenage motherhood is associated with increased economic and social problems, including a higher incidence of premature birth, and concerns are frequently expressed about the quality of parenting skills in this group. American nursing researchers Spieker and Bensley (1994) studied 197 adolescent mother–infant pairs to identify factors that influenced their parenting. They found that infants were more likely to be securely attached if their mother lived independently with their partner, but also received a high level of social support from their mother (the child's grandmother).

Sasha was only 16 when Lee was born and had no further contact with the father. Her parents would not tolerate the disgrace and Sasha was forced out into temporary accommodation where Lee cried a lot, while Sasha became very depressed and unresponsive. The health visitor observed this and also noticed signs of insecure attachment in Lee's behaviour. After discussion with the social worker, Sasha was put in touch with a mature registered childminder so that she could obtain support from an experienced mother. This also allowed her to continue with her education and attend parenting classes. She eventually met up with Jo and moved in with him. Although four years older, Jo still tended to be rather feckless. But Sasha built up a secure relationship with Jo's mother who provided much-needed **emotional support**, without interfering with the way she was bringing up Lee. This enabled Sasha to build her self-confidence as a mother and also build up a closer relationship with Lee.

It is important to note that the quality of the attachment relationship reflects a two-way interaction. The temperamental disposition of the child may affect the mother's behaviour, just as the mother's behaviour may affect the responses of the child. For example, some babies cry a lot and resist being held and cuddled, which can make it difficult for the mother to form a close relationship.

The influence of parenting styles on development

It is evident from the previous sections that home is the centre for children's learning, and relationships within the home offer a template for the development of future behaviour and interpersonal relationships. Distinct styles of parenting have been identified, based on a series of studies originally conducted by Baumrind 1967, 1971). Each of these has been shown to have a different influence on the development of the child (Boyd and Bee 2006).

- *Authoritative parents* are characterized as setting reasonable standards and enforcing them firmly and consistently without the need for physical punishment. They expect the child to conform to standards, but provide explanations, guidance and feedback, and encourage

self-direction. Children brought up in this way show higher levels of self-esteem, self-confidence, achievement and internal locus of control (Chapter 5). They are more independent and altruistic, while also most likely to comply with parental values.
- *Authoritarian parents* expect obedience, show less warmth and use less communication. They set absolute standards, often using physical punishment. They attempt to control the attitudes as well as the behaviour of the child and discourage argument. Teenage offspring tend to obtain poorer school grades, have more negative self-concepts and are less able to regulate their own behaviour.
- *Permissive parents* are indulgent towards the child's impulses, desires and actions and make little attempt to regulate the child's behaviour. They attempt reasoning, but avoid any exercise of control and make few demands on the child. Children tend to be immature and less able to take responsibility. They do worse in school and may be aggressive, if the parents are permissive towards aggressive behaviour.
- *Uninvolved parents* are neglectful. Infants show insecure avoidant attachment and later show disturbed, impulsive and antisocial patterns of social relationships.

A more recent longitudinal study by Baumrind (1991) suggested that parents who use an authoritative style may be more successful in protecting their children from problem drug use, as opposed to casual recreational use, in adolescence.

Cohen *et al.* (1994) conducted a large four-year prospective survey of preadolescents to identify which specific parenting behaviours were associated with the onset of alcohol and tobacco use. They found that children who claimed their parents spent more time with them and communicated with them more frequently had lower rates of alcohol and tobacco use. The findings indicate strong influences of parental monitoring and positive relationships on adolescent vulnerability to peer pressure and subsequent substance use. As a result, the authors recommend that parenting education with respect to substance use should take place before their children reach adolescence.

In addition to these characteristics of parenting, other positive attributes may include consistency and fairness. There have emerged clear links between parenting and adolescent and adult behaviour, suggesting that parenting education may have an important contribution to offer. However, it appears from the literature that further research is needed to identify key attributes of such programmes.

Development in adolescence

Adolescence refers to the period between childhood and adulthood. As such, it is a key time of development but one that was overlooked by major stage theorists including Freud and Piaget – perhaps because it is difficult to define and understand. The onset of adolescence, if defined as the onset of puberty, is subject to variation between cultures and within the same culture over time, due to environmental influences such as diet. Entry to adulthood, in contrast, is culturally determined. Some cultures have initiation rights that determine the end of childhood and give access to the rights and privileges of adulthood. In western cultures, there are many markers by which adulthood may be defined: biological markers such as the attainment of ultimate height and completion of pubertal changes; legal markers such as attaining the right to have legal sexual intercourse, get married, smoke, drink alcohol, hold a credit card and vote; status markers such as marriage, having a family and home ownership. Between these markers lie many contradictions. For example, it may be possible to get married or join the British Army, but not buy alcohol or vote. And in an age when young people are encouraged to attend university, many remain financially dependent on their parents until well into their twenties and some into their thirties.

Different individuals mature in different ways at different rates and the situation is further complicated when they have a learning difficulty that delays cognitive and moral, but not physical, development. These issues create confusion for the adolescent, and pose dilemmas for those providing services that were designed for either children or adults, or which transfer from one to the other at a fixed age. For example, within health care, neither children's wards nor adult units are best suited to the needs of adolescent patients, while automatic discharge from social care at age 18 can have damaging consequences for a group who are not sufficiently mature to cope without support. Dealing with the transition from adolescence to adulthood poses particular problems for those who have a severe learning difficulty, for whom there appears to be a prolonged period of childhood and delayed adolescence.

Todd and Shearn (1997) interviewed the parents of adults with moderate to severe learning difficulties who were aged between 17 and 44 years, in order to address the issue 'when is an adult not an adult?' The conflict is summed up by one parent as: 'He looks and sounds like a man. But when you look and listen more carefully you realize he's just a child. You've got to treat him like an adult in one way, and like a child in another.' One mother observed of her 32-year-old son: 'I think he's going through his adolescence now. He's beginning to find his feet.' The study highlights some of the conflicts of the adult body and child's mind. Those with learning difficulties appear torn between being dependent and wanting to be independent; wanting to do normal things, such as get married, but being rejected as 'different' by others.

In Vygotskian terms, adolescence may be regarded as a time of intense social, intellectual and behavioural learning; a period of apprenticeship for the autonomy of adult life and the responsibilities that go with it. It is also a period during which youngsters attempt to discover their identities and roles in life, socially and at work. It is a time when adolescents rebel against parental constraints and values and seek to establish their own identities within peer groups (Chapter 2). We have already focused on some aspects of parenting that facilitate successful transition. In defining 'success' we have been guided by government and societal concerns about the incidence of teenage depression, suicide and pregnancy; substance misuse, including binge drinking, smoking and opiate use; and antisocial behaviour.

A review of the literature on these issues confirms that they are all closely linked to parenting before and during adolescence. Emotional warmth and parental involvement are associated with secure attachment (see above) and have been shown to be particularly important in protecting against adolescent depression (Taris and Bok 1996).

A longitudinal study by Waatkaar *et al.* (2004) in Norway sought to establish a causal link between stressful life events and teenage depression. They confirmed that depression was indeed associated with broken friendships, death or serious illness of a close friend, parental divorce, problems with a teacher, family member in trouble with the police and drug/alcohol problems within the family, most of which appeared to impact more on girls who reported more depressive symptoms than boys. But a more sophisticated analysis appears to show that the presence of depression early in the study predicted negative life events later in the study, *not the other way round*. They point out that life events do not occur 'out of the blue' but are often the consequence of family lifestyle.

Studies such as these confirm the importance of warm, secure relationships early in life. Such parenting will help to establish good role models with respect to substance use, prepare adolescents to avoid unnecessary risks, resist negative peer pressure and deal with difficulties as they arise. Adolescents who live in deviant, chaotic or disrupted families, or who lack family support, are more likely to develop low self-esteem and mental health problems. They are also more likely to link up with peer groups that encourage antisocial and risk behaviours. A review by Asarnow *et al.* (2001) suggests that interventions for adolescent depression should begin with assessment and management of such issues as substance misuse, family dysfunction and maternal depression, while the management of the youngster's depression should combine cognitive behaviour therapy (CBT, see Chapter 6) with antidepressant medication.

Risk behaviours in adolescence include those that pose long-term **threats** to health and well-being, such as substance misuse (including alcohol and tobacco) and unprotected sex. Steinberg (2004) provides a useful review of this aspect of adolescence, arguing that teenagers are more likely to be influenced by emotional considerations than practical ones when faced with choices. High arousal, whether due to excitement or substance use, together with peer group pressure, impairs 'rational' decision-making.

There is some indication in the literature to suggest that gender differences may explain some variations in engagement in risk behaviours. For example, Taris and Bok (1996) found that involvement of the father in young adulthood was linked to taking personal responsibility for one's actions (internal locus of control – see Chapter 5) while over-involvement of the mother had the opposite effect. They observed that young people who felt unable to influence what happened to them were more likely to feel depressed. Griffin *et al.* (2002) showed that parental monitoring is associated with lower levels of alcohol use in boys, but not girls. This means that interventions may need to be different for boys and girls.

Prevention is better than cure, and Greenberg *et al.* (2003) in the USA found strong evidence that long-term school-based and youth development programmes, which are student-focused and relationship-orientated, are capable of improving social behaviour, school attendance and performance, and mental health in adolescents. However, the message is that it is best to start such programmes before youngsters start to experiment with risky behaviours. As health and social care professionals, an important role is to find ways to listen to, support and encourage youngsters and youth groups to find adaptive ways of dealing with important issues.

Development in adult life

People continue to develop throughout their lives and not just during childhood as the developmental theories of Freud and Piaget might have us believe. Erikson and Levinson both proposed stage theories of lifespan development. Levinson *et al.* (1978) described a series of life transitions that reflect common patterns of changing family and work roles across the lifespan. For example, young adults move away from home, make and break new friendships, establish and negotiate sexual relationships, get a job, start a family. In early middle life, people may have to reappraise life goals in the light of achievements, or the failure to achieve previously determined goals. This might include having or not having children, career progression or change, adjustments in lifestyle or expectations, maintaining relationships or separations, dealing with success or failure. Later middle life often includes physical changes associated with the menopause for women, the demands of caring for older parents, loss of parents, children leaving home (or staying at home), separation or divorce and increasing concerns about health.

Many of the major life changes faced by adults are included in the Holmes and Rahe (1967) list of major life events (Chapter 8), designed as a measure of exposure to stress though now somewhat out of date. However, neither stage theories nor the measurement of stressful life events explain *how* adults are able to negotiate successful transitions between different roles and circumstances. A theory that attempts to address this was put forward by Paul and Margaret Baltes in 1990 (Coleman and O'Hanlon

2004). They called it 'selective optimization with compensation' (generally referred to as SOC, but not to be confused with **sense of coherence**, see Chapter 8). Based on goal theory, Baltes and Baltes proposed three fundamental processes by which individuals actively manage their lives: *selection* refers to developing and committing to a set of personal goals that focus the acquisition and use of effort, skills and resources; *optimization* refers to the effort, skills and resources the individual invests in achieving these goals; *compensation* refers to finding alternative means to achieving goals when previous means are no longer available (Bajor and Baltes 2003). In the face of life changes or losses, a further process of selection is required to re-evaluate existing goals and identify new ones (see Chapter 9 for examples in relation to chronic illness). Some indicators of these processes are given in Table 3.1. You will find similarities between these responses and locus of control (Chapter 5).

Wiese *et al.* (2002) found evidence that these processes are predictive of well-being in the context of both family and work. In many ways, they resemble the active **coping strategies** designed to gain and maintain control, referred to in Chapter 8. But it is important to note that seeking help is identified as a positive strategy if this is used to assist the individual to achieve personally relevant goals. This model is potentially of considerable use in practice, both for our own benefit and that of those we care for:

- If there are goals – are these realistic? Or is help needed to review and modify them?
- If there are no goals – what help is available to help identify goals and motivate action?

Table 3.1 Examples of selection, optimization and compensation strategies (based on Bajor and Baltes 2003)

Positive	*Negative*
Selection When I think about what I want in life, I commit myself to one or two important goals	I wait and see what happens instead of committing myself to just one or two particular goals
Optimization I keep working on what I have planned until I succeed	When I don't succeed right away, I don't try other possibilities for very long
Compensation When things don't go as well as they used to, I keep trying other ways or seek help	When things don't go as well as they used to, I accept it
Loss-based selection When I can't do something important the way I did before, I look for a new goal	When things don't go as well as they have in the past, I still try to keep all my goals OR I just wait and see

- Is it necessary to prioritize and focus more energy on certain achievable goals?
- Is it necessary to gain new skills or resources to help achieve goals?
- How can the individual be encouraged to persevere in the face of setbacks or deal with losses?

Some of the challenges likely to emerge during the adult lifespan are dealt with elsewhere in this book, notably in Chapter 8 on stress and coping and Chapter 9 on health and well-being. A challenge identified as particularly likely to lead to stress and the development of stress-related illness is the transition from being a son or daughter to the role of carer of a parent.

Ted recently moved to live with his son Mark and wife Janice. He had always relied on his wife to do all the household chores and expected his daughter-in-law to do the same. Janice had worked hard to train Mark to assist with these, but now even he was starting to copy his father. Janice was busy working and this led to considerable tensions. Anna became aware of the reasons for these difficulties as a result of her nursing lectures and set up a family meeting to review roles and responsibilities. This resulted in an agreement that Ted would help with light housework and vegetable preparation, but would need help with cleaning the bathroom and floors, and changing bed linen.

Much depends on the nature of the relationship that exists between the parties and in the above example Ted is amenable to this type of negotiation. But it is possible to predict that an authoritarian style or insecure attachment relationship may make it more difficult to deal with this type of transition. Particular burdens also arise when caring for a parent who has experienced serious mental decline (see Chapter 8).

Development in later life

Old age has been categorized as a separate life stage since antiquity. For example, Faulkner and Luce (1992) noted that the Greeks and Romans characterized old age as a time of physical and mental deterioration, social marginalization and closeness of death. From this, it would appear that ageist stereotypes have a long history. Nowadays, the majority of those requiring medical care and hospitalization are 'elderly'. Therefore the needs of this group deserve particular consideration. But how should 'old age' be defined?

Theories of age and ageing

Old age is often defined in chronological terms and the age of retirement at 60 or 65 is still commonly used as a convenient point of entry. But these days, people choose to retire at any time from the age of 50, while the official age of retirement may, in some countries, eventually rise to age 70. People now live so long that it is common to distinguish the old from the 'old old' at age 80. The health of those aged over 50 is very variable. Some develop chronic diseases at a relatively young age due to genetic and life-style reasons, while others remain fit and active into their nineties. Some feel old in their fifties, others never feel old. Therefore both objective and subjective transition points are very variable and chronological age is not a particularly useful concept. Functional age may seem somewhat easier to define in terms of the activities that people are able to undertake. However, these activities are often limited by cultural, legal and economic con-straints, as well as individual emotional, cognitive and physical limitations. Overall, old age remains difficult to define.

Traditionally, theories of old age focused on the notion of gradual decline. Cumming and Henry's disengagement theory (1961) used to be a prominent theory of old age. Based on an American study of people aged 50 to 90 reported in 1961, the researchers noted that retirement and other events such as death of a spouse led to restrictions in lifestyle. Subsequent researchers have pointed out that these changes were often forced on people, particularly those who were poor. Certainly many people experi-ence decline in physical strength and function as they grow older. Yet in twenty-first century western societes, older people are generally fitter, better off financially and able to enjoy a longer period of active retirement with far more choices available to them. Improvements in the management of dis-eases such as arthritis, heart disease and cancer mean that there is generally a shorter period of decline prior to death. It is inevitable that older people are more likely to be exposed to illness, disablement and loss. It is not necessarily inevitable that they will respond to these differently from those who are younger, though multiple health problems (co-morbidities) make this more difficult.

So how should 'successful' ageing be defined and how can professions support it? Erikson (1980) characterized the final life stage as one that brought either integrity or despair. Successful ageing refers to successful completion of previous life stages including:

- 'hope' resulting from the sense of trust developed in childhood;
- 'will', 'purpose' and 'competence' gained through childhood experiences;
- 'fidelity', referring to sense of identify and set of values gained during adolescence;
- 'love' and 'care' resulting from intimacy and relationships in adulthood;
- 'wisdom' resulting from attaining 'ego integrity' in old age – this enables people to maintain a positive sense of self in spite of a decline in bodily and mental function.

In contrast to Cumming and Henry's predictions, Coleman and O'Hanlon (2004) presented evidence that in general people are at least as satisfied with their lives, more positive about themselves, and no more anxious, depressed or fearful as they get older. Reasons offered for this include the flexibility to adapt to changed circumstances and re-evaluate and, where necessary, modify personal goals. There is a minority who approach the end of their lives in despair, but it may never be too late to change for some.

Anna went on a home visit with a health visitor to see a lady, aged 90, who seemed very depressed. She talked of her early life. After a difficult childhood, she had married at an early age to someone who turned out to be married already. She left him, but never admitted the reason to others, even to her own mother, who had died at the age of 94. As a result, she had never married nor had children of her own. But by the time Anna and the health visitor left, she seemed much more cheerful. Being able to talk this through with non-judgemental nurses really seemed to help her to make sense of these experiences in the context of the time and culture in which they had happened.

Older people who have not successfully achieved Erikson's state of integration tend to complain more about everything and are likely to be among the 'unpopular patients' referred to in Chapter 2. This leads to responses such as avoidance that reinforces feelings of sense of isolation, resentment and despair. This is unhelpful and can lead to aggressive responses (see Chapter 7). Such people can be very challenging to care for, but are likely to be more in need of a listening ear than others who are a pleasure to care for.

Approaching life's end

As people approach the end of their lives, whatever their age, they seem naturally to reflect on their accomplishments and try to find a sense of meaning or purpose in past problems or failures. Butler (1974) termed this natural process as 'the life review'. People who approach the end of life with a sense of accomplishment or satisfaction at having achieved certain life goals are generally less anxious and depressed, while those who have a sense of regret report more anxiety, depression and anger (Walker and Sofaer 1998). Life goals may be quite modest ones related to holding down a job, rearing children to be independent, having grandchildren, or dealing successfully with small challenges. Everyone experiences some failures, but generally goals may be reset to allow for achievements that balance these. Some people need opportunities to review these issues, find meaning from difficult lives, or deal with 'unfinished business' before their life end.

Life review therapy is a structured form of **narrative therapy** (see Chapters 1 and 6) through which the individual is encouraged to review, reorganize and re-evaluate the overall picture of their life, and gain a sense of meaning and coherence. This has been confirmed as an effective therapy for depressed older people (Bohlmeijer *et al.* 2003). It can be emotionally painful remembering situations associated with shame or guilt, but Coleman (1999) has suggested that life review therapy has a 'confessional' dimension that encourages reconciliation.

Haight and Olson (1989) developed a structured format for life review therapy for use by nurses and home aides. The intervention consists of six one-hour sessions during which the older person reviews happy and sad events in childhood, middle life and finishes with a reappraisal of these events. Structured life review has been shown to lead to improvements in life satisfaction, well-being and self-esteem, and decreases in depression.

Life review therapy should not be regarded as the preserve of old age, but may be helpful for others who have experienced important losses or face a terminal illness. It is part of a growing tradition of narrative psychology (see Chapter 1).

Coping with dementia

The processes described above are based on an assumption of normal development. But increasing numbers of people experience premature cognitive decline due to dementia or Alzheimer's disease. The prevalence of dementias in Europe ranges from about 1 per cent at age 60–64 years to almost 25 per cent in those aged 85 years and over (Ferri *et al.* 2005). Prevalence in the older age group is higher in North America and much lower in the developing countries – which may reflect different reporting systems and/ or the availability of medical and social services to support survival. It is also important to note that the rate of dementia is very much higher, for genetic reasons, in people who have Down's syndrome who are increasingly reaching retirement age. Dementia is considered a psychiatric diagnosis, made using the Mini Mental State Examination (MMSE) which tests orientation in time and place, recognition, attention, recall and language. The MMSE with instructions for use can be found on the website of the Alzheimer's Society (see chapter end), where advice on management for carers is also to be found. These tests are inappropriate for people with learning difficulties. Diagnosis is difficult in this group, though family carers may report increasing forgetfulness. Dementias are often accompanied by depression, which could be explained by the growing sense of uncertainty and loss of control (including bodily control) that inevitably accompanies memory loss. Changes in routine and environment worsen agitation and make the challenges of caring more difficult.

Kitwood (1997) noted that the main problems faced by those with dementia relate to **depersonalization** (being treated as objects and not as individual people) and include:

- *treachery* – using deception to distract or manipulate, or forcing them to comply;
- *disempowerment* – not allowing the individual to use the abilities they retain or failing to assist them to complete actions they have initiated;
- *infantilization* – treating and talking to them as if they were a young child;

- *intimidation* – use of threats or physical power;
- *labelling* as the main basis for interaction and explaining behaviour;
- *stigmatization* – treating the person as if they were a diseased object.

Professional carer behaviours that have been observed to have negative effects include: carrying on conversations as if the person was not there; refusing to give asked-for attention; blaming the person for actions or failures; crudely interrupting thoughts or activities; mockery, humiliation and disparagement. Kitwood refers to these actions in terms of 'malignant' social psychology (see Chapter 7). Approaching people who have dementia in these ways is demeaning and demoralizing for all concerned and should play no part in professional caring. In contrast, effective communication can be life-enhancing and satisfying. In Chapter 4 we illustrate how positive communication with people with dementia can help them to retain their sense of personhood and their dignity. In Chapter 8, we demonstrate the importance of providing support for family carers in order to avoid stress-related illness and family breakdown.

Anna was working on night duty on a busy medical ward where an elderly patient with early symptoms of dementia was constantly interrupting their work by attempting to leave the ward with the intention of going home. In desperation, the staff nurse sent for the doctor, anticipating that she would prescribe a tranquilizer. Instead, the doctor sat down with the patient for half an hour, listening carefully to his concerns and talking with him. At the end of this time, he had calmed down, got into bed and went to sleep. Anna learned that attending to dementia patients is time-consuming. But it probably takes less time in the long run to build up a relationship of trust than it does to engage in physical restraint. Drugs appear to offer a short-term solution, but cause further disorientation and confusion (Kitwood 1997), and make matters worse once the patient is discharged to family or long-stay care.

Summary of key points

- Stage models of cognitive development offer some guidance to children's understandings at different ages, but there are wide individual variations.
- It is necessary to ask the child to talk about their existing understanding of health and illness, so that it is possible to help build on and extend this through demonstration and play as well as talk.
- Secure attachment relationships that involve parental warmth, involvement and monitoring, are important for normal adult psychological development and reduction of behaviours that pose risks to health.
- When considering development across the lifespan, it is helpful to consider common challenges and demands within their environmental and

cultural context, using frameworks such as loss, stress and coping (Chapters 6 and 8).
- Listening to older people's stories and valuing their individual life experiences has therapeutic value.

Exercise

See after Chapter 10.

Further reading

Berger, K.S. (2005) *The Developing Person: Through the Life Span*, 6th edn. New York: Worth.

Boyd, D. and Bee, H. (2006) *Lifespan Development*, 4th edn. Boston, MA: Pearson.

Cassidy, J. and Shaver, P.R. (eds) (1999) *Handbook of Attachment: Theory, Research and Clinical Applications*. New York: The Guilford Press.

Coleman, P.G. and O'Hanlon, A. (2004) *Ageing and Development*. London: Arnold.

Kitwood, T. (1997) *Dementia Reconsidered: The Person Comes First*. Buckingham: Open University Press.

Web address for Alzheimer's Society: www.alzheimers.org.uk.

MEMORY, UNDERSTANDING AND INFORMATION-GIVING

- **What influences what we remember?**
- **Why do we forget important information?**
- **How is our understanding influenced by our existing knowledge?**
- **What are the main causes of memory loss and confusion in older people?**
- **How can we give information in a way that improves memory and understanding?**
- **What are the best ways of breaking bad news?**

Introduction

Health professionals rely heavily on verbal and written information in order to inform patients about their diagnosis and treatment, and members of the public about ways in which they can take personal action to promote their own health and prevent future adverse health consequences. Much of this activity it based on an assumption that the recipients will remember and/or understand what they are told. We have all experienced frustration when people appear to have taken no notice of the instructions they were given and even deny ever having been told. This chapter examines reasons for this, based on memory theory and research, and offers evidence-based recommendations to improve information-giving.

Memory

Memory involves receiving, processing, encoding, storing and retrieving information. Memory loss or forgetting may occur at any stage, although most information appears to be lost at the receiving, processing and retrieval stages. Memory theory is based on the assumption that there are two distinct types of memory: short-term and long-term memory. Short-term memory (otherwise known as primary or working memory) holds a limited amount of unprocessed information for a short time. Following that, information is selectively processed and transferred into long-term memory for permanent storage. Even then, information is subject to bias during recall. Some knowledge of these processes can help health and social care professionals to ensure that their patients or clients have a correct understanding of important information. To illustrate this, we present a situation in which Lillian is being given the results of a biopsy she recently had taken from a lump in her neck.

> *Doctor:* Well, Lillian, the tests show that you have a type of cancerous growth called a lymphoma. This type of tumour normally responds well to treatment. We will get you into hospital next week to remove the lump and then organize some follow-up treatment in the form of chemotherapy.

We review the effects of this style of information-giving and consider others in due course.

Arousal and attention

In order to receive any type of information, we must pay attention to it. In other words, the information must stimulate our interest and arrest our attention. This implies a state of arousal, which refers to the arousal of the autonomic nervous system and release of adrenaline that prepares the body for action (Chapter 8). Based on research over many years, it is well established that cognitive performance, including memory, is related to our level of arousal. But this relationship is not linear. There appears to be an inverse U relationship between arousal and cognitive performance which is termed the Yerkes-Dodson Law (see Figure 4.1). Since arousal is frequently associated with feelings of anxiety, the Yerkes-Dodson Law applies equally to levels of anxiety. This is explained below.

A low level of arousal reflects a state of apathy or disinterest. If Lillian is in this state, she may not be taking the situation seriously and is unlikely to be attending to the information being presented. Therefore her memory encoding is likely to be minimal and she will be unable to recall what she was told.

An extremely high level of arousal is associated with a high level of anxiety

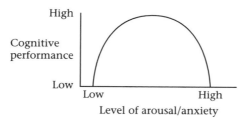

Figure 4.1 The Yerkes-Dodson Law of the relationship between arousal and cognitive performance

or panic. If this were the case, Lillian would probably be unable to attend properly to any type of cognitive task and her memory encoding is likely to be poor. Her attention may focus solely on the most salient aspect of the information received and this is not necessarily the main point the doctor wished to convey.

The best cognitive performance is obtained if Lillian is aroused, slightly anxious, alert and her attention clearly focused upon the task in hand. This would enable her to concentrate on and encode what was being said, and recall more accurately the information she was given. This highlights the importance of noting the patient's emotional state when trying to give important information. Time needs to be taken to listen to, and calm someone who is highly anxious, or alert someone of the importance of an issue if they are totally unconcerned. If doctors or others use euphemisms for cancer, such as 'tumour' or 'growth', the patient may not be alerted to the significance of the information being given.

Short-term memory

Short-term memory is also referred to as working memory since remembering at this level is an active and conscious process. Ebbinghaus and Wundt, in the nineteenth century, asked people to recall a series of nonsense syllables and showed that people could normally repeat about seven of these. Miller (1956) confirmed that short-term memory has a processing capacity that is limited to 7+/−2 bits of information. The combination of seven letters and numbers in the British car number plate was determined by this psychological research. But a 'bit' is not the same thing as a letter or number. You will note that it is easy to remember a number plate such as LIM1T, which effectively reduces five digits to one meaningful chunk of information. In contrast, the number plate that reads NMG3P, each of the five digits is a separate, unrelated bit of information.

How many separate chunks of information are commonly given to patients during a single consultation? In the short extract from Lillian's consultation, it is possible to identify at least nine separate bits of information that may make it unlikely that Lillian will remember all of it:

Well, Lillian, the tests show that you have

1 a type of cancerous growth
2 called a lymphoma.
3 This type of tumour
4 normally responds well to treatment.
5 We will get you into hospital
6 next week
7 to remove the lump
8 and then organize some follow-up treatment
9 in the form of chemotherapy.

The holding of information in short-term memory, and transfer to long-term memory, is facilitated by repetition and association. If we wish to remember a telephone number, we keep repeating it until it has 'sunk in'. If we are distracted during this process, we often have to start all over again. When we are given a series of important items of information in a short space of time, there is no opportunity to repeat or reflect on each one. This helps to explain why much of it is promptly lost. Lillian's consultation is time-limited and is likely to cover a lot of information, most of which will never reach her long-term memory.

It is possible to improve memory by using memory-enhancing devices such as **mnemonics**. Mnemonic techniques are useful ways of organizing discrete bits of information into a meaningful chunk. For example, if I wish to remember the number plate NMG3P, I might make up a little saying, such as 'No Man Gets 3 Pence'. This would be even more memorable if it was accompanied by a visual image of a man picking up coins. Mnemonics are commonly used to assist with remembering medical information. For example, a common mnemonic for remembering the first letters of the 12 cranial nerves is: 'On Old Olympic's Towering Tops, A Fin And German Viewed Some Hops'.

In the case of treatment regimes, patients could be encouraged to repeat their instructions several times and relate them to daily events, such as meals, in order to retain the information. When trying to remember which tablet is for what, white for water, blue for blood, yellow for yawning (sleep) might prove memorable if the colours of the tablets were obliging enough to conform to this mnemonic. It is probably best if patients invent their own, but they may need some encouragement to do so. Some people prefer verbal mnemonics while others prefer visual ones. Of course, the best way of ensuring that something is not forgotten is to write it down. It would be helpful if Lillian was given written information about her condition and treatment plan so that she could take it away and read it at her leisure.

Familiarity, salience and selective attention

Even when people are attending to what is being said to them, their attention will tend to focus upon things that are familiar or important to them. In other words, people tend to pay attention to what they know about or expect to hear and not necessarily to the things that health professionals feel are important. In Lillian's case, the salient aspects of information are highlighted in bold below.

Doctor: Well, Lillian, the tests show that you have a type of **cancer** called a lymphoma. This type of tumour normally responds well to treatment. We will get you into **hospital** next week for an **operation** to remove the lump and then organize some follow-up treatment in the form of **chemotherapy**.

Lillian is likely to hear certain key words during her consultation, of which 'cancer' is probably the most important to her. This may interfere with her ability to hear other important details, such as 'the tumour normally responds well to treatment'. Furthermore, you may have noticed that Lillian's problem is referred to in four different ways: cancer, lymphoma, tumour, lump. Lillian may or may not realize that these terms refer to the same thing.

Selective attention is an important problem in relation to health promotion. There is a danger that those most likely to attend to health messages are those already engaging in healthy lifestyles, since the information serves to vindicate their existing attitudes and behaviour. Those whose behaviour is contrary to the advice being given tend to regard it as irrelevant.

Primacy and recency effects

When people are given several pieces of information in sequence, they are most likely to remember the thing they are told first (the **primacy effect**) and the thing they are told last (the **recency effect**), and forget most of the rest. One of the reasons for this is that they have more opportunity to mentally rehearse these items. In the case of Lillian's information, this means that she is most likely to remember the fact that she has cancer and will have to have chemotherapy.

Well, Lillian, the tests show that you have

1   a type of **cancer**ous growth
2   called a lymphoma.
3   This type of tumour
4   normally responds well to treatment.
5   We will get you into hospital
6   next week
7   to remove the lump
8   and then organize some follow-up treatment
9   in the form of **chemotherapy**.

Conveying useful information

Health professionals can use memory research to try to ensure that they give the most important information first and repeat it last. Thus if the doctor really wishes to convey to Lillian the good news that her lump is likely to respond to treatment, it would be better to approach this by reordering the sequence of the information given to Lillian:

Well, Lillian,

1 **Your tests indicate that you have something that is likely to
   respond well to treatment**
   . . . pause
2 You have a form of cancer
3 called a lymphoma.
4 We will need to bring you into hospital
5 next week
6 to remove the lump
7 and then give you some further treatment
8 in the form of chemotherapy.
9 **Fortunately, the outcomes of this treatment are good**.
   . . . pause

Presenting positive information first and repeating it last emphasizes the likelihood of a successful treatment outcome. The pauses also allow time for important information to be attended to and facilitate transfer from short-term into long-term memory. In this case, Lillian is much more likely to go away feeling positive about her results. Even where an outcome is not so positive, this approach can be used to highlight the fact that everything possible will be done to ensure the well-being of the individual. In practice, Fallowfield and Jenkins (1999: 1592) recorded that 'many patients leave consultations unsure about their diagnosis and prognosis, confused about the meaning of and need for further diagnostic tests, unclear about the management plan and uncertain about the true therapeutic intent of treatment'. An important example is the use of the term 'positive' when referring to test results. From a medical perspective, this means finding cancer cells. From the patient's perspective, it implies good news about negative test results.

Long-term memory

Long-term memory has been the subject of much research and theory development in psychology, assisted more recently by the introduction of brain scanning and imaging techniques. Once transferred from short-term to long-term memory, memories are stored in the brain according to series of complex linkages between language, meanings, emotions, images, sounds and responses that are still not fully understood. Long-term memory is normally divided into three distinct types:

1 Procedural memory is concerned with motor skills, rules, habits or sequences, such as riding a bike.
2 Semantic memory is concerned with general knowledge, or knowledge for facts, and is heavily dependent on language.

3 Episodic or autobiographical memory is concerned with memory of events from the past and is strongly associated with sensory images.

Procedural memory is related to habit formation (see conditioning, Chapter 4), and is extremely enduring. Semantic memory may be subject to interference and is commonly affected during dementia. Autobiographical memory tends also to be very enduring and it is common to find that even older people with severe Alzheimer's disease are able to retain memories of emotionally important events from their past. This may be because emotionally arousing events are more easily or strongly embedded within our long-term memories and become more memorable. McGaugh (2003) reminds us that autobiographical memories are what connects our past to our present and help us to predict the future. This aspect of memory is fundamental to our sense of self (Chapter 2) and to the way we cope with loss and other stressful events (Chapters 6 and 8).

Understanding

Remembering is not the same as understanding. For example, Anna was able to recall the list of cranial nerves for her examination, but found it difficult to organize and present these in a coherent way because she had not fully understood their functions. Lay people are often disadvantaged in health care settings by their limited knowledge and understanding of their bodies (see also Chapter 3 on children's understandings). It is only fairly recently in evolutionary history that adult humans have had much idea about the nature and function of internal organs, and many adults today have little idea about how their bodies actually work. As health professionals, we should not take for granted that patients understand the names, functions and locations of essential organs, or that they necessarily wish to know. Adults may sometimes suffer unnecessary illness or disability as a result of incorrect beliefs about their bodies and body functions. For example, people with back pain often avoid activity or exercise because they believe that pain signals damage (see Chapter 10). Those working in the field of health care take biomedical explanations for granted, but those working in complementary therapies have totally different explanations for symptoms such as pain, while lay people draw on a range of understandings to explain aches, pains and other symptoms, including family and folk lore. It is essential to check out patients' understandings rather than assume that they share the same explanations.

Mental schemas and scripts

Recent memory research has focused on the fact that individuals tend to encode information in relation to their own framework of understanding, which is referred to as a mental schema (schemas were also mentioned in Chapter 2 in relation to the self-concept, see also Vygotsky's theory of development in Chapter 3). Schemas enable us to organize and process large amounts of information, but their existence implies that memory encoding and recall involves a certain amount of selectivity and reconstruction.

A classic experiment by Bartlett (1932) studied what happens when a complex and mysterious legend or story is passed from one person to another in the same way as 'Chinese whispers'. He selected a North American folk tale, 'The War of the Ghosts' that contained a number of features that were strange and difficult to make sense of for those in twentieth-century western cultures. He found that the story changed in certain predictable ways as it was passed on. The story became shorter, more coherent and more conventional, to fit in with common cultural ways of understanding. The study is easy to replicate and demonstrates that while distinctive and familiar events are retained, less familiar information is altered to fit in with the framework of understanding of the individual.

Bartlett's work highlighted that memory schemas are strongly influenced by shared social and cultural understandings. When a patient is given medical information by word of mouth, they tell their friends and relatives, framed in ways that all can understand. The facts as well as the story are thus transformed in the telling. It is not unusual for professionals to note that a patient or client reports a completely different version of events from that recorded, or that their understanding appears quite incorrect. It is essential for professionals to take time to encourage each patient or client to share their understanding so that misapprehensions can be corrected at an early stage. Basic misunderstandings can lead to unnecessary, incorrect or inaccurate treatments. Time spent listening and checking is often time saved in the long run.

Jo's friend, Kris, had suffered from a painful back condition, ankylosing spondylitis, since he was a teenager. Although he had learned to cope quite well, his doctor referred him to the local pain clinic where he was offered a course of acupuncture. While Kris was waiting for the doctor to place the needles, the nurse asked him what effect he thought acupuncture would have. He said that the needles would untangle his nerves and cure his pain. When it was properly explained to him (see Chapter 10), he decided that it was not necessary and opted not to have any further treatment.

Mental scripts and autobiographical memories are gaining increasing attention within the relatively new fields of narrative psychology and narrative medicine. Receiving medical information is not just a matter of remembering a list of facts. Finding out that one has a disease changes an individual's life story, confronting them with a different future to the one that they had anticipated. This is often referred to as biographical disruption (see Chapter 2). As patients are receiving news about their disease and treatment, they may be trying to make sense of this in the context of an unexpected and important change to their anticipated life story.

When Lillian heard the doctor tell her she had cancer, she started thinking about the much longed-for holiday she was due to go on with a friend in two months' time. It was her first long distance holiday and she had spent so much time planning and looking forward to it. Logically, her health was far more important, but why this and why now? All she could think about was that it could not possibly be happening to her. Perhaps she would wake up in the morning and find that it was all a bad dream. As she considered this, she realized that she had missed most of what the doctor was saying. She did not like to ask the doctor to repeat it, even when asked if she had understood everything, because the doctor was obviously very busy.

Finding out that one has diabetes or heart disease is a lot to take in at a single brief consultation, particularly when it involves learning a new medical language. It is hardly surprising that people are often upset or confused and fail to recall important details.

Recall and false memories

Recall involves far more than remembering facts. It is a reconstructive process that is subject to a variety of external influences. Experimental research into memory has shown how it is relatively easy to 'plant' memories by the use of prompts, probes or other devices (see review by Loftus 2005). If you wish to find out what a patient has remembered it is better to ask an open question like, 'What did the doctor tell you last time?' rather than a closed question such as, 'Do you remember the doctor telling you [facts]?'. Asking a closed question plants information and ensures that the answer cannot be relied upon to be true.

There have been accusations in the media that psychotherapy can lead to the recovery of false memories about events such as childhood sexual abuse. Memories associated with events that cause emotional arousal are usually better embedded in memory. So is it possible that someone can forget such an important event? Clinical psychologists sometimes refer to lack of memory for a traumatic event as 'dissociation', which implies that memory has become cut off from conscious thought as a form of self-protection. Alternatively, applying the Yerkes-Dodson Law, it is possible for intense physiological arousal during trauma to eliminate memory processing. Drawing on either explanation, it is very hard to know if someone has 'recovered' a memory for a real event or if the 'memory' has been acquired by some other means.

Elizabeth Loftus, one of the leading researchers in this field of study, reviewed a range of experimental and 'real-life' evidence in which so-called 'recovered' memories were subsequently refuted by incontrovertible evidence (Loftus 2002). Some of her examples were associated with gross miscarriages of justice. She concluded that there is *no way* of distinguishing true from false memories. If practitioners encourage recall, it is essential they do not provide prompts or leading information that can lead to false reconstructions. Further, Loftus asserted that it is dangerous for mental health practitioners to assume that the failure to recall childhood trauma implies that these memories have been repressed and therefore need to be excavated. Such assumptions are based on a psychodynamic model for which there is *no substantiated evidence*.

Context-specific memories

Certain memories are context-specific, which means that they are aided by a return to the environment or emotional state in which the event or incident originally took place. This is because the memory was encoded into a schema that included strong environmental information. You have probably had an experience where a certain piece of music or smell triggers a memory of a forgotten incident. In the same way, patients may have entirely forgotten an instruction or piece of advice until returning to the sight and smell of the hospital. Only then do they remember what they should have done, but may be too embarrassed to admit that they didn't do it.

Forgetting

Memory loss is rarely due to the decay or loss of memories, but is more often caused by problems in transferring information from working (short-term) memory into long-term memory, or in retrieving information from long-term memory. Research by Anderson (2003) suggested that it may be difficult to encode new information that threatens to disrupt existing patterns of belief or ways of behaving. This lends support to Festinger's theory of **cognitive dissonance** (Chapter 7), but there may also be a structural explanation. De Beni and Palladino (2004) studied working memory between the ages of 55 and 75 and found that older people had greater difficulty accommodating new information into their existing memory schemas. This reinforces the need to check out a patient's understanding of new information, as in the case of Lilian.

> Lillian, perhaps you would like to tell me what you understand about what is wrong and what the plan is for your treatment?

It may be that a patient's apparent failure to grasp what they were told is caused by their inability to update existing schemas, or by the threat to their existing belief systems or narrative structure. It is always best to start with what they already know or believe and build gradually on this, taking account of the coping strategies available to the individual (Chapter 8). This can be demanding in terms of time and patience, but it is pointless for the health professional to try in vain to bombard the patient with advice and instructions that cannot be assimilated. Practitioners are failing in their duty of care if they persist in attempting to do this.

It is often assumed that older people are less likely to adhere to medication use than younger people because of poorer memory. But this appears to be a stereotypical belief for which there is little evidence.

> Park *et al.* (1999) created an age-stratified profile of individuals with rheumatoid arthritis and studied factors that influenced adherence to medications. They assessed cognitive function, disability, emotional state, lifestyle and beliefs about the illness. They found that older adults made the fewest adherence errors, and middle-aged adults made the most. Despite strong evidence for normal, age-related, cognitive decline, most older adults had sufficient cognitive function to manage medications. A busy lifestyle was the strongest predictor of non-adherence and this was more likely to occur in middle life.

Health care professionals should not assume that older adults are more likely to forget to take their medications, unless there is good reason to suppose that they are suffering from memory loss.

Memory loss

Sudden memory loss, confusion and disorientation in older people is commonly due to simple medical conditions, such as respiratory or urinary tract infections, anaemia, or self-neglect associated with malnutrition or dehydration. Medical treatment for these conditions usually results in memory restoration unless permanent toxic brain damage has occurred. In later life, confusion is also a relatively common response to certain drugs or anaesthetics. Correctly assessing the cause of the problem and initiating appropriate treatment should reverse memory loss in most cases. Many older people can remember details of adverse events long afterwards, even though they appeared totally confused at the time. The following scenario illustrates how important it is to explain to people who are in a temporary confused state what is happening.

> Ted's friend Violet, aged 81, described what had happened the day after an operation she'd had three months previously. She recalled seeing snakes crawling over the lady in the bed opposite and remembered trying to climb out of bed to remove them. She was aware of becoming more and more agitated as nurses kept dragging her back, until finally one of them explained that these were hallucinations caused by the anaesthetic. She remembered the relief at receiving this explanation.

Dementias

A study by Sliwinski *et al.* (2003) found no direct statistical relationship between memory loss and chronological age. Instead, they found that the progression of pre-clinical dementia was the most important predictor of memory loss. Alzheimer's disease is probably the best-known form of long-term memory loss and confusion, and is the most common cause of dementia. It is a progressive brain disease that involves loss of memory, confusion, and problems with speech and understanding. The number of people with dementia increases dramatically with age (Chapter 3). The main risk factor for Alzheimer's disease is genetic and for reasons that are partly genetic but not yet fully understood, people with Down's syndrome are at greater risk of dementia at a much earlier age. Another common type of dementia, vascular dementia, is associated with the same genetic and lifestyle factors as other vascular diseases, including smoking and heavy drinking.

Many people remain undiagnosed until the later stages of dementia. This is partly because of difficulties in diagnosis and partly due to the stigma associated with the disease. The most commonly used test for dementia or Alzheimer's disease is the 'Mini Mental State Examination' (MMSE) (Folstein *et al.* 1975) – see Chapter 3. A test score of less than 24 out of 30 is indicative of dementia. Some authors have drawn attention to the possibility of cultural bias in these types of test, particularly where items involve the use of language or lack cultural relevance (Teresi *et al.* 2001). This means that older members of some immigrant groups are vulnerable to false positive testing using standard measures.

There is no cure for most types of dementia, including Alzheimer's disease, though some drugs have been developed that can temporarily improve quality of life. In the early stages, simple memory aids such as writing reminders and making lists can help to overcome forgetfulness. Later, the aim of treatment is not simply to improve memory, but to enable patients and their families to manage and come to terms with the problems of dementia. Depression and anxiety are commonly associated with dementia but it is difficult to distinguish between cause and effect. Confusion and forgetfulness are likely to increase distress and agitation, while increased anxiety and agitation make the memory problem worse. In terms of psychological approaches, cognitive retraining has been shown to improve learning, memory, activities of daily living, depression and self-rated general functioning (Sitzer *et al.* 2006). It consists of learning new problem-solving strategies to cope with memory loss and repetitive techniques to improve memory.

The caregivers of those with Alzheimers are particularly at risk of stress-related illness (Chapter 8). Agitation and aggression are hard to deal with, while memory problems make reciprocal communication very difficult and take great patience and understanding. It is also tempting to think that once a person's memory has gone, the individual inside has also gone. Many caregivers experience great distress because the person they love no longer remembers who they are, or may mistake a spouse for a parent or a daughter or son for a deceased wife or husband. People with dementia may ask the same question again and again and never appear to take in the answer. This can become very frustrating and makes the sufferer susceptible to abuse from relatives. It is not easy for professionals either. But aspects of autobiographical memory, particularly those related to emotionally salient events, often remain intact until the very late stages of Alzheimer's disease. Encouraging the person to remember events from their past can be informative as well as rewarding.

Marie Mills (Mills and Walker 1994) studied institutionalized older patients who had severe dementia, during which she encouraged them to talk about their past. She recounted how one particular man, Mr Fellows, initially appeared confused and depressed. Nevertheless, he described detailed episodes from his childhood which his wife, to her surprise, confirmed as accurate. One day he told Marie how he had once lost his school cap, which meant his mother had to buy another (they were very poor). This made sense of the fact that Mr Fellows would often wander round the ward in an agitated state saying, 'Where's my cap?'

Later on, Mr Fellows confided how ashamed he was of being incontinent and how annoyed he was because the chiropodist had not come to attend to his feet. It emerged that he actually had quite a lot of awareness of his current feelings and needs. As the study progressed, Mr Fellows started to cheer up and became less agitated and depressed. The best explanation for this is that the staff began to respond to him more as an individual with an interesting life history. Mills recommended that a social history should accompany older patients, particularly those needing longer-term care, so that staff are encouraged to treat each person as a unique individual.

Autobiographical accounts can be encouraged while engaging in personal care, which helps to make better use of this time. Alternatively, it may help to involve volunteer 'listeners' to record this information. It does not matter if the events recalled are happy or sad, provided the professional is willing to listen and tolerate the shedding of a few tears. Recalling early memories helps the individual to regain some sense of coherence within their lives (Chapter 2). It also helps care providers to gain a sense of the individual as a person in their own right, rather than drawing on stereotypes to classify them as another forgetful old person.

Brain injury

Certain types of brain injury caused by trauma or stroke can lead to particular types of memory loss. This comes under 'abnormal' psychology and we are unable to cover this in depth. Accidental brain damage may cause complete loss of short-term memory and encoding, such that the individual fails to remember anything that has occurred since the onset of the disorder or trauma. Total memory loss or **amnesia** is actually rare. More common are specific types of memory loss associated with damage to different parts of the brain. For example, it is fairly common following cerebral vascular accident (stroke) to find that the individual has unilateral neglect. This means that the patient 'forgets' that they have a left or right side to their body until they are reminded. The arm or leg functions perfectly well when they make a conscious effort to move it, but in the course of trying to walk or feed themselves, they fail to attempt to use it. Some people actually fail to see objects on the left or right side. This may be caused by a breakdown in the ability to integrate visual, perceptual and motor information and may respond to a programme of re-education.

Communicating effectively with patients

Volumes have been written about the importance of effective communication in health care. It is well established that lack of information is strongly associated with patient dissatisfaction but studies such as that by Oterhals *et al.* (2006) indicate that there is still plenty of room for improvement. Philip Ley's classic work (Ley 1997) drew on the principles of memory research to propose a number of ways in which client–health care professional communication can be improved.

- Improve the environment (avoid delays, be friendly, allow the patient to explain things in their own words).
- Find out what the patient believes and encourage feedback.
- Stress the importance of particular content and repeat it.
- Give important information first and repeat it last.
- Check that you are using language that the patient can understand.
- Give specific, rather than general or vague advice.
- Provide written back-up material, but ensure that this is written and presented so that people can understand it.

Ley (1997)

Ley (1997) provided a comprehensive research-based analysis of problems of poor communication, much of which is quite old but nevertheless relevant. For example, he explored reasons for taking incorrect medication including not taking enough, taking too much, incorrect dose interval, incorrect treatment duration and taking additional medications. He found, for example, that patients were often unable to understand quite simple written or verbal instructions. Even instructions such as 'consult your doctor if symptoms persist' were poorly understood by large number of people. In high-school students, words such as 'fatal' and 'misuse' were poorly understood. Among the general public, the words 'infection' and 'cancer' were understood by most people, but the terms 'metastasis' and 'prognosis' were not. Boulos reported that even the most readable patient information leaflets on diabetes required a reading age of 11 to 13 years, compared to the average reading age of the British public of 9 years (Boulos 2005).

Ethical principles of autonomy and non-maleficence (do no harm) are central to research governance. Beaver *et al.* (1996) wanted to find out about children's understanding of the type of written information typically given to those invited to participate in a randomized controlled trial (RCT) of a new drug (DoH 2001a). Specifically, they wanted to test understanding of randomization (whether they would get the real or the dummy drug), safety and effectiveness (whether the drug would make them better), voluntariness (refusal would not affect their normal treatment) and redress (what would happen if something went wrong). The information was given to schoolchildren aged 9 to 11, who had higher than average educational achievement, in three different formats: question and answer, block text and story. Overall understanding of written information ranged from 54 to 63 per cent, with the story format improving overall understanding, possibly because it was most familiar to them. The question-and-answer format was least understandable. Interestingly, willingness to participate in such research was reduced by over 10 per cent using the story format. If this was a result of better understanding, it would have worrying implications for researchers.

Those preparing to design patient information leaflets will do well to read Ley's book for simple tips on how to improve the chances that patients can read and understand the information. They include using shorter words and shorter sentences. Standard tests of readability may help to ensure this. But perhaps the most important way of improving written information is to involve representatives of patient or user groups (expert patients) in developing and presenting relevant and appropriate content in a way that is meaningful and accessible to the people who really matter. It is important when giving written or verbal information for practitioners to understand patients' priorities in terms of the information they are likely to wish to receive. The manner in which information is given, as well as its content, is important.

Hall *et al.* (2003) reported that, following antenatal genetic testing, women who were given information about the presence of chromosomal abnormalities accompanied by negative statements were far more likely to undergo termination than those who were given information in a neutral or positive way. As a result of their study, the authors recommended that staff adhere to standard protocols for giving sensitive information.

Information is very easily biased when given in a negative or apologetic way, and choices are manipulated by the ways in which professionals convey information. Compare the following ways in which Sasha might be told that she will have to have her baby in a consultant obstetric unit instead of the midwife-led unit for which she originally booked.

Compare the impact of the following statements:

- Well, Sasha, I'm afraid that we will have to transfer you to the consultant unit.
- Well, Sasha, we will need to transfer you to our friends over in the consultant unit.

Subtle differences in the ways that information is conveyed can make a lot of difference to the way that it is perceived. For Sasha, it could make the difference between acceptance and disappointment or fear.

Breaking bad news

The analysis of Lillian's experience of being told about having cancer highlights just how difficult it is for people to remember information when being given bad news about their diagnosis. Lesley Fallowfield was the first psychologist to study the effects of offering patients a tape recording of the 'bad news' consultation (Hogbin and Fallowfield 1989) so that they could listen again at their leisure. This does not suit everybody, but those who have elected to do this have found it extremely helpful in gaining a better understanding of the whole situation, and in explaining it to close family or friends. Fallowfield has since investigated other aspects of the bad news consultation.

Fallowfield and her co-researchers observed that health care professionals often censor information in an attempt to protect patients from potentially distressing information. However, she argued that the well-intentioned desire to shield patients from the reality of their situation usually creates even greater difficulties for patients, caregivers and members of the health care team, since it leads to a conspiracy of silence and heightened state of anxiety and confusion. 'Ambiguous or deliberately misleading information may afford short-term benefits while things continue to go well, but denies individuals and their families opportunities to reorganize and adapt their lives towards the attainment of more achievable goals, realistic hopes and aspirations' (Fallowfield *et al.* 2002: 297).

Gaston and Mitchell (2005) undertook a **systematic review** of the information needs of cancer patients and found evidence that these changed over the course of the cancer journey. Desire for information was generally strong, but they found evidence of widespread misunderstanding of disease course, prognosis and treatment aims. Ambiguous information contributed to misunderstanding, for example, 'response to treatment' could be interpreted as meaning cure.

A good way to establish people's needs and wishes for information is to undertake some 'what if' explorations at an early stage, as in the scenario below.

When Lillian originally went for her biopsy, her doctor explained that the results would show whether or not she had cancer. The doctor asked her how she might feel if she did have cancer, and what sort of information she would wish to be told. When the results came through, the doctor reminded Lillian of what she had said and asked her if she had changed her mind. She was then given the sort of information that she was best able to cope with.

Walker (1989) asked older people 'if you had something seriously wrong with you, would you like to know all about it, even if the outlook was not good?' Eighty per cent said that they would wish to know, indicating that 'you can only deal with what you know about'. Ten per cent were unconcerned and only 10 per cent said that they would not wish to know, so that they could keep their dreams and hopes. Some commented that they might not have been so keen to know when they were younger.

Forgetting bad news

A number of explanations for forgetting bad news have already been given. Freud argued that painful memories are repressed, or forced out of the conscious mind. According to Freud, repression is one of several mechanisms that defend the ego, or sense of self, against harsh external realities. Denial is another. Denial is generally used to refer to the failure of people to acknowledge the reality of a situation that causes great anxiety. This may offer protection in the short term, since the individual does not have to face up to the difficult realities. Some argue that denial is an effective coping mechanism when death is imminent, as in a terminal illness. But it can lead to problems of communication between patient, caregivers and professionals, as observed by Fallowfield *et al.* (2002). Nevertheless, it is important to ensure that patients' information needs are respected.

Individualized information-giving

It is difficult to judge the amount and type of information that an individual person wants or needs. The best approach, as illustrated above, is to elicit what the patient already understands, find out what they wish to know, and check afterwards what they have understood. When faced with the possibility of having to give bad news, it is preferable to negotiate information needs with the patient before investigations are carried out and results received. At that point, it is possible to find if people want to know every detail of the causes and likely consequences of their illness, or not. For example, Beaver *et al.* (1996) trialled the use of preference cards to allow women with breast cancer the opportunity to identify the extent to which they wanted to be involved in decision-making, from full involvement to none at all. This seems rarely to be done in practice and can lead to unfortunate consequences. It is not uncommon for relatives to try to protect their loved ones by requesting that they should not be given bad news. This is not only unethical, but can in many instances interfere with communication. People often change their minds during their illness journey and good communication requires frequent renegotiation. Good practice in information-giving starts, continues and ends with listening.

Summary of key points

- Remembering verbal information is hard, but can be enhanced by reducing the amount of information given, the order it is given in, and emphasis given to key issues.
- People are unlikely to remember information if it does not fit with their existing framework of understanding (schema). Therefore it is important to take time to find out a patient's current understanding and then to build on it.
- When dealing with patients with severe memory loss, taking the time to explain what is happening can reduce anxiety and agitation.
- People's need for information varies and it is helpful to find out what and how much people want to know when embarking on a course of investigation or treatment.

- Listening to individuals to elicit their understanding is an essential component of care.

Exercise

See after Chapter 10.

Further reading

Ley, P. (1997) *Communicating with Patients: Improving Satisfaction and Compliance*. Cheltenham: Stanley Thornes.

CHAPTER FIVE

LEARNING AND SOCIAL LEARNING

- **How can we learn without being aware of it?**
- **What influences ways we learn to respond to different situations?**
- **How can we apply learning theory to treat fears and phobias?**
- **What is 'learned helplessness' and how might this account for depression?**
- **How can we use learning theories to help manage our own lives and improve the health and well-being of others?**

Introduction

This chapter focuses on theories of learning developed from behavioural psychology. These theories direct attention to situational influences on behaviour which are amenable to change. Behavioural theories can be helpful in understanding how a range of health-related behaviours and emotional responses are acquired and maintained, and how they can be managed or treated. These theories have been used to develop evidence-based approaches to behaviour and lifestyle management in a variety of health and social care settings.

In this chapter we describe aspects of behavioural and social learning theory that are relevant to health and social care. We seek to demonstrate how these theories help to explain the development of adaptive and mal-adaptive responses, and how they can be used to enable people to improve their own lifestyles as well as those of patients and clients. The theory and research that forms the basis of this chapter is quite old but nonetheless relevant to current practice

Types of learning

It is tempting to confuse learning with memory because most learning in educational settings appears to involve memorizing. However, much of what we learn in life does not involve deliberate activity. For example, learning how to make relationships, learning new skills, learning how and when to avoid difficult situations, learning how to behave in different social settings and learning how to ride a bike. Some of these behaviours might be described as innate, some involve trial and error, while others develop by watching and copying others. Some skills can be learned from books or manuals or are taught by others, but a surprising amount of learning takes place without our being aware of it and continues throughout our lives. In this chapter, we focus particularly on conditioning theories and social learning theory because these have particular relevance in health and social care. 'Learning theory' in this context refers specifically to theories that were developed by behavioural psychologists and were originally referred to as theories of conditioning.

Background to the development of learning theory

As a background to understanding conditioning theory, it is helpful to have some insight into the thinking behind it. Philosophers and psychologists have tended to subscribe to one of two views about the nature of human learning: **nativism** or **empiricism**. Nativists believe that humans have a unique set of innate abilities that enables them to acquire and organize knowledge in a special way. Language is cited as a good example of this because children learn very quickly how to apply rules of grammar. In contrast, empiricists believe that we are born 'tabula rasa' (literally 'blank slate') and that all knowledge is gained from experience. Empiricists prior to the twentieth century believed that learning took place by association. Association might be because objects or situations are in important ways similar to each other; or because events occur together at the same time; or because one event always precedes another, implying a relationship of cause and effect. Behaviourism grew out of empiricism.

Behaviourists were the first psychologists to engage in the systematic study of learning processes, based mainly on animal experiments. With encouragement from Darwin's theory of evolution, they made no distinction between the learning processes of animals and humans, and claimed that theories derived from animal studies could be applied to human beings. Behaviourists did not concern themselves with mental processes. Although they did not deny the existence of thought processes, they claimed that these are 'private events' that cannot be studied objectively. They argued that the only legitimate way to demonstrate that learning had taken place was to observe the ways living organisms (such as dogs, rats, pigeons and humans) respond to external stimuli. This attracted the name stimulus-response theory or S–R theory. Initially, behaviour change was used as evidence that simple learning (called 'conditioning') had taken place. However, in the latter part of the twentieth century, more sophisticated methodologies enabled psychologists to reinterpret conditioning theories in terms of a set of underlying beliefs or expectations (cognitions). This has enabled behavioural principles of learning to be incorporated into cognitive psychology and, more recently, cognitive science. These principles have made important contributions to contemporary cognitive behaviour therapies.

Conditioning theories

Conditioning refers to a simple form of learning-by-association. Two types of conditioning were identified during the last century, **classical conditioning** and operant conditioning. Classical conditioning refers to learning that involves changes in reflex responses over which we have little or no conscious control. **Operant conditioning** refers to learning that involves changes in voluntary responses (those over which we normally have conscious control).

Classical conditioning

Classical conditioning is the simplest form of associative learning. Ivan Pavlov first recorded the phenomenon of classical conditioning during studies of the digestive systems of dogs. Dogs, like humans, salivate when they see food; it is a natural physiological reflex response. But Pavlov demonstrated that a signal, such as a bell, if presented immediately prior to giving the dog food, would eventually lead the dog to salivate at the sound of the bell, even when no food was present. Salivation to a bell is a 'conditioned' or learned response. This type of learning has clear implications for health and health care. A typical illustration involves the child who 'learns' to be afraid of the doctor (see Figure 5.1).

> When he went for immunization, Lee was quite happy to see the doctor. Then the doctor gave Lee his immunization, which hurt a lot. Now Lee associates the doctor with pain and howls with protest as he approaches to the doctor's surgery.
>
> At a cognitive level, Lee has learned that going to see the doctor predicts the possibility of having a painful injection. Therefore he cries and protests whenever he approaches the surgery.

Prevention is always better than cure. One way to reduce the impact of an injection for the pre-verbal child is to distract their attention while they have the injection, and reward them immediately afterwards with a treat. Hopefully, they will then come to associate the doctor with something pleasant, rather than the painful injection.

Adults, too, are susceptible to conditioned responses in health care settings.

> Lillian felt very sick after her first chemotherapy treatment. As she approached the hospital for her second treatment, she started to feel sick again.

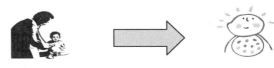

The child is happy in the presence of the doctor

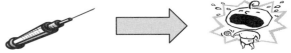

The doctor gives the child an injection that hurts

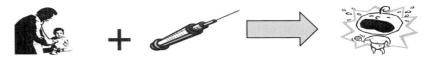

The child now associates the doctor with the painful injection

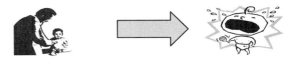

So the child screams when the doctor appears

Figure 5.1   Classically conditioned fear of the doctor

Many patients undergoing chemotherapy feel nauseous at the sight or smell of the hospital. This is a classically conditioned response. It is difficult to gain conscious control over this type of reaction once it has become a conditioned response. Therefore, it is important to prevent the development of the response by giving the patient a pre-emptive anti-emetic drug that aims to inhibit nausea before it actually occurs.

Another example of classical conditioning is the triggering of an asthmatic attack. Asthma is caused by the constriction of the bronchus in response to an allergen. So how is it that someone who is allergic to the fur of a cat or dog finds that their asthmatic attack is triggered by the sight of a cat or dog in the distance, or even by a picture of a cat or dog? It used to be believed that this type of response indicated that asthma was a psychogenic disorder (all in the mind). But medical research has shown conclusively that asthma is caused by an allergic response. The best explanation is that classical conditioning has taken place.

For years, Jo believed that his symptoms of hay fever were caused by allergy to cats. He experienced itchy eyes and runny nose when his cat

entered the room. More recently, he discovered from skin tests that he is actually allergic to house dust mite but not cats. House dust mite cells are present in bedding and allergic responses are often worse on waking. The appearance of the cat first thing in the morning, when symptoms were at their worst, was probably sufficient to generate an association between the cat and the hay fever symptoms. Thus hay fever symptoms came to be triggered by the sight of the cat.

Other reflexes amenable to classical conditioning include anxiety, fear or panic, urinary and anal sphincter control, hunger, thirst, sexual arousal, facial ticks and other involuntary body movements or mannerisms.

The principles of classical conditioning have led to the development of a number of important and widely used therapeutic interventions. One example is the use of a pad and bell to stop bed-wetting in children, once they are old enough to understand and manage it themselves:

- the child normally sleeps soundly and fails to recognize or wake to the urge to urinate;
- two sensitive pads are placed under the sheet and wired to a bell;
- the bell sounds as soon as urine makes a connection between the pads and wakes the child up;
- the bell eventually prompts an association between urination and waking;
- over a period of time, the urge to urinate becomes sufficient to wake the child in time to get to the toilet.

There are two important points to remember when applying the principle of classical conditioning.

- A conditioned response is not under conscious or voluntary control. For example, asthma sufferers are quite incapable of using willpower to stop themselves from having an attack in response to the picture of the cat.
- All autonomic responses (those involving the arousal of the sympathetic and parasympathetic nervous systems) are capable of this type of conditioning.

Conditioned emotional responses

Anxiety and fear involve autonomic responses that cause breathing, pulse rate and blood pressure to increase and muscles to tense. In an extreme form, this gives rise to a panic attack. Because emotions such as fear and anxiety involve these autonomic responses, they are very susceptible to classical conditioning. Classical conditioning theory was shown a long time ago to explain the development of fear responses to non-threatening stimuli.

Watson and Rayner demonstrated in 1920 that an 11-month-old child named Albert, who had previously shown no fear, was conditioned to be

> frightened of a white rat. This followed a period in which each time the rat was held in front of the child, the researcher made a sudden loud bang on the cot. This elicited a strong startle response and over a number of repetitions the rat became associated with a fear response. More important, little Albert subsequently showed a fear of anything that was white and furry. The transfer of the conditioned fear response from one object to other similar objects is called 'generalization'.

Most associations take repeated experiences to develop. However, exposure to a single intense **stimulus** that leads to strong autonomic arousal can sometimes be enough to cause a conditioned fear response. For example, someone who has been in a very frightening road or rail accident may be too scared to get into any type of moving transport after that, even though they are well aware that the chance of it happening again is extremely low. This type of conditioning may be a contributory cause of post-traumatic stress disorder (PTSD) (Chapter 6).

The importance of fear-reduction in hospital settings

Classically conditioned fear or anxiety responses are troublesome and difficult to treat. Therefore prevention is always better than cure. In hospital settings, this can be achieved through better patient preparation for planned procedures. For example, nurses, doctors and therapists can help patients to anticipate potentially frightening or painful stimuli (injections, procedures etc.) so that they do not experience sudden or unexpected fear, pain or other unpleasant experiences. It is often claimed that it is not necessary to concern patients by telling them about the likelihood of experiencing pain or discomfort, since this could lead to a self-fulfilling prophecy. But there is no evidence to support this and plenty of evidence that good preparation about what to expect and how to deal with it is important (Chapter 10).

> Lee needed to go to hospital for a planned procedure. The staff on the unit recognized the importance of preparing Lee for this. They had a pre-operation clinic where Lee could see the surroundings, meet other children, and watch a video showing what procedures he would experience. Staff encouraged Lee to rehearse these with a doll. This reduced the likelihood of a conditioned fear response and also reduced Sasha's anxieties about Lee's operation.

Classically conditioned responses occur at a subconscious or unconscious level. Reasonable or rational argument is not effective for someone whose fear response has already been conditioned. In fact, fears and phobias acquired in this way are often described as 'irrational' because the individual has no logical reason to be frightened.

Fear, avoidance and phobias

One way some individuals deal with situations that cause them to feel frightened or anxious is to avoid them. For example, many people avoid going for dental checks because of their fear of the dentist. But conditioned responses remain strong even in the absence of the stimulus that caused them. Fear of movement following an episode of back pain is an example of this (Chapter 10).

One way of overcoming this type of fear is 'exposure therapy', where the individual is deliberately exposed to the feared stimulus until the fear response is no longer elicited. Boersma *et al.* (2004) tested out this treatment approach with a small group of patients who had severe functional limitations as a result of back pain. Working with each individual in turn, the researcher assessed which movements were feared, demonstrated that they could safely engage in these movements without causing any damage, and encouraged them to do exercises at home on a regular basis. They found that for most patients, fear-avoidance beliefs were largely extinguished over a period of two to three months.

Phobias arise when the fear of a specific object or situation leads to the deliberate avoidance of those objects or situations. For example, agoraphobia refers to a fear of open spaces. In many cases, the individual has experienced a panic attack (sudden intense arousal of the autonomic nervous system) while in a public place and is afraid of this happening again. This leads them to avoid going out of the house and has serious social consequences. The best-known therapeutic approach to the treatment of fears and phobias, such as agoraphobia, is a gentle form of exposure therapy called systematic desensitization (Wolpe 1958).

Systematic desensitization

The patient is first taught techniques of relaxation and controlled breathing that oppose autonomic arousal. They then learn to apply these techniques when confronted with a 'hierarchical' series of situations that are graded in terms of threat, starting with the mildest stimulus. For example, first they might be asked to imagine a mild fear-producing situation while practising relaxation. Once they can achieve this without experiencing any arousal, they are asked to imagine more severe fear-producing situations. They then progress to looking at pictures or films, then to thinking about approaching the actual situation, and finally to exposure to the feared situation in the company of the therapist. The precise programme will vary according to the nature and severity of the problem. At each stage, the individual must demonstrate complete control through relaxation before proceeding to the next stage. This ensures that any association between the feared stimulus and autonomic arousal is eliminated.

Systematic desensitization has a long history of successfully treating a wide variety of incapacitating and long-standing conditioned fear and anxiety responses. Wolpe recognized that many fears and phobias occur in response to social demands or situations. Therefore, he recommended assertiveness training as an additional means of helping people to gain control over anxiety-provoking social encounters. This means training them to stand up for themselves in a non-confrontational way. It remains an important component of cognitive behaviour therapy (CBT) treatments (Chapter 6).

Operant conditioning

According to the theory of operant conditioning, behaviour is dependent on its consequences. Operant conditioning applies to voluntary actions – those over which we normally have conscious control and can therefore choose whether or not to do. Most health-related behaviours, including smoking, eating, exercising and having sex, are included in this category.

Operant conditioning theory proposes that learning takes place as a result of reinforcement and punishment. For example, I learn from experience that eating strawberries is pleasurable, so I eat more. In this case, the strawberry is termed a reinforcer because it increases the likelihood that my behaviour (eating them) will be repeated. Alternatively, if I touch a hot iron, I learn that I will burn myself so I don't touch it again. In this case, the hot iron is termed a punisher because it decreases the likelihood that I will repeat the action.

The terms reinforcement and punishment have particular meaning for behaviourists, for whom reinforcement does not necessarily mean the same as reward.

When the new baby was born, Lee became much naughtier. Sasha scolded him, believing that this was a punishment. However, Lee viewed the scold as attention and repeated the naughty behaviour to gain more of his mother's attention. Therefore, in behaviourist terms, the scold is defined as a reinforcer.

- A primary reinforcer is something that fulfils basic needs, such as food, drink or sex. Substances such as nicotine and crack cocaine may also be regarded as primary reinforcers because they satisfy basic psychological and physiological needs.
- A secondary reinforcer is one that can be used to gain primary reinforce-

ment. Social security benefit may be regarded as a form of secondary reinforcement because it allows the individual to buy food etc. Some illness behaviours, such as complaining of pain, are described as achieving secondary gain because they elicit help from others and thus enable the individual to avoid difficult or painful tasks (see later in this chapter and also Chapter 10).

The psychologist famous for the development of the principles of operant conditioning was B.F. Skinner. Operant principles were derived from animal laboratory experiments and used such equipment such as the 'Skinner box'. This was a cage in which a light or sound was used to signal to the animal or bird that, if it pressed a particular lever or pecked a particular key, it would receive a reward in the form of food or drink. Thus animals were trained to respond to different types of stimulus or cue and the effect on the animal's behaviour of different patterns or schedules of reinforcement could be measured. Below, we have illustrated some operant concepts and principles that are useful in practice.

Schedules of reinforcement or punishment

The term 'schedule' refers to the pattern or sequence of reinforcement or punishment. For example, reinforcement may be continuous (occurs every time) or intermittent (occurs only occasionally). Sometimes an occasional intense reward or punishment can influence behaviour more strongly than continuous but less intense ones. Gambling is a good example of how one large win (or even the possibility of one) can provide strong motivation to continue for a very long time. The intense effects of crack cocaine may help to explain the speed of addiction. Similarly, one intense unpleasant experience may act as a deterrent (as in the principle of the short, sharp shock).

Continuous reinforcement may lead to satiation. For example, if we always praise someone, this is eventually taken for granted and ceases to enhance their performance. Certain drugs, such as opioid analgesics, if taken regularly over a long period of time lead to increased tolerance. This means that people with chronic pain gradually have to increase the dose in order to achieve the same effect.

The subjective perception of reinforcement and punishment

Reinforcement is not necessarily the same thing as reward. Food is only reinforcing if someone is hungry and likes the food on offer. The child who receives little adult attention may behave badly to provoke punishment as a source of attention. Therefore one person's punishment is another person's reward. Smoking is a good illustration of this. Smoking may seem a disgusting habit to a non-smoker, but it has a number of immediate and highly reinforcing consequences for the smoker. These include:

- immediate pleasure/satisfaction;
- relaxation/stress management;

- maintaining alertness;
- social bonding;
- time out from demanding or difficult situations;
- having something to do with the hands.

Graham (1993) conducted a qualitative research study to find out why working-class women smoked when they could ill afford to. She found that smoking provided 'time out' from their dreary and demanding lives. One woman explained that when she lit her cigarette, it was a cue for the children to leave her alone. The cigarette provided her with personal time and space in a difficult and demanding life.

It is clear that, in cognitive terms, reinforcement and punishment are based on subjective perceptions. In other words, actions are influenced by perceived outcomes for the person engaging in them. As health or social care professionals, we need to be very careful not to assume that our own or our professional preferences and values are the same as those of a patient or client. In the above example, the professional may see smoking as a dirty, dangerous and expensive habit, while the smoker sees it as offering a pleasurable refuge. In order to help the smoker give up smoking, it is necessary to explore all of the reinforcing effects of smoking *for them*. Only then is it possible to help them plan how to substitute for the effects of each of these (see the programme at the end of this chapter). You will note that few of the benefits are a direct consequence of nicotine. Therefore using nicotine patches or chewing gum is only part of the solution.

The immediacy of consequences

Generally, the more immediate the consequence, the more powerful is its effect. Small children will normally choose to have a small chocolate bar now, rather than wait for a large one later (assuming they like chocolate). As we grow older, we learn to delay gratification, but the effect of an immediate reward is still powerful.

Consider the list of reasons why smokers smoke. You will notice that the consequences are all immediate. On the other hand, the likelihood of adverse consequences of smoking on health, particularly for younger people, are located in the distant future, if at all. This may be an important reason why smokers are not persuaded to give up smoking for health reasons, unless or until they experience symptoms of illness.

Punishment frequently fails to work because it is administered long after the crime was committed and any effects of conditioning are lost. Chastising a child when a misdemeanor is discovered, rather than when it was committed, is unlikely to have the desired effect unless accompanied by a clear explanation about what they had done wrong. In the absence of the explanation, the child is likely to interpret the displeasure as directed at them, meaning 'I am a bad person', rather than realizing that the punishment is directed at their behaviour.

Some consequences are not weakened by delay. For example, experiments have shown that rats made ill by poison will subsequently avoid the type of food or drink that contained the poison, even though there is a substantial delay between eating the food and being ill (Garcia *et al.* 1966). This type of association clearly has survival value and has given rise to the argument that some responses are innately primed or 'prepared' (Seligman 1972). An alternative cognitive explanation is that in spite of the delay, there is only one likely cause of the problem – in this case the most recent thing eaten or drunk, especially if the flavour or smell was in some way distinctive.

The certainty of the consequences

In order to have any impact on behaviour, the reinforcing or punishing consequences must be either certain or very likely to occur. In cognitive terms, this is referred to in terms of the perceived probability of an occurrence. An important reason why punishment fails to eliminate or reduce crime is because the chances of getting caught are believed to be small. The same applies to the perceived probability of getting ill.

> Janice tried to persuade Jo to cut down on his smoking and drinking for health reasons. But the reinforcing consequences of smoking and alcohol were all predictable and certain. In contrast, Jo could see no certainty that he was likely to get ill as a result of smoking or drinking. He cited the example of his uncle who smoked and drank heavily but had lived to a ripe old age.

This leads to the conclusion that healthy people are less likely to take preventative health advice because they have never been ill and therefore don't associate their behaviour with illness. Many people fail to take action until symptoms occur and this may be too late. The perceived probability of getting ill becomes greater as one gets older. This may be one reason why more people attempt to change their lifestyles as they grow older, compared to young people who feel invulnerable to disease.

Cues

Individuals quickly learn that particular actions have certain consequences only in specific situations or contexts that act as cues.

> Sasha scolded Lee when he attempted to go near the fire. This stopped him from approaching the fire in her presence so she assumed that it was

now safe to leave him alone in the room when the fire was lit. However, as soon as Sasha left the room, Lee attempted to poke the fire. He had learned that he must not touch the fire when his mother was present, but not when she was absent.

Many health-related behaviours are described as under '**stimulus control**'. That is to say, they are automatic responses to environmental cues, just as in classical conditioning.

Jo lights up a cigarette automatically as soon as he sits down to drink a cup of coffee. Lighting up a cigarette is normally considered to be a conscious or voluntary response, but becomes automatic in certain situations. Similarly, someone may get into the habit of pouring a drink when they arrive home from work.

An important reason why health-related behaviours, such as smoking, fail to respond to health promotion or health education is because in many situations they are not the product of conscious thought. Rather they are habits that involve automatic responses to particular environmental or internal cues. Once someone has expressed the desire to give up smoking, it is necessary to interrupt these habitual routines and bring the behaviour back under conscious control.

Lifestyle and behaviour

Behaviours such as smoking, eating, drinking and taking exercise play important roles in filling time in our lives. If someone wishes to stop one of these behaviours, it is necessary to replace it with something that is equally rewarding. This means that the reinforcing consequences of smoking, drinking or drug-taking need to be taken into account if a programme of lifestyle change is to be effective (DiClemente 1993).

Jo enjoys drinking seven or eight pints of beer with his mates at the pub. This is not because he is thirsty, but because it is a relaxing social activity that occupies a pleasant evening out. Sasha wants him to cut down on his drinking. But if he wants to spend the same amount of time with his mates, he will need to find an alternative that provides similar sources of reinforcement. A low alcohol lager may seem a reasonable alternative, but is more expensive, does not taste the same, and does not have the social approval of his drinking companions. It is very difficult to address individual behaviour in a binge-drinking culture.

Taking up a new health-related behaviour such as exercise requires extra time and space within an individual's lifestyle, therefore another activity will need to be displaced. For example, if exercise is to be maintained, it must be more reinforcing for the individual than alternative ways of using their time. It is often more likely that an individual will persevere with an exercise programme if they engage in it with others, so that there are beneficial social as well as health consequences.

Behaviour modification

Behaviour modification means changing behaviour by deliberately manipulating its context and/or consequences. It is based directly upon the operant principles of B.F. Skinner. During the 1970s, behaviour modification became a popular way to control socially undesirable or obsessive behaviours in long-stay institutions, using a 'token economy'. This meant that socially desirable behaviours were reinforced by immediately giving tokens that could be exchanged for primary reinforcers of the patient's choice (sadly, this often took the form of cigarettes). Punishment had no place in Skinner's approach to behaviour modification. Therefore, antisocial behaviour was ignored and not punished. Behaviour modification fell from favour during the late twentieth century, largely because behaviourism was seen to deny the possibility of free will and the deliberate manipulation of others' behaviours posed ethical problems. However, there remain many applications in common use, for example, in education the principles of classroom management are generally based on giving attention for good behaviour and ignoring bad behaviour.

Principles of behaviour modification, such as the use of a 'star chart' are often used to change children's behaviour. For example, this can be used to help cure bed-wetting, once the child is capable of achieving bladder control. Every dry morning, a star is placed by the child on a specially prepared chart. Once an agreed number of stars has been acquired, these can be exchanged for a gift or treat of the child's choice. The child is rewarded for having a dry bed, but is not chastised for a wet one. Similar approaches can be used to eliminate temper tantrums or other challenging behaviours, provided the child is able to understand the process (see cognitive development, Chapter 3).

It is worth noting that behaviour modification does not always work as intended.

Janice's friend had a 9-year-old child who was reluctant to eat, so his parents started rewarding him with money each time he finished a meal. The child gradually increased the tariff and, to his parents' dismay, quickly saved enough money to buy a television set for his bedroom. By that time he refused to eat at all unless he was paid to do so.

Therefore, before embarking on a programme of behaviour modification, it is worth considering the possibility of unintended or adverse consequences.

Functional analysis of behaviour

Functional analysis of behaviour is an important part of behaviour modification and involves monitoring the ABC (Antecedents – Behaviour – Consequences) of the problem behaviour. Behaviourists recommend that before any programme of behaviour change is started, the frequency of the problem behaviour should be recorded in a diary, together with the immediate cues to the behaviour (the antecedents) and immediate consequences (sources of reinforcement). This process is termed functional analysis of behaviour. It can be applied to any behaviour and used by anyone, for example, by someone planning to give up smoking, or a parent who wishes to eliminate their child's temper tantrums, or someone who wishes to improve their timekeeping. The process and the principles are illustrated in relation to Lee's tantrums.

Baseline measures

- Sasha recorded exactly when and how often the tantrums occurred during the course of a week.
- Identify stimulus cues. In addition to recording the occurrence of tantrums, Sasha recorded what was happening at the time each tantrum started.
- Identify reinforcers or punishers. Sasha also recorded what happened as an immediate consequence of Lee's tantrums.

Having collected this information, Sasha identified that Lee's tantrums usually occurred when he was tired or when her attention was directed towards the baby or housework. As a result, she was able to plan ways of distracting him from situations likely to lead to a tantrum, and doing certain chores when he was having a rest or otherwise occupied. She introduced a system of 'time out' (removing him from the scene) or ignoring him when he was having a tantrum, and giving him more attention at other times when he was being good. This effectively reinforced good behaviour.

Measurement of change

- She continued to monitor the frequency of Lee's tantrums to provide feedback on progress.

Over a period of three weeks, Lee's tantrums had reduced dramatically. By this time, Sasha felt much more confident in dealing with his behaviour.

Dixon *et al.* (2001) tested the use of functional analysis of behaviour in conjunction with behaviour modification in the case of a 25-year-old young man with a dual diagnosis of mental retardation and psychosis, including auditory hallucinations. The aim was to reduce inappropriate or offensive talk. During assessment using functional analysis, it was observed that inappropriate talk was reinforced by attention. Behaviour modification involved ignoring inappropriate talk and attending to alternative appropriate talk and behaviours. As predicted, this led to a decrease in inappropriate talk and increase in appropriate behaviours.

These types of intervention are most appropriate where the therapist, caregiver or parent is in a position to manipulate the consequences of behaviour for the individual concerned. This naturally raises ethical concerns in some situations, though the principles undoubtedly work.

Self-modification

The principles of functional analysis and behaviour modification can be used to help us change all sorts of aspects of our own behaviour. For example, being late for work or being short-tempered with our partner or spouse. It involves the following steps:

1 Decide which aspect of behaviour needs to change.
2 Monitor the frequency, causes and consequences of the behaviour.
3 Study the pattern of behaviour and identify persistent cues or consequences.
4 Plan to alter routines or respond differently to stimulus cues.
5 Substitute reinforcers for undesired behaviour with rewards or treats for desired behaviour.
6 Measure the change in frequency of the behaviour.
7 Maintain change with treats or self-praise to reinforce successful behaviour and boost self-esteem. Quite often the improvement is sufficient to maintain the change, but treats help as a reminder.

Anna was finding it difficult to get out of bed in the mornings. She was missing lectures and on two occasions arrived late in practice. She needed to address this urgently. She decided to get in some special treats for breakfast to tempt her out of bed.

Illness behaviours

The term illness behaviour was introduced by Mechanic in the early 1960s to describe the different ways that people perceive, evaluate and act on their illness, much of which is determined by what is culturally acceptable. Illness behaviours include engaging in self-care activities, seeking help, advice and reassurance, or doing nothing and ignoring the problem. But the term is usually used to describe abnormal or maladaptive ways of responding. Therefore much of the research into this concept seeks to describe how the behaviour of the patient deviates from that which appears to be justified by the extent of their illness. For example, if medical help-seeking seems excessive, the patient may be stigmatized as a hypochondriac or malingerer (Chapter 2) and regarded as a nuisance.

Illness behaviour is more likely to occur in those who are anxious (Rief *et al.* 2003). This is probably because uncertainty about the nature or consequences of an illness prompts the individual to persist in seeking help until they find an answer (Chapter 8). There appear to be cultural differences in the level and duration of symptoms that people from different countries expect to experience and this, too, will have an effect on help-seeking behaviour (de Melker *et al.* 1997).

There are also behavioural explanations for illness behaviours. Many are behaviours that have been reinforced by the responses of others. Chronic pain provides a useful example of this. Pain produces expressive 'pain behaviours', such as crying, wincing and other non-verbal expressions of pain and distress. Craig (2004) described how these attract the attention of others who recognize suffering and respond by offering help and protection. It is natural to want to help someone you love and protect them from pain. But if a caregiver responds by taking over the recipient's former tasks or roles, the person in pain gradually becomes less active and more dependent, pain behaviours become more exaggerated and the pain gradually becomes chronic (Chapter 10). Crane and Martin (2002) showed how parental reinforcement of illness behaviours in childhood can still exert some influence on responses to illnesses in adulthood. For example, people are more likely to adopt the sick role by taking rest and staying away from work when they have a cold if these responses were reinforced during childhood. Established patterns of belief and response may be amenable to change using principles of behaviour modification.

William Fordyce (1982), an influential figure in chronic pain research during the 1980s, developed a programme of treatment for patients with chronic pain who had given up work and most other activities. It required caregivers to recognize and ignore pain behaviours, while giving encouragement for any kind of activity. Although this did not necessarily improve self-reports of pain, patients showed a significant improvement in function.

This approach seems rather harsh, but some of these principles have been incorporated into cognitive behaviour therapy (CBT) for chronic pain, in which patients and caregivers learn to recognize the negative consequences of responding in an attentive way to pain behaviours and change their responses through a process of self-modification.

Reinforcement or control?

For years, behaviourists focused experiments on the effects of reinforcement and punishment in the belief that these were responsible for maintaining or changing behaviour. It therefore came as something of a surprise when researchers faced experimental results that could not be explained in terms of reinforcement or punishment alone. Rather, behaviour maintenance and behaviour change was found to be a consequence of the degree of control the animal or human had over positive or negative outcomes in their lives. This originated with the idea put forward by DeCharms (1968) that one of the key motivators of human behaviour is to gain mastery over our environment. It has clear implications in the contexts of health and social care.

Experiments conducted during the 1960s and 1970s led to a large body of research into the concept of control. Experimental evidence accumulated to show that humans are able to tolerate higher levels of discomfort if they believe they have some means of controlling it (see example in Chapter 10 on pain). This explains why, for example, we enjoy the fresh air when we open the window ourselves, but complain about the draught when someone else does so! Meanwhile, behavioural psychologists discovered a direct association between loss or lack of control and depression.

Learned helplessness, uncontrollability and depression

For many years it had been noted that some experimental animals showed symptoms of what was termed experimental neurosis. Basically, they cowered in a corner and could not be persuaded to participate in further experiments. Seligman and Maier (1967) demonstrated that this behaviour was caused by uncontrollability.

Two dogs were administered a series of identical minor electric shocks. One (called the executive dog) was able to terminate the shock by pressing a panel with its muzzle. This immediately stopped the shock delivered to itself and the other dog, so that both dogs received exactly the same intensity and duration of shock. The only difference was that one dog had control over the shock, while the other had none.

Each dog was then transferred to another experimental environment called a shuttle box. The dog was placed at one end and minor electric shocks were delivered through the floor. Both dogs could easily escape by jumping over a low barrier to safety. In this situation, the executive dog quickly learned to jump to safety. In contrast, the other dog made no attempt to escape. The 'helpless' dog demonstrated a motivational deficit (it made no attempt to move), a cognitive deficit (it failed to recognize a simple escape route), and an emotional deficit (it appeared very miserable). Seligman termed this 'learned helplessness'.

According to Seligman, learned helplessness means learning that one's actions have no influence over outcomes. Seligman (1975) noted that the motivational, cognitive and emotional deficits he observed are all symptomatic of human depression, and proposed learned helplessness as a theory of human depression. The theory of learned helplessness predicts that people become depressed because of exposure to situations or events that they are unable to control. Subsequent researchers have applied this in different types of situations, including social settings.

Lack of control over important aspects of life has been suggested as a reason for the higher incidence of depression among the unemployed, those on low pay, those with less education, and women. Sociologists John Mirowsky and Catherine Ross (2003) argued that depression among these groups is caused by their powerlessness in society and not by personal depressive tendencies that had brought them down the social scale.

Learned helplessness has much intuitive appeal. It highlights the dangers of depriving people of control, focuses on situational causes of depression and implies that what has been learned can be unlearned. In contrast, cognitive theories of depression emphasize the importance of pessimistic belief sets that lead people to feel they have little control. These points of view are in fact complementary since what really matters is *perceived* control, not actual control. This explains why in similar circumstances, some people become depressed while others do not.

Mark started feeling quite depressed after he retired from work due to ill health. He had experienced one previous bout of depression which had lifted when he changed his job (Chapter 8). Now, he felt that he had lost control over his life and felt helpless. Other people envied his freedom to do other things, but he could not be bothered. He demonstrated the motivational, cognitive and emotional deficits typical of learned helplessness: he made no effort to do anything, did not believe that he was capable of achieving anything more in his life, and felt depressed.

Since the 1970s, learned helplessness has been subject to a number of critiques and reformulations using attribution theory (Chapter 2) and ultimately challenged by the academic community as a theory of depression. Nevertheless, there is still powerful evidence from social psychology and psychoneuroimmunology to support the relationship between uncontrollability, depression and health outcomes (Chapter 8).

Undoing learned helplessness

Seligman and his colleagues (Seligman and Maier 1967) experimented with helpless dogs and found that they could be cured if the experimenter physically dragged them across the barrier on numerous occasions to demonstrate that it was possible to escape from the shock. This observation was used to develop behavioural interventions for depression.

Mark was referred to a clinical psychologist who invited him to review his skills and identify some achievable goals that would motivate him and restore his sense of control. Mark focused on cooking. Janice worked with him to identify suitable recipes and ingredients and soon Mark was preparing some lovely healthy meals. Success breeds success and Mark's depression decreased as he started to regain control over some aspects of his life and feel useful, rather than helpless.

The concepts of perceived control and controllability have enabled learning theory to be integrated into cognitive science, where terms such as reinforcement are no longer used. Nevertheless, the behaviourist principles outlined above have been incorporated into CBT for the management of depression (Chapter 6).

Social learning theory

The behavioural experiments and treatments so far described are to a great extent focused on the individual in isolation from their social context. But humans are social beings who live in complex social worlds. It might seem obvious that the majority of human learning takes place in a social environment, but most early behavioural experiments failed to take account of this. Social learning theory emerged in response to this criticism during the 1960s.

There are two important strands to social learning theory. One is attributable to Albert Bandura and focuses on the concepts of observational learning and self-efficacy. The other is usually attributed to Rotter (1966) and concerns the concept of locus of control. More recently, these two strands have been brought together under the general heading of 'social cognition' (Chapter 9).

Observational learning

Albert Bandura is one of the great original thinkers in psychology. Starting out as a behavioural psychologist, he became interested in social influences on behaviour. He conducted a series of classic experiments in the 1960s to study influences on aggressive behaviour in children, during which children were shown to imitate, without prompting or incentive, aggressive adult behaviour towards a large blow-up doll (Bandura *et al.* 1961). This raised fears that have never been resolved that children might mimic aggressive or violent behaviour seen on television.

Bandura's experiments demonstrated that children don't just learn from the consequences of their own actions, but are capable of copying or modelling their behaviour on that of others. Further, he showed that they are capable of judging the likely consequences of their own actions by observing what happens to others in similar circumstances. Bandura's work on modelling or imitative learning has filled important gaps in explaining the speed of human learning. It also highlighted the importance and influence of the social environment on behaviour. The following example illustrates how student nurses model their dress as well as their behaviour on those of experienced staff (these changes are also influenced by pressures to conform, see Chapter 7).

When Anna went on her first surgical ward placement, she had little idea what to expect. She had previously spent time as a health care assistant on a medical ward and had received training in basic nursing skills, but still felt very nervous. Almost without thinking, she observed what other members of staff were doing: the way they made beds, took observations, communicated with patients, responded to other members of staff, the way they wore their uniform and even the way they walked. She needed to be very careful not to model actions that she knew not to be best practice.

The concept of modelling goes some way to explaining the process that sociologists refer to as socialization. It can be seen in the way that children and adults learn new social skills and competencies. This is why practical learning is so important and why social or organizational behaviour patterns are particularly resistant to change.

Self-efficacy

Bandura (1977a, 1977b) was critical of Skinner's assertions that all human behaviour is passively driven by external forces, although he acknowledged that these are influential. He argued that we learn to monitor our own performance and reward ourselves by internal praise for good performance. According to Bandura, our sense of self-esteem is based primarily on our beliefs in our ability to achieve control, either individually or collectively, over our everyday lives. The failure to recognize and reward ourselves for good performance can lead to depression. He suggested that talented people often become depressed because they set themselves standards of achievement that are too high.

Bandura proposed that once children have learned to imitate a new skill, they are capable of monitoring and adjusting their own performance through a process of self-regulation, by comparing their own performance with that of others. Through this active process, they achieve a sense of self-efficacy. This refers to the fact that they have mastered the task and feel confident to do it again. Bandura defined perceived self-efficacy as 'beliefs in one's capabilities to organize and execute the courses of action required to produce given attainments' (Bandura 1997: 3). Self-efficacy therefore sits comfortably with the concept of perceived control.

A survey of nearly 300 people with either rheumatoid or osteo-arthritis, measured arthritis self-efficacy (confidence in the ability to manage pain and other symptoms) and health status. The researchers (Cross *et al.* 2006) focused on people with these conditions because the pain is difficult to treat or control. The findings showed that high reports of self-efficacy were associated with better control over pain, stiffness and function and better physical and mental health. Low self-efficacy was associated with more visits to the doctor and greater costs.

Bandura has written extensively on the concept of self-efficacy, which has emerged as a key mediating belief in a variety of health-related situations. Self-efficacy is not just an important predictor of health outcomes, but has been shown to be amenable to change. It has therefore become an important focus for intervention in health education and self-management programmes for people with chronic health problems (Chapters 9 and 10).

Locus of control

Locus of control (LOC) refers to a relatively stable set of beliefs about responsibility for control over outcomes. It combines the behavioural emphasis on the importance of outcomes with principles of attribution theory (Chapter 2). Rotter (1966) is well known for the development of the first LOC measurement scale, which placed beliefs about control on a single bipolar dimension: internal versus external. Internal LOC refers to the belief that I am responsible for the things that happen to me. External LOC refers to the belief that things that happen to me are a consequence of luck, fate, chance or someone else. This was quickly applied in health care situations. It was used, for example, to judge the likelihood that an individual would want to take responsibility for their own health and manage their own illness.

Levenson (1974) argued that there are three independent dimensions to

LOC: internal, external (powerful others) and external (chance). Accordingly, in the 1970s, Ken and Barbara Wallston and colleagues developed a multi-dimensional health LOC measure (Wallston *et al.* 1978).

- Internal LOC reflects the belief that my health is a consequence of my own actions.
- External (powerful others) LOC reflects the belief that health and illness are the responsibility of others such as doctors.
- External (chance) LOC reflects the belief that being well and getting ill is a matter luck, fate or chance.

This led to many studies to test the prediction that internal LOC is associated with better health outcomes. To some extent the prediction was upheld. For example, a longitudinal six-year study (Wallhagen *et al.* 1994) found that internal LOC was related to placing importance on good health. However, most other studies have proved weak or inconclusive.

It soon became evident that control beliefs are not necessarily generalizable to all situations, but need to be judged in relation to specific situations or medical conditions. For example, I may believe that my headache is under my control, but my abdominal pain is a matter for the doctor. Therefore, a variety of condition-specific LOC measures have been devised for the purposes of research. Examples include addiction, diabetes, cancer, pain and heart disease LOC (Walker 2001).

It has also become apparent that LOC should not be regarded as a personality variable, but as a set of expectations that can and do change with experience. LOC is a useful concept in clinical practice since it gives some indication of the likelihood of people's wishes and intentions to take responsibility for their health or manage their illness. It can often be detected by observing what people do and the way they speak.

Janice likes to be well informed and searches the internet for information before seeking medical treatment. She likes to know what she can do to help herself and feels quite angry if her needs for information and explanations are not being taken seriously by the doctor. She likes to take responsibility for self-managing her symptoms when she is ill, but does not always follow the doctor's advice if she does not agree with it. This pattern suggests that Janice has a strong internal LOC which may be problematic if she refuses to follow sound medical advice.

Margaret seeks medical advice whenever she has a slight illness. She always follows the doctor's advice, but finds it difficult to adhere to medication in the longer term. This pattern suggests that Margaret has strong external (powerful doctor) LOC, but needs help to develop the internal LOC needed to take personal responsibility for maintaining her own health in the longer term.

Mark tends to be fatalistic about his illnesses and believes that what will be will be. This illustrates external (chance) LOC which is associated with lack of motivation to follow health advice. He is not good at monitoring his

> diabetes or other symptoms and, as a result, is at risk of a poorer health outcome. He needs interventions designed to improve his sense of self-efficacy and encourage him to take personal responsibility for his own health.

> An American psychology team (Williams-Piehota *et al.* 2004) confirmed the prediction that people are more likely to respond to information that matches their LOC. They showed that women with internal LOC were more likely to respond to an invitation entitled 'The Best Thing You Can Do For Your Health – Mammography'. Women with external 'powerful other' beliefs were more likely to respond to one entitled 'The Best Thing Medical Science Has to Offer for Your Health – Mammography'.

It seems logical that internal LOC is preferable in situations such as attending for mammography, where the individual has control over attendance. On the other hand, external powerful others LOC is desirable in situations where medical help is essential for survival or future quality of life. Those with external chance LOC have been shown to respond less well to health education, though Holt *et al.* (2000) found that people with external chance LOC did respond to tailored information with counter-arguments (Chapter 7). We return to these concepts in Chapter 8 on stress and coping.

Applying behavioural principles to designing a health education programme

Behavioural principles can be used to change health-related behaviours. An example of such a programme is the 'Quit for life' smoking cessation programme designed and tested by David Marks (see Marks *et al.* 2005). The programme incorporates issues raised earlier in this chapter, including principles of counter-conditioning (substituting reinforcing alternatives), stimulus control and reinforcement management. The key assumptions on which it is based are as follows.

- Nicotine has immediate positive reinforcing consequences for the smoker.
  - It is relaxing, increases alertness and improves cognitive performance (because of these effects, smoking provides a useful way of coping with stress).
- Smoking a cigarette fills time.
  - This provides thinking time for problem-solving, and 'time out' from difficult situations.
- Smoking suppresses appetite.
  - Eating often replaces smoking, but leads to weight gain (many people relapse because they gain weight).

- Smoking is a social activity and the smoker is often under peer pressure to smoke.
  - Peer approval is reinforcing; peer disapproval acts as a punisher.
- Lighting up is a habit that takes place in certain situations without thinking (e.g. when having a cup of coffee after a meal).
  - Smoking is under stimulus control.

The following techniques were designed as part of the programme to address these points. Willpower plays no part in this programme and the individual does not pledge to stop smoking. Smoking behaviour declines naturally as the programme is implemented.

1 Interrupt the habitual element of smoking by putting a rubber band round the packet that must first be removed. Reduce the association of cigarettes with pleasure: place a personal message under the rubber band and read it out each time a cigarette is drawn out. For example:

> This cigarette is making me ill
> I do not like this cigarette
> I do not wish to smoke this cigarette

The individual *must* then take out a cigarette and smoke it so that a subconscious association is gradually built up between the cigarette and something unpleasant or unwanted.

2 Reduce the habitual effect by identifying the situations in which the smoker tends to light up without thinking and placing another message under the rubber band to read out before lighting the cigarette in that situation:

> Just because I have had a meal, I do not need to smoke
> Next time I finish a meal, I will not want to smoke

3 Find new ways of keeping the hands occupied, such as doodling or worry beads.
4 Build in an exercise and weight-control programme to prevent excessive weight gain.
5 Rehearse assertive skills for saying 'no' to peers.
6 Find social support from others who do not smoke. Marks included a 'buddy' system. Each participant was paired with another person in the programme that they could phone if they were findings things too hard or felt they might give in to temptation.
7 Find alternative methods of stress management, for example relaxation or yoga.

The success rate at the end of a year for the self-help version of this programme was reported to be 25 per cent, making it 26 times more cost-effective that nicotine replacement therapy.

Summary of key points

- Behaviour and behaviour change is influenced by its antecedents and its consequences, provided these are desirable, immediate and certain.
- Classical conditioning theory may help to prevent, explain and treat many common fears, phobias and other symptoms such as nausea or allergic responses that are associated with intense physiological arousal.
- Many health-related and illness behaviours appear to be habits that are under 'stimulus control', rather than cognitive control.
- The theory of learned helplessness suggests that depression is caused by perceived loss of control.
- Self-efficacy is an important predictor of positive health outcomes; chance locus of control is an important predictor of adverse health outcomes.
- Behavioural principles can be applied in a variety of contexts to improve health and well-being.

Exercise

See after Chapter 10.

Further reading

Behavioural theory is described and elaborated in all basic introductory psychology texts (see further reading, Chapter 1).

Bandura, A. (1997) *Self-efficacy: The Exercise of Control*. New York: W.H. Freeman.

Marks, D.F., Murray, M., Evans, B., Willig, C., Woodall, C. and Sykes, C.M. (2005) *Health Psychology: Theory, Research and Practice*, 2nd edn. London: Sage, Chapter 8, Tobacco and smoking, pp. 154–72.

UNDERSTANDING ANXIETY, DEPRESSION AND LOSS

- **What is an emotion?**
- **What do we mean by anxiety and how can it be managed?**
- **What are the main approaches to the assessment and management of anxiety and depression?**
- **What is post-traumatic stress disorder and what advice can be given to help patients deal with this?**
- **How do people deal with loss and how can they be helped to deal with this?**
- **How can health and social care professionals promote positive well-being?**

Introduction

In this chapter, we focus predominantly on anxiety and depression because all health and social care professionals encounter these states to varying degrees in their professional and personal lives. It is important, therefore, to understand how different interpretations lead to different psychological approaches to management. We start from the premise that anxiety and depression are normal responses to adverse conditions, particularly those involving loss but may, in some cases, develop into a more severe mental health problem. This chapter is directed primarily at generalist care professionals who need to be able to recognize and respond to common emotional problems and be able to offer immediate reassurance and advice to those they suspect might benefit from further mental health advice and support.

What is an emotion?

An emotion is an affective (mood) state that involves each of the following:

- A subjective experience
  - an event or situation that impinges on us.
- Cognitive appraisal
  - we interpret the experience in the light of our knowledge or experience.

- Physiological change
  - a range of internal bodily responses mediated in the short term by the autonomic nervous system and in the longer term by the endocrine system.
- Behavioural response
  - involuntary responses, such as moving away, crying.
  - coping strategies to reduce sense of threat.
- Affect
  - sensation, feeling, mood.

It seems 'common sense' to assume that cognitive **appraisal** of the subjective experience precedes physiological and behavioural responses and gives rise to feelings, as illustrated in the following scenario.

> Janice remembers picking up the phone to be told that her mother had died. She felt initially numb. As she started to comprehend the news, she felt sick, then burst into tears, overwhelmed by feelings of sadness.

In this scenario, the experience of learning that her mother had died was followed by realization, then by a physiological response, then the behavioural response and intense emotional feeling. However, a classic experiment showed that physiological changes can lead people to label their emotional feeling in accordance with the circumstances in which they find themselves. This suggests that the association between events, thoughts and feelings is not always straightforward.

> Schachter and Singer (1962) conducted an experiment in which participants were given an injection of either adrenalin (to trigger a bodily state of arousal) or saline (inert placebo), and were then subjected to situations likely to provoke either elation or anger. They found that identical states of arousal could lead to either elation or anger, depending on the situation in which the individuals found themselves.

Health and social care workers are likely to encounter many occasions when people in a high state of arousal incorrectly label their bodily feelings, sometimes with unfortunate consequences.

> Jo was taken to the accident and emergency department after he injured himself at a rave while 'high' on drugs. The state of arousal caused by the drugs made him very sensitive to cues in his environment. Quite out of character, he attempted to assault a member of the nursing staff who, he thought, 'dissed' him.

We address issues related to the management of aggression in Chapter 7. It is also important to remember that certain medical conditions, and some prescribed drugs, can produce physiological symptoms that may be incorrectly attributed to anxiety. In presenting different models, we refer back to Figure 1.1 (Chapter 1) which shows how these complement each other.

What do we mean by anxiety and how can it be managed?

Using the definition of 'emotion', anxiety may be described in terms of:

- *subjective experience:* exposure to new, strange, threatening or potentially uncontrollable events or situations;
- *cognitive appraisal:* perceived uncertainty about what is happening or how best to respond (Chapter 8);
- *physiological changes:* arousal of the autonomic nervous system leads to raised heart rate and systolic blood pressure, sweaty palms, shaking, feelings of 'butterflies' in the stomach or nausea, urinary or faecal urgency, tightness in the chest or difficulty breathing; other symptoms include insomnia (early waking and worrying);
- *behavioural responses:* including: agitation, obsessive checking, avoiding situations likely to provoke anxiety (or avoiding thinking about them), seeking help or support;
- *affect:* tense, nervous, worried.

Anxiety is a normal response to stress (Chapter 8) but can, if extreme or persistent, have a serious negative impact on an individual's quality of life. Explanations of anxiety and psychological approaches to its management vary depending on the approach to psychology used (for an overview see Chapter 1). Consider the following scenario involving Anna.

> In the first year of her nursing degree, Anna had to give a presentation to her tutor group. Although other students seemed nervous, they all delivered their presentations without too much fuss. Anna delayed until last, but as the day approached, she became panic-stricken and felt physically sick. She was even thinking about giving up her course because she could not face doing this. At this point, she sought help from the university counselling service.

Counselling and psychology services offer different types of therapeutic approaches, often depending on the training and approach of the therapist. Therefore Anna might have encountered any of the following approaches to help her manage her anxiety.

Cognitive approach

A cognitive interpretation would be that Anna's appraisal of the situation is distorted or dysfunctional (Beck 1976, Beck 1995). Anna is clearly as capable as the others of preparing and giving the presentation, but possibly under-estimates her own ability or has set herself too high a standard. As part of a cognitive approach to the management of anxiety, the therapist would help Anna to challenge automatic negative thoughts, such as 'I can't do this, I am not clever enough', and replace these with adaptive responses (Beck 1995: 113) which might be: 'this is difficult because it is the first time I have done it, therefore I need some guidance'. The cognitive therapist might encourage Anna to seek advice from her academic tutor to help her set about preparing more realistically for the task.

Behavioural approach

A behaviour therapist might seek to explain Anna's anxiety in terms of the outcomes of past experiences in similar situations. For example, she may have felt humiliated while giving a presentation at school. However, rather than dwell on these beliefs, the therapist would focus on her present reactions to the task. Anna might be taught relaxation skills to counteract feelings of anxiety. Then she might rehearse her presentation, first in the safe environment of the counselling room and then in an empty classroom with a few friends. This would gradually increase her sense of self-efficacy and reduce her anxiety so that when she finally has to give the presentation to her tutor group she feels more relaxed and confident.

Psychodynamic approach

A psychodynamic therapist or counsellor might be interested to find out why Anna is an anxious person. In exploring her childhood experiences, they might find, for example, that Anna's father was very strict and crit-ical and had set very high standards, while her mother put pressure on Anna to train as a nurse because she had not had that opportunity her-self. As a result, Anna has found herself under a lot of pressure to suc-ceed. The psychodynamic counsellor might seek to explore the origins of these feelings with her and, in so doing, seek to release her from her anxiety.

Humanistic approach

A humanistic psychologist or counsellor would help Anna explore reasons for her anxiety by encouraging her to talk about her thoughts and fears. If, for example, she sees herself as less competent than others at giving presen-tations, they would encourage her to explore why this might be, so that she could develop a more realistic appraisal of her task and her ability to achieve it. They would aim to improve Anna's sense of self-worth and self-confidence and support her to find suitable solutions to the problem in a non-directive way.

Influences from social psychology

All forms of therapy might also wish to take account of the social aspects of giving a presentation in public. Presentation is not just about content but about personal appearance and self-presentation. Much anxiety is generated because we are afraid of what other people will think of us. Drawing on the work of Goffman (Chapter 2), we might suggest that Anna make use of 'props', such as a new hair-do, make-up or outfit, to improve her self-confidence. She might also practise social presentation skills, including voice projection, to build her confidence.

Comparing different approaches to anxiety and its management

It can be seen from these brief analyses that different psychological approaches vary in their explanations and interpretations of the same phenomenon. It is not that one is right and one is wrong, rather as illustrated in Figure 1.1 (Chapter 1), they focus on different aspects. In reality, it is unlikely that 'one size fits all' in terms of management. Different approaches suit different people, depending on the type of problem they face and the way they prefer to deal with it.

- Humanistic counselling is probably the most common approach and is particularly useful for those with tangible problems, such as stress at work, marital difficulties or coming to terms with bereavement, where non-judgemental listening can facilitate problem-solving.
- Cognitive-based therapy is likely to be helpful for those whose anxieties are more persistent, but largely unfounded or exaggerated.
- Behaviour therapies such as systematic desensitization (Chapter 5) have been shown to be particularly successful in the treatment of fears and phobias.
- Psychodynamic psychotherapy is particularly helpful in promoting understanding for those with persistent anxiety related to unresolved issues or difficulties in establishing relationships that developed early on in their lives.

Currently, the most popular as well as the most effective approach to anxiety-related problems is cognitive behaviour therapy (CBT). The National Institute for Health and Clinical Excellence (NICE) in the UK recommends CBT as the main treatment for anxiety disorders (NICE 2004a). CBT combines a cognitive interpretation of the problem with cognitive and behavioural management strategies, such as those identified in Chapter 5. In reality, many therapists use an eclectic approach in which they select tools from each or any of the psychological approaches, as appropriate to the person and the problem.

You will note that we have referred throughout to anxiety 'management' and have made no reference to pharmaceutical treatment. Drug 'treatments' do not cure anxiety. They may provide temporary respite from the feelings of anxiety, but do not address the cause or offer effective coping strategies. The most common anxiolytic (anti-anxiety) drugs are the benzodiazepines, such as diazepam (Valium), which are now known to be potentially highly addictive. It is normally recommended that they should not be used continuously for more than two to four weeks. Patients taking anxiolytic drugs for longer than this may experience withdrawal symptoms and are advised to seek advice and support if they wish to stop taking them.

Anxiety as a mental health disorder

Ways of thinking and behaving that underpin emotions such as anxiety can become part of the individual's automatic pattern of responding to situations and life events and are then termed 'traits'. Anxiety traits such as 'neuroticism' are sometimes used (often incorrectly) to describe part of an individual's personality. In extreme cases, anxiety traits are associated with persistent emotional or behavioural disturbances and labelled as a psychiatric disorder. Examples include obsessive-compulsive disorder, in which anxiety leads people to engage in repetitive ritualistic behaviours, and phobias such as agoraphobia which can lead people to fear leaving the safety of their home. Assessment and diagnosis of these 'conditions' are conducted in accordance with either the *DSM* IV (*Diagnostic and Statistical Manual of Mental Disorders, 4th edn*, APA 2000) or the *ICD* 10 (*International Classification of Diseases*, 10th revision, WHO 2006), though it is important to note that there have been a number of dissenting critiques to this psychiatric approach, for example, Szasz (1996) and Beutler and Malik (2002). In general health and social care contexts it is unsafe to label people as having an anxiety trait, such as neuroticism, or any other form of mental health disorder, unless or until they have had a proper assessment by an appropriately trained mental health professional. Even within mental health care, it is important to remember that labelling someone as having a mental health disorder can lead to stereotypical attitudes and discrimination towards the individual even after the symptoms have been alleviated, affecting future health care and job prospects.

Dealing with an anxious patient or client

Most people get anxious when faced with uncertain or potentially threatening life situations (Chapter 8), particularly if they have had a bad experience in a similar situation in the past or are ill equipped with the coping skills or resources to deal with it. The concerns of patients about their illness and its implications for their ability to work, maintain personal relationships or meet obligations in their daily lives is quite sufficient to cause anxiety. But for some, an illness or event that appears relatively trivial may be 'the straw that broke the camel's back' in an already troubled life, for example, in those who have recently been bereaved or lost their job or experienced a marital break-up or have financial problems. Others may appear to have a level of anxiety out of all proportion to the problems they face because of inadequate or maladaptive coping skills. For example, they may have role-modelled anxious responses from a parent, or never learned effective ways of dealing with the type of situation they find themselves in. Others have literacy or communication difficulties or inadequate social skills that make it difficult to deal with situations outside the confines of their home and family, or to gain help from others when they need it.

If a patient or client is observed to be tense or anxious, it is often helpful to say: 'You seem rather [bothered/upset/tense]. Is there anything special worrying you?' This opens the way for them to share their concerns and feel that they are supported. You can then ask: 'Is there anything I/we can do to help you feel better?'

Many if not most nurses admit to avoiding asking these types of question, or even avoiding contact with anxious patients because, they say:

1 There is insufficient time to engage with the patient at this level.
2 There is no privacy to discuss personal issues.
3 They fear 'opening the flood gates'.
4 They fear an obligation to 'do something' about the problem disclosed.
5 They fear they lack the skills required to facilitate and then close successfully this kind of conversation.

The issue of time is important. If you suspect that the patient has problems, agree a time limit so that the patient can judge how much to share: 'I can see that you are [worried/concerned/upset]. I have ten minutes to spare – is there anything you would like to share?'

Wherever possible it is preferable to offer a private room, but where this is difficult, why not apologize for the lack of privacy and leave the patient to make the decision. With respect to points 3, 4 and 5, health care professionals (in contrast to social care professionals) need to be reminded that by inviting patients to share their feelings or emotions the primary task of the professional is to *listen*. It is important to listen fully to patients' or clients' concerns before jumping in with advice and suggestions. Having understood the problem, you might offer advice if you are confident you know the answer, or you could offer to find out more information or refer the individual to appropriate sources of assistance. But the responsibility for managing their problems and their emotions remains with the patient or client. No patient could or would reasonably expect a busy hospital nurse to sort out their employment difficulties, resolve their marital disharmony or offer bereavement counselling because this is not what they are trained to do. But patients do have a right to expect empathy and understanding. If an individual becomes upset or tearful, never leave them in this state. Place a comforting hand on the shoulder or arm until the tears have subsided, then ask: 'Is there anything you would like me to do right now?' The answer is normally, 'No, there is nothing you can do', together with an expression of gratitude as they pull themselves together. The main benefit is that they now feel confident that they are in the care of people they can trust (Walker *et al.* 1998) and this will reduce their anxiety. If the patient shares information that indicates the potential for harm to themselves or others, or has implications for their future care, it is ethical to advise them that you will need to record this information or pass it on to someone in authority.

What do we mean by depression and how can it be managed?

Using a similar framework as that used for anxiety, depression can be described in terms of:

- *subjective experience:* which may be conceptualized as uncontrollability or powerlessness in the face of life events, situations or even life in general;
- *cognitive appraisal:* sense of hopelessness or complete helplessness which may be accompanied by recurrent negative and possibly suicidal thoughts;
- *physiological changes:* including fatigue and general sluggishness, poor sleep quality, loss of concentration, poor appetite with weight loss or compulsive eating and weight gain, immune dysfunction which can lead to increased susceptibility to physical illness;
- *behavioural responses:* including social withdrawal, inactivity, lack of self-care;
- *affect:* persistent low mood, general loss of interest and pleasure, irritability, low self-esteem.

Depression is very common and most episodes of depression resolve without intervention. It is normal to feel emotionally low and hopeless when we experience a loss or when things go badly wrong. But when these feelings become persistent and are accompanied by other symptoms from those listed above, it may be classified as 'major depression' (clinical depression) and diagnosed as a mental disorder. Severe depression can be totally incapacitating and in a minority of cases leads to suicide. It is important to note that suicide is the third most common cause of death among adolescent males worldwide (Wasserman 2006), while suicide among the general population is often associated with untreated depression. Therefore it should not be minimized or ignored.

As with anxiety, explanations for depression vary, depending on the approach to psychology used. Consider the following scenario.

Anna's friend Marie found it increasingly difficult to cope during her second year at university. She became progressively unable to sleep or eat properly, could not concentrate on her academic work, and lost interest in social events and activities such as swimming that she previously enjoyed. Anna noticed that she was becoming withdrawn and uncommunicative and she made frequent excuses to avoid social contact. During the first term of that academic year, she stopped wearing make-up, took little care of her hair and clothes, did not join friends for meals in the refectory and appeared to have lost weight. She appeared to spend more and more time in bed, but was irritable with others when challenged about this. Lecturers noticed that her attendance at seminars was increasingly poor and she failed to hand in her assignments on time. She was asked to see her academic tutor who identified that she might be suffering from depression.

Within psychiatry, the diagnosis of clinical depression is based on criteria from the *DSM* or *ICD*, using an assessment such as the History and Mental State Examination (Nunes and Cutler 2000). Questionnaires such as the HADS (Hospital Anxiety and Depression Scale, Zigmond and Snaith 1983), BDI (Beck Depression Inventory, Beck *et al.* 1961) or the CES-D (Center for Epidemiologic Studies Depression Scale, Radloff 1977) may also be used to measure depression in research and clinical practice.

Vulnerability, triggering and maintaining factors in depression

Gilbert (2005) reviewed a number of ways in which stress is linked to depression including:

- learned helplessness (Chapter 5) in which depression may be seen as a response to total loss of personal control;
- loss of attachment or social affiliations (see this chapter on loss);
- subordination (being treated as inferior or worthless) and loss of self-esteem (Chapter 2).

Within each model, depression is influenced by the interaction of personal vulnerabilities (personality, past experiences) with exposure to certain types of stressful life events or situations.

- *Vulnerability factors* are those that predispose people to becoming depressed and include:
  1 Genetic. Depression that occurs in recurrent cycles appears to indicate some kind of genetic predisposition.
  2 Biological. Hormone disruption, such as thyroid dysfunction, may predispose to depression, especially in interaction with other factors.
  3 Drugs. Some prescribed drugs, including anxiolytic drugs such as diazepam, if taken over a long period may cause depression, as may long-term use of other mood altering substances such as alcohol.
  4 Season. There is growing evidence that some people are affected by lack of daylight, as in seasonal affective disorder (SAD).
  5 Negative life events, changes or circumstances that involve uncontrollability or loss, often in combination.

- *Trigger factors* are those that can precipitate depression but, unless overwhelming, require vulnerability factors to do so – for example not everyone who loses their job becomes depressed.
- *Maintaining factors* are those such as poverty, poor coping skills and/or lack of social support that conspire to maintain depression.

Theories of depression and approaches to management

As with anxiety, approaches to the management of depression are based on different explanatory frameworks, depending on different psychological approaches, though there are commonalities among these.

Cognitive approaches to depression and its management

The cognitive model of depression, developed by Aaron Beck in the 1960s, is probably the most widely accepted framework for understanding and managing depression. Beck (1976) assumed that our emotions directly reflect our beliefs and perceptions (cognitions), therefore depression is a direct consequence of distorted thought processes. He held that a depressed person has an unduly pessimistic interpretation of events and their ability to deal with them. This may be due to innate or genetic differences in outlook; or to persistent negative feedback in early life (such as being told that 'you're no good'); or to the scale and extent of negative life events to which they have been subjected, particularly when combined with a lack of coping skills or adequate social or spiritual resources to be able to deal with them, or to any combination of these.

From a critical perspective, a number of researchers have demonstrated that in fact 'normal' people (those who are not depressed) have a systematic positive cognitive bias which leads to an unrealistic sense of optimism and tendency to 'look on the bright side' (Taylor and Brown 1988). This is achieved by selective attention to positive feedback, attribution of successes to personal competence rather than chance, and the tendency to see themselves as better, or better off, than others. In contrast, people who are depressed are often quite realistic in their appraisals of negative events or the awfulness of their lives. This clearly suggests that their problems are not 'all in the mind'. Nevertheless, people benefit from finding positive alternative ways of interpreting and managing their situation, particularly when combined with an anti-depressant drug that helps boost their mood and motivation.

Beck (1976) originated cognitive therapy as a way of changing negative thought patterns into more positive ones. Based on this approach, cognitive therapy sessions for Marie included the following (Beck 1995).

The therapist explained the cognitive model of depression, assessed Marie's mood using the Beck Depression Inventory, asked Marie to think about important goals that she would like to achieve and set some 'homework' to refine her goals, remind herself that she is not stupid, and read the therapy booklet.

As part of the following 6–12 sessions, Marie agreed that her main goal was to complete her course. She was encouraged systematically to identify and monitor automatic dysfunctional thoughts such as:

'I am not clever enough to write this essay.'
'I am not good enough to be at university.'

Marie was asked to keep a log of her emotions (Beck 1995: 99), as illustrated in Figure 6.1 With the therapist, Marie re-evaluated her responses to these emotions, which were mainly avoidant – she tried to avoid thinking about her assignment and therefore failed to address her problems. Finally, she learned to challenge her core belief that she was not good enough to be at university.

Angry	Upset	Anxious
I got poor marks for my first essay even though I did a lot more work than the others	I can't afford to go out clubbing with the other students	I can't find time to write my essays while I am in practice
My new (second-hand) printer packed up	My placement was not really what I wanted	I feel panicky going into lectures on my own

Figure 6.1 Extract from Marie's emotional log

When Marie first went to the therapist, she thought that the problem was that she was a failure in academic and social terms. She thought that everyone else was much more confident than she was and having a better time. As the sessions progressed, she began to see that she was just as capable as the others, but set herself impossibly high standards. As part of her 'homework' she contacted an old friend to repair her printer and saw her academic tutor for feedback on her approach to essay writing and found that she was then able to help others, which made her popular with fellow students. It was difficult to work out a balance between work and social life, given her financial constraints, but eventually she and Anna set up a weekly essay-writing/study group which when combined with a shared meal and bottle of wine served an academic as well as an economical social function. Now she was really enjoying university and got really good marks.

The cognitive model is undoubtedly dominant at the start of the twenty-first century, but other models still have an important contribution to our understanding and management of depression. Some key elements of these are briefly summarized here.

Behaviourist models of depression: learned helplessness or lack of positive reinforcement?

There are two distinct accounts of depression based on behaviourist principles. The best known is Seligman's learned helplessness model of depression, covered in some detail in Chapter 5. Since its original inception this has undergone a number of revisions, most recently as the hopelessness (rather than helplessness) model of depression. However, it retains some attraction as an easily understood model of depression.

A second model (Lewinsohn 1974) was based on reinforcement theory (Chapter 5). Lewinsohn observed that people who are depressed have little positive reinforcement (pleasure) in their lives. Since this is normally gained from social activities, Lewinsohn proposed that people who are depressed lack the social skills to elicit positive reinforcement in social contexts.

> When Marie went to university, she found it difficult to make friends because she lived at home. The students who lived in the university halls of residence had formed friendship groups and she didn't know how to engage with them. As a result she found herself sitting alone in lectures and feeling unsupported in seminars. The therapist worked with her to identify strategies for approaching other students. This led to the setting up of the study group which provided a springboard for developing her social confidence.

There is no doubt that people who are depressed are difficult to engage with socially. Whether poor social skills are a cause or a consequence of their depression is unclear, but it is apparent that developing or improving social skills can be an important part of therapy. Even emailing and texting have a social etiquette that needs to be adhered to in order to elicit friendly responses, and these are skills that can be taught if deficits are recognized.

Psychodynamic approaches to depression

According to Gilbert (1992), Freud proposed that loss was central to what he termed 'melancholia'. However, in attempting to account for the lowering of self-esteem and suppressed anger commonly found in people who are depressed, Freud's explanations focused on the role of structures of the unconscious mind. The role of the therapist, according to the psychoanalytic model, is to promote the cathartic unleashing of inhibited negative emotions. Melanie Klein focused instead on the importance of relationships in early life, their power to define the self as good or bad and to deal with separation. She retained Freud's notion that memories associated with negative feelings are 'repressed' from consciousness. The work of Bowlby and others on attachment (Chapter 3) has added insights into the impact of early relationships on psychological functioning throughout life.

According to psychodynamic theory, insight is the main vehicle for change and the role of the therapist is to help the individual interpret 'hidden' motivations and understand the nature and influence of these early experiences. But although psychodynamic psychotherapy is a popular form of therapy, there is no evidence that it is more successful than other therapies (Roth and Fonagy 1996) and its often long duration makes it less attractive for the funders of health care.

Humanistic approaches

Humanistic approaches to the management of depression are enshrined in person-centred counselling, in which the therapist works though empathy to assist the individual in discovering their own route to personal development and self-actualization (Chapter 1). In support of this, there is evidence that therapist warmth and positive regard, and the establishment of a therapeutic alliance, increases patient confidence and disposition to change (Keijsers *et al.* 2000).

Cognitive behaviour therapy (CBT)

CBT has become the most popular psychological intervention for anxiety disorders, depression and medical conditions such as chronic pain that have a psychological component. One of its attractions for health care funders is that it is structured and time-limited. CBT, as the name suggests, combines cognitive and behavioural management strategies to recognize, interrupt and change automatic negative thoughts and maladaptive ways of responding. CBT programmes may be offered as individual therapy, but most involve group therapy. CBT assessment is based on its own version of 'ABC' (Lam and Gale 2000) which is quite different from the ABC of behaviour modification (Chapter 5):

A refers to **a**ctivating or triggering event(s)
B is the individual's **b**eliefs about or interpretations of the event(s)
C represents the individual's emotional or behavioural responses or **c**onsequences

According to cognitive principles:

* A does not cause C: i.e. events are not responsible for emotional responses;
* B is largely responsible for C: i.e. emotions are a consequence of the individual's beliefs about the events (Chapter 8).

Therapy therefore focuses on changing dysfunctional beliefs and recognizing and changing maladaptive behavioural responses. CBT is typically a brief intervention that involves six to ten sessions of one to two hours of problem-focused intervention. Group therapy using CBT has been shown to be more effective than other forms of group psychotherapy or even individual therapy (McDermut *et al.* 2001). However, although group therapy is more cost-effective, individual therapy needs to be available for people who are unable or unwilling to attend group sessions (see the case study in Chapter 10).

In addition to depression, CBT has been shown to be effective in the management of a range of disorders and conditions such as asthma and chronic pain (Chapter 10) that have an emotional or psychological component. Cochrane reviews have demonstrated its effectiveness for such problems as post-traumatic stress disorder (PTSD; Bisson and Andrew 2006), anxiety disorders in children (James *et al.* 2006), bulimia nervosa (Hay *et al.*

2006) and chronic fatigue syndrome (Price and Couper 2003). There is good evidence that it can be used effectively with all age groups, including adolescents and children (Christie and Wilson 2005). There is also increasing evidence that internet and computer-based applications of CBT offer a cost-effective alternative for moderate depression (Wright 2006).

NICE (2004b, 2005a) provides detailed guidelines for the assessment and management of depression in adults and children. Based on the most recent evidence, CBT should be offered to adults with moderate to severe depression who fail to respond to antidepressant therapy. Interpersonal psychotherapy may be offered if this reflects patient preference, although the evidence base is not so strong. CBT should be offered as the intervention of first choice for children and adolescents with moderate to severe depression.

Post-traumatic stress disorder (PTSD)

According to the *DSM* IV, PTSD may occur if the person has been exposed to a traumatic event in which the person experienced, witnessed, or was confronted with an event or events that involved actual or threatened death or serious injury, or a threat to the physical integrity of self or others, and responded with intense fear, helplessness or horror. PTSD has been recorded in response to a variety of events including assault, accident, disaster and medical treatment. Symptoms of PTSD include:

- Recurrent and intrusive distressing recollections of the event, including images, thoughts, and/or perceptions. In young children, repetitive play may occur in which these or other aspects of the trauma are expressed.
- Recurrent distressing dreams of the event. In young children, there may be frightening dreams without recognizable content.
- Sense of reliving the experience, illusions, hallucinations, and/or flashbacks, including those that occur on awakening or when intoxicated. In young children, trauma-specific re-enactment may occur.
- Intense psychological distress and/or physiological reactivity on exposure to internal or external cues that symbolize or resemble an aspect of the traumatic event.

According to the *DSM* IV, diagnostic criteria for PTSD include persistent avoidance of stimuli (images or situations) associated with the trauma, and general emotional numbing. People suffering from PTSD may use alcohol or other substances as self-medication in an attempt to avoid or eliminate intrusive memories. Other symptoms include at least two of the following:

- difficulty falling or staying asleep;
- irritability or outbursts of anger;
- difficulty concentrating;
- hypervigilance (constant wariness);
- exaggerated startle response (reacting to the slightest noise or disturbance).

Symptoms may occur immediately following the trauma, or may be delayed. Most recover within a few weeks or months without treatment, particularly if there is good family support.

Explaining PTSD

A number of possible explanations for PTSD have been offered. The first is that it is a conditioned emotional response (Chapter 5), brought about by the strength of emotional reaction to the event and maintained by avoidance. Other researchers have focused on memory. Ehlers and Clark (2000) suggested that memories of the traumatic event are poorly encoded in long-term memory because things happened so quickly. As a result, victims are unable to control their responses or make sense or meaning out of what happened. They are therefore unable to integrate the event or their response to it into biographical memory. Brewin *et al.* (1996) and Dalgleish (2004) have suggested that memories for traumatic events may be encoded in different ways, rather than as a single schema. Some of these may be accessible and others not, so people may be unable to talk about memories that nevertheless do exist (Chapter 4). The jury is clearly still out on these complex issues.

It is commonly assumed that PTSD results from exceptionally threatening or catastrophic incidents (NICE 2005b). But the literature indicates that PTSD can occur following a wide range of medical interventions such as cardiac surgery in children (Connolly 2004) and childbirth (Walker 2000). Professionals need to be alert to this and recommend that anyone with manifest symptoms of PTSD ask for help from a specialist psychologist. The following example is based on a real situation.

> One day, Janice felt ill in the night and went to the bathroom where she suffered a severe attack of vomiting and diarrhoea. Mark found her unconscious on the bathroom floor in a dreadful mess and called an ambulance. Janice came round in hospital, unwashed in the same night clothes. Mark told her what had happened. For several months after this she suffered flashbacks and nightmares based on mental images of her experience. She constantly monitored herself for feelings of nausea and never went anywhere without checking out the availability of toilets. She experienced panic attacks when she tried to go out alone and was afraid to be left in the house on her own. It was several months before she felt able to return to work.

The trauma in Janice's case was the total unexpected loss of bodily control and subsequent fear that her own body would let her down again.

Treatment of PTSD

It was originally believed that immediate counselling was important in the prevention of PTSD. However, a meta-analysis of all studies of psychological debriefing indicated that debriefing *increased* the risk of PTSD nearly three-fold (Rose *et al.* 2004). Therefore the current advice is that compulsory debriefing after trauma should stop. That is not to say that people should be discouraged from talking about the event to family, friends or a confidant if they wish to do so. Those most likely to benefit from counselling support soon after a traumatic event are those who have experienced previous traumas or lack emotional support (Litz *et al.* 2002).

Health care professionals need to warn people who have experienced a traumatic incident that it is possible they may at some time in the future experience flashbacks associated with feelings of panic. If so, they can be reassured that most of the symptoms will disappear within three months. If they don't, their doctor should refer them for treatment to a clinical psychologist who specializes in PTSD. Current guidelines (NICE 2005b), based on all the available evidence, recommend trauma-focused CBT as a primary method of treatment for all age groups, including children. Systematic desensitization (Chapter 5) is likely to be a component. This requires the patient to consciously hold images of the trauma in their minds until sympathetic arousal has subsided and they feel calm. When done repeatedly, the fear response associated with traumatic memories is eliminated.

An alternative recent psychological treatment, for which there is currently no agreed theoretical explanation, is eye movement desensitization and reprocessing (EMDR, Shapiro 1996). As in systematic desensitization, the individual is asked to hold traumatic images, but in this case while watching the therapist's finger move back and forth. After a series of repeats over several sessions, the traumatic image disappears. For all these therapies, it is suggested that it is helpful if people talk about the event after treatment to prevent recurrence.

Some people continue to experience PTSD long after the event, for example, there are many examples in the literature of World War II veterans who still manifest symptoms. Both CBT and EMDR are effective no matter how long after the traumatic event they are offered.

Dealing with loss

Experiencing losses is an inevitable part of life. When we make choices about careers, relationships or places and ways to live, choosing one inevitably involves loss of the other. Transitions like marriage, promotion at work or having a baby bring both gains and losses. Some losses occur as part of a traumatic event. Other losses may be not of actual things or people, but of potential experiences, roles or relationships, and it is therefore possible to lose something that you have never had. This type of loss is experienced by many infertile couples, for whom the role of parent cannot be realized. Certain experiences such as unemployment, homelessness or loss of a body part or function are associated with multiple actual and potential losses.

Kelly (1998) reviewed the multiple losses associated with chronic pain and illness. Concrete losses include loss of mobility, energy, comfort, physical activity and lifestyle. Personal and interpersonal losses include loss of privacy, body image, human relationships, independence, sense of self, family roles, work roles, sexual fulfilment, ideal life and loss of life as it used to be. It can be seen from this that loss can take many forms and chronically ill or disabled patients need opportunities to come to terms with these.

The death of someone we love is generally recognized as one of the most serious adverse life events, yet loss of a pet or other attachment object can be almost as traumatic. Attachment bonds are important throughout our lives and the disruption or breakdown of close relationships is an important source of loss, sometimes leading to physical and psychological illness including impaired immune functioning (Chapter 8), accidents, substance abuse, suicide, depression and other forms of psychopathology (Hazan and Zeifman 1999). Nurses encounter death more frequently than most other people, but many still have a high level of anxiety about it. Payne *et al.* (1998) found that those working in emergency care settings had higher levels of death anxiety than those working in palliative care settings, possibly because they had less opportunity to discuss their feelings. The next sections consider theories that account for people's responses to loss. The following definitions clarify different aspects of response:

- bereavement is the process surrounding loss;
- **grief** is the reaction associated with loss;
- **mourning** is the behavioural and emotional expression of grief.

Mourning is strongly influenced by cultural norms. For example, the rituals that occur after a death, such as laying out the body, the type of funeral and type of clothing worn by mourners are all very much dependent upon culture norms. In the USA, it is common practice to have open coffins. This used to be common in Britain, but not now. The funeral is often followed by a family or community gathering where the deceased individual is remembered and aspects of his or her life celebrated. It is probably helpful to have well accepted rituals because they direct people how to behave and how to respond to each other during a time when it is difficult to make informed decisions. Rituals, such as state funerals, both contain and allow public expression of feelings. Rituals also mark the status change of individuals, such as a wife becoming a widow. They provide an opportunity to demonstrate emotional support, and enable grieving people to derive comfort from others.

Traditional theories of loss and grief

Traditional theories of loss, like attachment, were derived from psychoanalysis, because the key theorists emerged from that tradition. Central to these is the concept of 'ego defence', which means that some things that happen are so threatening that the conscious mind, the ego, cannot cope with them. Freud introduced the notion of **defence mechanisms**, which are unconscious ways of coping. Defence mechanisms, such as denial, may be helpful in allowing us to continue functioning in very stressful situations, so that we can 'work through' problems at a later stage. Freud suggested that in order to recover from loss, we need to confront our fears and feelings in a conscious process that he called 'grief work'. Freud suggested that failure to do this might lead to prolonged or pathological types of grief. Freud's ideas influenced later theories of loss, including Bowlby's work on separation and loss and psychodynamic approaches. The notion of 'grief work' is still very prevalent, even though there is actually little evidence to support it.

Two of the best-known models of bereavement are those described by Elizabeth Kübler-Ross and Colin Murray Parkes. These models were both based on clinical observations. Kübler-Ross (1969) based her model of loss on her clinical experiences with dying patients who were confronting their own loss of life. She described how patients who were given a life-threatening diagnosis, like cancer, appeared to pass through four stages: denial (not me), anger, bargaining (for more time) and depression, before reaching psychological acceptance of death. The model is popular with nurses and other caring professions because they frequently encounter these types of reaction. The 'Kübler-Ross' stages provide a framework for understanding aspects of adjustment to loss although there is no evidence that people go through a series of invariant stages. Reactions to loss are very variable and it is often unhelpful to categorize dying people in terms of stages.

Parkes (1972) developed a model of bereavement loss based on clinical observations of those who had experienced major losses such as the death of a spouse. He suggested that all significant losses result in a major and rapid change to people's taken-for-granted world (their schemas), which is threatening and frightening. He noted a number of common responses, many of which are similar to those noted by Kübler-Ross. The following list of grief reactions is drawn from observations of Kübler-Ross, Parkes, and Stroebe and Stroebe (1987). Some of these are similar to the manifestations of depression, perhaps because both tend to involve perceptions of loss.

- *Initial reactions*
  - Numbness, disbelief, unreality or denial
  - Alarm reaction (Chapter 8): experienced as anxiety, restlessness and fear
- *Common emotional and psychosocial responses*
  - Feelings of failure, regret or guilt
  - Yearning and pining for the lost one
  - Continuing to interact with the deceased, for example, feeling their presence and talking to them as though they were still there
  - Feeling alone or abandoned
  - Anger
  - Sorrow, despair, pessimism, rumination
  - Loss of purpose, feelings of loss of the self, loss of enjoyment, sense of worthlessness
  - Difficulty in maintaining social relationships

- *Physical symptoms*
- Insomnia
- Feelings of fatigue, lethargy, reduction in activity
- Slowed thinking, poor concentration
- Loss of appetite

Challenging traditional assumptions about loss

Stroebe and Schut (1998) proposed a 'dual process' model of grief, illustrated in Figure 6.2. Instead of proposing a linear trajectory towards resolution, this identifies a process of oscillation between the feelings of grief and thoughts, feelings and behaviours directed towards restoration. Over time, grief experiences diminish while restoration activities increase. Restoration experiences include doing new things, finding sources of distraction and eventually finding new roles, identities and relationships. The rate at which this occurs is very variable. Some people orient themselves towards restoration at an early stage, such as undertaking activities in memory of the person who has died. Examples include fundraising in aid of a charity associated with the illness experienced by the person who died, or involvement in a self-help group for those who have experienced similar losses. Some people remain focused on the loss and those who engage in excessive rumination about their loss, long after the event, usually require professional help.

Wortman and Silver (1989) challenged other common assumptions about bereavement loss:

1 *Is distress or depression inevitable?* Studies of bereaved people show that depression affects only 10 to 15 per cent of those who are bereaved

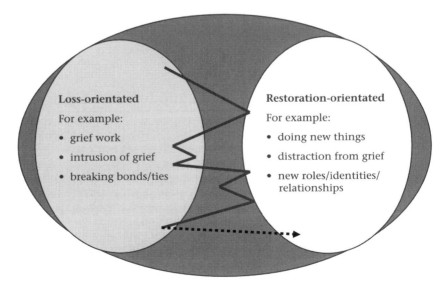

Figure 6.2 The dual process model of grief (adapted from Stroebe and Schut 1998)

(Bonanno 2004). Research with widows conducted by Vachon *et al.* (1982) indicated that those who were most depressed in the early stages where also the people most likely to be still depressed after two years. Bonanno challenged Bowlby's assumptions that an absence of grief is pathological or that it indicates a superficial attachment to the deceased. Rather he suggested it is relatively common for people to show great resilience in the face of trauma and loss, and the ability to continue functioning (this may relate to hardy personality characteristics and/or effective coping strategies, see Chapter 8). Bonanno called for a re-evaluation of basic assumptions about responses to loss and more research into human fortitude.

2   *Is it important to 'work through' feelings of loss?* It used to be assumed that resolution of grief requires cognitive-emotional processing (grief work) and this is an important aim of interventions like psychotherapy or bereavement counselling. Yet studies suggest that people who exhibit high levels of yearning or pining tend to have a poorer outcome in the long term, regardless of intervention. Jordan and Neimeyer (2003), having studied the literature on bereavement intervention, concluded that the scientific basis for accepting the efficacy of grief counselling appears weak. Bonanno's (2004) review of the evidence went further to indicate that, as with PTSD debriefing, grief therapies can actually make matters worse, other than for those with chronic (prolonged) grief responses. Professional carers should not automatically assume that all people require, or will benefit from, one of the 'talking' therapies; rather, people should be allowed to decide for themselves if and when they need this type of support.

3   *Do all people resolve their grief?* All models of loss assume that the final outcome of grieving will be a return to a normal psychological state. But Wortman and Silver (1989) suggested that, for a minority of individuals, grieving may continue over many years. This would not be considered abnormal or a problem unless it interferes with the individual's ability to function normally.

It might be assumed that the stronger the marital relationship, the greater the sense of loss when the partner dies. But Van Doorn *et al.* (1998) found that those who had had insecure attachment or dependent relationships were more likely to experience traumatic grief following the death of their spouse.

Ted was devastated when Laura died. They had known each other since school, and had recently celebrated their golden wedding anniversary. She died of cancer after a relatively short illness and Ted was quite unprepared for this. It was clear that he would find it difficult to look after himself because Laura had done all the housework, but he refused help. He could not bear the thought of leaving the house or of anyone else touching Laura's things. He sought refuge in his greenhouse and in the evenings felt Laura's presence by having all of her things around him. The family were concerned, but he refused all offers of help. Eventually, he developed bronchitis and moved in with Mark and Janice on a temporary basis. When he felt better, he visited his home and was able, with help, to start clearing a few things out. After a little longer he started making plans for the future and look forward to the birth of his next great-grandchild.

Grief can be seen to have many components and is best thought of as a holistic response to loss. Grief is a normal process, not a state, and does not involve a series of stages. Grief is painful and affects almost all aspects of the person. Many people describe grief as physically painful and may need reassurance that they are not ill. Some people cope with grief by increasing their use of mood altering substances like alcohol, tobacco or drugs. Drugs or alcohol use may (as in PTSD) begin as a form of self-medication to blot out memories of the loss. This impedes successful adaptation and increases risk to health. It is known that there is an increased risk of death in the first few years after the death of a spouse. Loss leads to immunological suppression and increased susceptibility to infections and stress-related diseases (Chapter 8). In a minority who are vulnerable, depression following bereavement leads to increased risk of suicide. Interestingly, a study of district nurses found that only a small proportion felt it their responsibility to provide bereavement support for relatives after a cancer patient had died (Birtwistle *et al.* 2002).

A biographical approach to loss

A 'biographical' perspective on loss was put forward by Walter (1996), who applied this to all forms of loss, including changes in body image. His theory proposed that a person who has experienced an important change or loss needs to construct or reconstruct their identity in the light of the changes that have occurred. This reflects a growing interest in narrative psychology (Chapters 2 and 3). Bury (1982) introduced the concept of biographical disruption to explain the impact of losses. This means that many of the taken-for-granted aspects of daily life and future expectations are disrupted and the notion of 'self' has to alter to accommodate these changes. Borrowing the notion of schemas, some people are able to accommodate change within their existing schemas, while others cannot. Narrative psychologists (Crossley 2003) and gerontologists (Clark 2001) suggest that therapeutic work involves structuring chaotic and disruptive memories into a meaningful story. Coming to terms with losses requires that these events are integrated into continuing life, or mental health may suffer. According to Walter (1999), storytelling is the means by which people have traditionally achieved this. Kelly (1998) described how coming to terms with the changes brought about by these losses required what she termed 're-storying one's life'. It involves finding new goals and sense of purpose to one's life and requires the individual to construct a new and different ongoing life story. This is part of what is termed narrative therapy (Friedman and Combs 1996). Narrative interviewing is also gaining in popularity in qualitative research, providing powerful insights into the lived experience of illness and loss.

Asbring (2001) interviewed women with fibromyalgia to find out how their illness had affected them. Fibromyalgia is a painful condition that affects the muscles and for which there is no known effective treatment. Losses included the ability to work and one participant described her life as similar to that of a pensioner. The main finding was that the illness led to a radical disruption in the women's biographies and had a profound effect on their sense of identity, particularly in relation to work and social life. However, not all of the changes were negative and many of the women also experienced gains as a result of their illness. For example, they felt they had learned to place more value on small joys and less on material goods.

Conversations with friends, non-directive counselling, narrative writing and life review (Chapter 3) all provide therapeutic opportunities. This indicates that the most important task of the health professional, when faced with someone who is bereaved, is to be available to listen.

Walter (1996: 26) published this quotation from an anonymous source. We have reproduced it in poetic form to capture its full impact.

I am a student nurse. I am dying.
I write this to you who are, and will become, nurses
in the hope that by my sharing my feeling with you,
you may someday be better able to help those who share my
experience. For me, fear is today and dying is now.
You slip in and out of my room,
give me medications and check my blood pressure.
Is it because I am a student nurse myself, or just a human being,
that I sense your fright?
And your fears enhance mine.
Why are you afraid? I am the one who is dying.
If only we could be honest, both admit our fear, touch one another.
If you really care,
would you lose so much of our valuable professionalism
if you even cried with me? . . .
Then it might not be so hard to die
– in a hospital – with friends close by.

Anticipatory grief

Some diseases involve a protracted period of illness and illness-related losses prior to death which affect caregivers as well as the patients. For example, in

Alzheimers's disease, the spouse loses the person they married and loved, the friend, social companion, source of emotional support, lover, income-provider, car driver, person to argue with and so on. These losses may occur gradually over many years, each loss to be mourned and requiring adjustment. This is termed 'anticipatory grief'. Very extended periods of anticipatory grief are not necessarily adaptive for the caregiver of someone with a chronic illness because withdrawal of emotional involvement during this period can induce a sense of guilt after the death has occurred. But there are examples of how it can help people to say and do things they might otherwise regret not doing. This can help adjustment when the death finally occurs.

> This is an extract reported by (Evans 1994: 160): 'Some time after the death of her father, a young woman returned to the hospital ward on which he died to thank the nursing staff. She explained that, despite the distress and pain she experienced when informed of her father's terminal condition and his subsequent death, she was grateful for the time period between these two events. Amongst other things, it gave her time to resolve conflicts, express her love and say goodbye.'

This extract suggests that we are able to help people prepare for bereavement and start to mourn their loss before death actually occurs. Much of the care offered to relatives of dying patients is based on the assumption that 'grief work' can begin prior to the death. It may help relatives to realistically face up to their imminent loss. The grief experienced at that time will help to prevent subsequent abnormal bereavement. However, the research evidence about anticipatory grief is rather confused. Evans (1994) suggested that instead of focusing just on the death, we should be aware of the multiple stresses and losses that occur for patients and their caregivers during a terminal illness and support them while they deal with these.

Hope

Perhaps one of the reasons why many health care professionals find it so hard to confront death is because of their desire to maintain hope. Hope is what most of us live for, but when pain, illness, disability or any loss occurs, previously valued goals may seem, or may actually be, unattainable. This can engender hopelessness, bring acceptance or promote determination. Snyder (1998) presented a theory of hope in situations involving pain, loss and suffering. Paraphrasing Snyder, he defined hope as a combination of a determination to achieve a desired goal or end point and a plan for getting there.

A feature of those who maintain high hope is the ability to modify or change some of their original goals (see also Chapters 9 and 10).

This requires a willingness to change one's personal biography. Snyder identified that people with high hope have different goals within different life arenas. This means that they are able to switch to another goal when one appears unobtainable. He argued that grieving occurs when a previously attainable goal is no longer obtainable. However, following a period of mourning, people with high hope turn their attentions to substitute goals that are achievable. Health care professionals can help patients to face things one step at a time when faced with overwhelming challenges.

> During her third year of training, Anna had a placement in a hospice for people with all kinds of terminal illness. She was very anxious because she did not really know how to talk to people who were dying or how to approach other patients following a death. However, once she had started on the ward her mentor carefully discussed with her the philosophy of hospice care, the holistic approach and the emphasis on openness and sharing with patient, family and staff. The mentor helped Anna to understand her own reactions to death and dying. This enabled Anna to communicate in a positive way with others who were exploring their own issues in relation to dying. Anna was surprised to discover that, rather than being a place of sadness, there was a real sense of hope which focused on maximizing quality of life for the patients and their families.

Positive psychology: promoting wellness

In writing this chapter we are aware that we have focused almost exclusively on negative emotions even though, as we have pointed out, the majority of people feel positive most of the time. There has been a recent move in psychology, led by Martin Seligman who is better known for his work on learned helplessness, away from focusing solely on psychological problems and toward what is termed positive psychology. Seligman and Csikszentmihalyi (2000) define this as a focus on well-being and contentment, satisfaction with the past, happiness in the present, and optimism and hope for the future. To end on a positive note, Cowen (1994) suggested that ways of achieving this include:

- forming wholesome early attachments (Chapter 3);
- acquiring age- and ability-appropriate competencies (see self-efficacy, Chapters 5 and 9);
- engineering settings that promote adaptive outcomes (Chapter 9);
- fostering empowerment (Chapters 2, 7 and 8);
- acquiring skills needed to cope effectively with life **stressors** (Chapter 8).

Summary of key points

- Anxiety and depression may be explained from different psychological perspectives, each of which makes an important contribution to our understanding.
- Anxiety and depression are common human emotions which require assessment and management if symptoms cause an abnormal level of distress or interfere with the ability to lead a normal life.
- CBT is currently the intervention of choice in the management of anxiety and depression for children, adolescents and adults.
- PTSD is relatively common and easy to treat, but can cause considerable distress if not recognized.
- Grief is a normal response to loss, but an apparent absence of grief reactions is not indicative of long-term problems with psychological adjustment.
- The majority of people are resilient and maintain hope in the face of losses.
- Empathetic listening is the most important contribution that people who do not have special training can offer to people in emotional distress.

Exercise

See after Chapter 10.

Further reading

Arthur, A.R. (2003) The emotional lives of people with learning disabilities, *British Journal of Learning Disabilities*, 31(1): 25–31.

Harvey, J.H. (1998) *Perspectives on Loss: A Sourcebook*. Philadelphia, PA: Brunner Maazel.

Payne, S., Horn, S. and Relf, M. (1999) *Loss and Bereavement*. Buckingham: Open University Press.

Walter, T. (1999) *On Bereavement: The Culture of Grief*. Buckingham: Open University Press.

Wasserman, D. (2006) *Depression, the Facts: Expert Advice for Patients, Carers and Professionals*. Oxford: Oxford University Press.

CHAPTER SEVEN

SOCIAL INFLUENCE AND INTERACTION

- **What special techniques can be used to persuade people to change their beliefs and motivate them to want to change their behaviour?**
- **To what extent are we influenced by others when making important decisions and what are the implications of this in health and social care?**
- **Why are some people more likely to receive help than others?**
- **What is non-verbal behaviour and why is it important in communication?**
- **How do groups influence individual decisions and behaviour?**
- **What is the best way to deal with conflict and complaints?**
- **What influences effective interprofessional teamworking?**

Introduction

In this chapter, we explore social processes involved in interactions between care professionals and members of the public; between different groups of professionals; and between managers and members of the workforce. Much of western psychology has tended to focus rather narrowly on the individual when studying psychological influences on behaviour, yet these processes are strongly influenced by the attitudes and behaviour of those around us. In this chapter we explore these issues. To do so, we have integrated research and theory from a variety of classic and original sources, together with information taken from texts devoted entirely to social psychology.

Persuasion

Persuasion is central to the encouragement of others to change their behaviour, as in many health promotion and education activities. Therefore it is useful to know some of the principles that can be used to enhance persuasive techniques. In Chapter 4, we addressed how information can be conveyed in a form that people can understand and remember. But knowledge does not guarantee action. An important question to be addressed in this chapter is, 'How can people be persuaded to act on information they are given?'

There are several basic steps in the persuasion process. First it is necessary to identify the target audience and customize the message to their particular needs. In order for the message to be assimilated, the audience must:

- *See or hear the message.* The sender must select a medium (television or radio network, newspaper or magazine, leaflets) likely to ensure that the target audience has easy access to it. Placing leaflets in a doctor's surgery, while cheap and convenient, is rarely an effective way to achieve this.
- *Pay attention to the message.* Attention is selective, so the format of the message must be eye-catching. Presenting health information in a leaflet that is not eye-catching or attractive will ensure that people do not pick it up and read it. Also, the audience must see it as relevant to them. For example, an ongoing study of osteoporosis in men has observed that leaflets on osteoporosis mainly feature pictures of women. This signals that it is not a male issue (which is not true).
- *Understand the message.* Hearing advice or reading information does not mean that everyone will be able to understand it. It is the responsibility of professionals to ensure that all people are able to understand the information given (Chapter 4). This can best be achieved by working with representatives of relevant patient or client groups when preparing information.
- *Accept the message's conclusion.* People are unlikely to accept a message if it conflicts with long-standing beliefs or personal experience (Chapter 4), or information gained from other sources that are seen as more credible.

  Factors likely to influence whether or not the message is accepted are considered below.

The source or sender of the message

Several factors have been identified as influencing a recipient's judgements about the source or sender.

- *Perceived credibility of the message-giver.* This does not always equate with the expertise of the message-giver. For example, nutritionists know most about diet, and physiotherapists about exercise, but the public may nevertheless see the doctor as a more credible source of information on these topics. Similarly, information on feeding practices given by a midwife or health visitor may prove less persuasive that that given by close family or friends who offer advice based on personal experience.
- *Perceived trustworthiness.* Is the sender seen to have anything to gain by persuading others? Health professionals are often seen as having a vested interest in health promotion, which might be seen as a source of bias. For example, UK doctors are paid for undertaking screening and giving immunizations. Evidence from social psychology suggests that messages may be more persuasive if the sender argues from a position that is apparently opposed to his or her self-interest. It could therefore be argued that a heavy drinker will take more notice of advice to cut down from a former alcoholic or heavy drinker rather than a health professional that does not drink.

- *Perceived attractiveness.* People may view the sender as a role model for the lifestyle being promoted and reject the message if they see them as unattractive or not 'cool'. It appears that the attractiveness of the communicator is more influential for relatively trivial messages than for serious ones. Nevertheless, health promoters may wish to pay attention to their personal appearance if they wish others to take note of them.

Each of these factors will vary according to the target audience. It seems logical that factors likely to influence persuasion in a young audience are quite different from those likely to persuade an older audience. Petty and Cacioppo (1986) also found the interaction between the source, the message and the audience is influenced by educational level. Those who are well-educated and think carefully about health and social issues are more likely to focus on the significance and content of the message. Those who are less well educated and motivated are more likely to be persuaded by superficial images such as the attractiveness of the presenter or the advertisement (see Figure 7.1).

This implies that those at greatest risk of health and social problems are among those least likely to be persuaded by the professional purveyors of unwelcome messages. It throws out a challenge to professionals to find more innovative ways of promoting 'better' lifestyles.

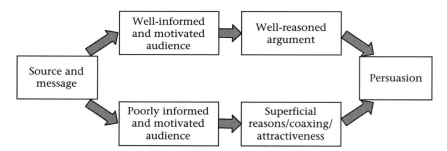

Figure 7.1   Dual process model of persuasion (based on Petty and Cacioppo 1986)

The nature of the message

Reason versus emotion

Many health promotion campaigns are designed to scare recipients into taking health action. A meta-analysis by Witte and Allen (2000) indicated that high fear appeals are effective only if the recipient is confident that they are able to achieve the behaviour change recommended. In those who are not confident of being able to take preventive action, high fear appeals result in avoidance rather than behaviour change. Messages must therefore be accompanied by clear and specific advice about simple and effective courses of action.

Most people find it easier to relate to personal stories or examples that have strong emotional appeal, rather than statistical or epidemiological evidence that has strong rational appeal. This is why many campaigns feature people with whom the target group are likely to identify. Television is a good medium for making emotional appeals since emotional images are stronger when they combine sight, sound and movement. The persuasive power of leaflets can be increased by including pictures that have emotional impact.

When trying to appeal to reason when conveying a serious issue, it is worth considering if only one side of an argument should be presented, or if both sides should be considered. A well-informed audience is more likely to be persuaded by two-sided arguments because they will be aware of the counter-arguments and will wish to see these addressed. A less well-informed audience is likely to be confused by two-sided arguments and it may be better to present them with a single point of view.

> Before Mark was diagnosed as having diabetes and hypertension, Janice knew that he was in a high-risk group because of his weight gain and high sugar intake. She warned him of the possible consequences if he carried on as he was, but he didn't listen, reasoning that nobody in his family had diabetes or heart problems and these were unlikely to happen to him. He was eventually persuaded by the diabetic consultant and nutritionist because they took the time to explain his condition to him and discuss the pros and cons of dietary and other lifestyle change.

Order of presentation

The importance of primacy and recency effects has already been discussed (Chapter 4). When presenting verbal arguments, health professionals often unwittingly influence client's decisions by the order in which the issues are presented.

Cognitive dissonance

Festinger (1957) observed that when an individual holds two or more beliefs that are inconsistent with each other, they experience a state of dissonance. For example, 'I am a healthy person' may conflict with the knowledge that 'I do not take enough exercise'. Therefore, when individuals are presented with messages that conflict with their current behaviour, this creates a state of cognitive dissonance. According to Festinger, this state is unsettling and needs to be resolved. Aronson (1988) suggested a number of ways people deal with this:

- change their opinion (and their behaviour);
- induce the communicator to change his or her opinion;
- seek support for their original opinion from others;
- convince themselves that the communicator is untrustworthy or uncreditworthy.

A good example is the use of cannabis in teenagers. The rational reasons for change are that it can have serious mental health consequences in the long term. But teenagers seek to justify its continued use on the grounds that all their friends do it and have not suffered any noticeable ill effects, and that older people are just determined to spoil their fun.

It has been found that the greater the discrepancy between the argument being presented and the individual's current attitudes, the less the extent of attitude change (this fits with the concept of the mental schema, Chapters 3 and 4). Therefore it is important to find out about the current beliefs of the target or audience and try to work out a solution that they can accommodate.

> Mark originally refused to listen to health messages because they contradicted a lifestyle that he enjoyed, notably eating crisps and chocolate and drinking beer. He thought that dietary advice was just a fad and 'they' would think of something else next week. When Janice tried to persuade him to change, he reasoned that she was not an expert on diet and sought support from his friends in the pub.

So what works? Individual change requires the professional to take time to understand the beliefs and attitudes of the person they are trying to persuade and then use arguments that fit with these belief sets. This is difficult if arguments contradict the views of the individual's reference group. Change within a population usually comes about gradually. It is a good idea initially to target trend-setters who are open to changing their attitude and behaviour and engage their help in promoting change.

Complexity and presentation of the message

Complex information cannot be assimilated quickly. It requires repetition and time. Therefore, where complex information is given to people, it should be provided in a written (or possibly taped) format that they can take away and study at their leisure.

> When Sasha attended her first antenatal check, when she was expecting Lee, she was asked if she wished to have a screening test for congenital abnormalities in her unborn child. Although the midwife explained the tests carefully, Anna had difficulty understanding the full implications. The choices she was asked to make were complex. If she had the screening done, what were the options if the tests proved positive? If she chose not have screening, what were the potential consequences for her and her family? She agreed to the tests because she did not want to waste the midwife's time or appear foolish. But she was quite uncertain about

the answers to these questions. When she became pregnant again, she made sure that she had read and understood the leaflets she was given at the doctor's surgery. She discussed them with Janice and with Jo before her first hospital antenatal check. This time she felt more confident and was able to ask questions to assure herself that she was making the right decision.

You might wish to review the sections on information-giving in Chapter 4.

Immediacy of action and endurance of the message

Change-promoting messages quickly lose their effect. The longer the gap between receiving the persuasive message and taking protective action, the more likely that other pressures will intervene. It is also more likely that the individual will find justifications and counter-arguments. Therefore, it is helpful if individuals are persuaded to make an immediate act of commitment, much in the same way that religious evangelists invite audience members to make an immediate declaration of commitment. This is why the salesman tries hard to get people to sign up to an immediate sale (and why the law allows a cooling off period). Clinical psychologists sometimes use contracts to confirm their client's commitment to an agreed behaviour change.

Once initiated, the new attitude must be sustained in order to preserve the behaviour change. Health promotion is more likely to be effective if the message or media image is maintained in the public domain over a long period of time. Mass campaigns are largely ineffectual unless the impetus is maintained.

When Mark was seen by the nutritionist, she reviewed his current diet and made a plan of change that would be achievable. He was asked to record his eating pattern and to see the diabetic nurse for a regular review. This made it more difficult for him to go home and forget or ignore what he had been told, or be tempted to cheat too drastically.

Sadly, regular reviews are not normally offered for reasons of cost. Research is urgently needed to test if regular reviews of behaviour change and management are more likely to improve long-term outcomes. Some support for this hypothesis is found in a review of self-management programmes for asthma in which those who did not receive regular reviews were reported to have more health centre visits and sickness days (Powell and Gibson 2003).

Audience influences and effects

Selective attention

It is well recognized that people tend to focus attention on issues that reflect their existing understanding or point of view (Chapters 3 and 4).

> In an old but relevant study, Kleinhesselink and Edwards (1975) asked university students to complete a questionnaire concerning their attitudes to the legalization of cannabis. They then listened to a broadcast, through headphones, that contained seven strong (irrefutable) arguments and seven weak (refutable) arguments in favour of legalization. Constant static noise made listening difficult, but students could press a button to reduce this. Those who favoured legalization pushed the button significantly more often when strong arguments were presented. Subjects who opposed legalization pushed the button significantly more often when weak (refutable) arguments were presented. The conclusion of this study was that individuals pay more attention to messages that support their own beliefs.

Festinger's social comparison theory (Chapter 2) proposed that individuals deliberately seek validation of their own attitudes and beliefs by attending to those who hold ideas similar to their own and distancing themselves from those who hold different beliefs or attitudes. This means that some social groups, such as teenagers, may be difficult to penetrate by those seen as outsiders. Health educators need to find novel ways of gaining acceptance if health messages are to be received and taken seriously.

> When Jo left school, he regularly took drugs including alcohol and ecstasy, as did all his friends. Janice tried to warn him that this was not a good idea, but this simply drove him out of the house to meet his mates, thus reinforcing his attitudes. When he met Sasha, he spent less time with these friends and started using alcohol and drugs less frequently.

Self-esteem and compliance

People with low self-esteem do not place high value on their own ideas and are therefore more likely to be compliant. But this means that they are more likely to give in to peer pressure if this conflicts with advice from professionals. People with high self-esteem are more likely to question and challenge, but may be persuaded by rational argument and are less likely to be influenced by peer pressure to do things they feel are wrong. Education provides people with essential knowledge and life skills and is an important source of self-efficacy (Chapter 5) and self-esteem.

Summary of persuasive techniques

Change-promoting messages, including health promotion and education, need to be tailored to the needs of the audience. Those who are well educated, well motivated and have high self-esteem are more likely to respond to full information and a well reasoned argument from a credible professional source. Although targeting this group may be regarded as preaching to the converted, these are people who may act as future trend-setters and are therefore an important audience. Those who are less well educated and have low self-esteem are more likely to respond to superficial but directive messages from attractive and emotionally appealing sources with whom they are able to identify. They are likely to be very susceptible to peer-pressure from other members of their reference group. Health messages that contradict prevailing social and cultural beliefs and behaviours, particularly those within cohesive subcultures, are likely to be resisted. These issues are best addressed by respected group members working from within.

Obedience

Persuasion appeals to reason, whereas obedience does not. Obedience means 'do as you are told without asking questions'. Stanley Milgram was a psychologist at Yale University in the 1960s who was interested to understand how Hitler was able to induce mass obedience to engage in extreme acts of cruelty during World War II. He set up a laboratory experiment that turned out to have implications far beyond his expectations.

Milgram advertised for volunteers to take part in an educational experiment at Yale University. On arrival, each volunteer was introduced to another participant and a draw took place to identify who would be the pupil and who the teacher in the experiment. In fact, the draw was fixed: the volunteer always took the part of the teacher while the other was a stooge who acted the part of pupil. The 'teacher' was told by the experimenter to press a button to give the 'pupil' an electric shock as a punishment if he made a mistake. The shocks gradually increased in intensity from 15 volts to 450 volts, the upper range clearly marked on the dial in red as 'danger'.

It came as a shock to all concerned that 26 out of the 40 'teachers' continued, on instruction from the experimenter, to give up to 450 volts of shock even though their 'pupil' had progressed through protests and

> screams and by this time appeared to be unconscious. Nobody stopped at below 300 volts (the British household voltage is 240 volts and the American voltage 110 volts).

The following features have subsequently been shown to influence obedience in this type of experimental situation:

- *The legitimacy or status of the authority figure.* When the experiment was repeated at a less well-known institution, obedience was less likely, although still occurred at an alarming level.
- *The proximity of victim.* Obedience was less likely when the victim was in the same room, rather than behind a glass screen.
- *The proximity of the authority figure.* Obedience was less likely when the experimenter was in another room and gave instructions by telephone.
- *Personal characteristics.* Some volunteers appeared to be more conformist than others and more obedient to instruction.
- *Habit.* Some people appeared to respond automatically to authority cues.
- *Social rules of commitment.* Having agreed to participate in the experiment, the volunteers felt obliged to do as they were asked.

Does obedience to authority happen in health care?

> A 'real life' experiment was conducted by Hofling *et al.* (1966). A drug clearly marked 'Astroten 5mg, maximum dose 10 mg' was planted in the drugs cabinet on a mental health care ward. The experimenter, purporting to be a psychiatrist, phoned the ward and told the nurse in charge to give a named patient 20 mg of Astroten. An observer intercepted the nurse before she (they were all female) reached the patient. Twenty-one out of 22 nurses complied with the instruction even though:
>
> - there was no written prescription
> - the drug exceeded the safe dose (11 claimed not to have noticed this)
> - none of the nurses had ever heard of either the drug or the 'doctor' beforehand.

Could this type of problem occur today?

> Anna had recently qualified and was working on a unit that undertook invasive investigations for which there is a long waiting list. The procedure required the routine administration of a drug one hour beforehand. The drug was harmless in the dose normally given, but could be harmful in higher doses. The rules stated that she was not allowed to give a drug

without a doctor's written prescription. On this occasion, a new registrar whom she had not yet met had forgotten to write up the drug for one of the patients who had been waiting for half an hour. He phoned to inform Anna that he was otherwise engaged. He was very nice and apologetic. He asked Anna to administer the drug and he would sign for it as soon as he could get away. What should Anna do?

- What if the patient was a well known figure likely to cause a scene at being kept waiting?
- What if the registrar expresses fear about the consultant's reaction to his mistake?

One of the main reasons for introducing diploma and degree level training for health and social care professionals is to raise awareness of these issues, encourage questioning and consider the potential consequences before accepting or giving orders.

Conformity

In the section on persuasion, we refer particularly to the importance of peer group pressure. The tendency to conform to the beliefs and behaviours of others is an important source of social influence. These are the 'social norms' which form a component of social cognition theories used to predict **health behaviour** (Chapter 9). Conformity, like obedience, has been shown to affect our behaviour in ways that can have serious implications for health and social care provision.

The extent to which people feel under pressure to conform was demonstrated in a classic psychology experiment by Solomon Asch in the early 1950s (Asch 1956). Male college students volunteered to take part in an experiment which they were told involved visual judgement. They were shown a line on a card and asked to match it with the length of one of three lines shown on a separate card (as shown in Figure 7.2). This is an extremely straightforward and unambiguous task. However, each student was unknowingly placed in a room with confederates of the experimenter who deliberately selected the wrong line. In this situation, a third of students gave the same 'wrong' answer as the one given by the confederates. In total, 70 per cent of students conformed at least once to the wrong answer. Only a minority remained independent in the face of this type of group pressure.

It appears that people are prepared to deny the evidence of their own senses if this is contradicted by the beliefs or behaviour of others.

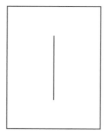 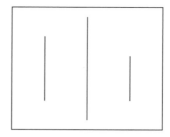

Figure 7.2 Presentation similar to that used in the Asch experiment on conformity. Participants were asked to match the length of the line on the left-hand card with one of the lines on the right-hand card

> Imagine you are a student nurse, like Anna, working on a first clinical placement. You are asked to take a routine blood pressure. You are not confident and are unable to take meaningful readings at the first attempt. What are you likely to do? You try again, and this time you are reasonably confident with the result. However, it is much lower than the patient's previous recordings. What do you do? The pressure is checked by another nurse who, having first checked the chart, confidently announces a pressure in line with previous recordings. You try again and obtain the same lower recording. How do you feel? What do you do?

Conformity to the views and behaviour of other people has been shown to be more likely in certain circumstances:

- when the task is difficult or the information available is ambiguous or sparse – this is true of many situations in health care;
- when the desire for social approval overrides other aspects of judgement;
- when contradicting the judgement of someone else might appear rude or discourteous;
- if others are perceived to have greater expertise – novices may be correct, but it is the views of experts which normally prevail;
- if the confidence, self-esteem and self-efficacy of the individual is low.

These conditions commonly apply in health and social care settings. They explain why patients or clients are reluctant openly to question or disagree with the advice they are given. They explain why patients give consent to procedures when they have not understood what they have been told. They explain why nurses and others may sometimes fail to question instructions.

It often takes considerable courage to stand up for one's convictions or question authority. Brehm *et al.* (2002) suggested that people are less likely to conform in individualistic societies that value self-reliance, and more likely to conform in collectivist societies that value cooperation and family and social allegiances. However, adherence to group norms is very strong. Non-conformity and non-compliance may be higher among those with a strong desire for self-expression, but this may be regarded by others as evidence of deviance, eccentricity or 'being difficult'.

The failure of individuals to act on their own beliefs can have very serious consequences. Reason (1990) undertook an analysis of a number of major disasters and identified that this was a significant contributory factor. In the case of the Chernobyl nuclear power disaster (1986), the local maintenance team appear to have assumed that the team of experts from Moscow knew what they were doing and were in control of the situation, even though they could see that the dials clearly registered danger levels. This is the very type of problem that has been highlighted in British health services, where junior colleagues and nurses have been reluctant to report errors and wrongdoings by senior consultants.

> Anna started work on a busy surgical ward and observed that a senior member of nursing staff was not conducting sterile dressings in accordance with hospital policy, as she had been taught. Anna recognized that this could have serious consequences for patients and drew this to the attention of the nurse involved. The nurse became quite angry and told her that there was not time to be fussy on this ward. Anna was faced with the choice of either being labelled 'difficult' or conforming with poor practice. What would you do in these circumstances?

It often takes a serious incident to draw attention to these types of practice, even though there is clearly an accident waiting to happen. It is difficult to deal with these types of situation alone, since 'whistleblowers' are often discredited (see also Chapter 2 on stigma). Ideally it is best to gain support from others, though this may be difficult.

Social desirability

Social desirability refers to the tendency to conform with the views of others. It is often used to refer to the tendency to answer questions in a socially approved manner. Many people are willing to lie in order to put forward a good impression of themselves. This is an important reason why patients do not always tell the truth about their lifestyle or adherence to their medications. It is also an important consideration for those collecting self-report information for research in health and social care. Individuals invariably try to interpret what is required of them and often modify their responses as part of their own impression-management (Chapter 2). This is why social researchers frequently have to use false cover stories. In social survey research, researchers sometimes use the Crowne-Marlowe Social Desirability Scale (Crowne and Marlowe 1960) to identify those whose responses are strongly influenced by the wish to portray themselves in a positive light.

In practice, it is important to ask open questions starting 'tell me . . .', in order to elicit people's own views or understanding, rather than asking questions that require a 'yes/no' answer. This approach to questioning gives less opportunity for conformity and compliance.

Helping others

This book is written for those working or training to work in the caring professions. But what is it that drives people to want to help others? Do some professionals help only because they are paid to do so? What motivates people to volunteer to help others?

There are both intrinsic and extrinsic rewards to be gained from helping others. Helping others may elicit social approval or praise and makes helpers feel good about themselves. Another explanation focuses on the notion of 'reciprocal altruism'. This reflects the belief that if I help someone else, they may help me if or when I need it. This applies to groups as well as to individuals. Self-help groups are often set up by people who have received help and wish to share their knowledge and experience.

Omoto and Snyder (1995) identified five reasons why people volunteered to work with AIDS patients.

- *Humanitarian values:* wanting to help others; being a caring person.
- *Curiosity:* the desire to learn more about illness or disability and to reduce personal fears and anxieties.
- *Personal and social development:* meeting new people, making new friends; gaining experience of dealing with difficult topics.
- *Social obligation:* out of particular concern for a particular underprivileged group in society.
- *Esteem/control enhancement:* to feel good, escape from other pressures, feel less lonely.

Most health and social care professionals, if we are honest, will admit to coming into the profession for at least three of these reasons, quite apart from other important issues of pay and career prospects.

Janice became a health care assistant after her children had gone to school because she needed something to do and wanted to get out of the house to meet new people. She was interested in helping others, particularly older people. But she was also curious to learn more about the treatment of various diseases and disorders that she had heard of, but knew little about.

Helping others is not always in the best interests of those who are being helped. In Chapters 8 to 10, you will find references to different types of social support: emotional support (listening, caring), **instrumental support** (doing things for people) and **informational support** (giving information and advice). Research referred to in those chapters supports the positive benefits of emotional and informational support, but demonstrates that doing things for people when they could or should be able to do them for themselves can, even when the individual wants or accepts the help, take away their autonomy and render them dependent or helpless. It is important when offering help to consider the potential for negative consequences. Sometimes it is better to be cruel to be kind.

> Margaret's friend, Sheila, had a stroke and was left with a weakness on her left side (she was right-handed). Her husband, Ron, was advised to encourage her to do as much for herself as possible. When Margaret visited, she found Sheila struggling to peel the potatoes for lunch and offered to take over. Margaret thought it cruel to see Sheila struggle. But Ron pointed out that these tasks made her feel useful. As a result, Sheila had not become depressed like her disabled friend of the same age whose husband had taken over all the chores.

Taking responsibility in an emergency

Social psychologists became interested in studying the phenomenon of 'bystander apathy' following an incident in the USA when a young woman, Kitty Genovese, was brutally murdered outside a block of flats. Her cries for help over a half-hour period were heard by a large number of people, yet no one phoned for the police.

This shocked the nation.

> Latané and Darley (1968) subsequently staged a series of 'emergencies' to explore the circumstances in which bystanders were more or less likely to intervene. A typical situation involved a man collapsed on a busy underground train. They identified quite a few factors likely to be influential in determining helping action.
>
> - People are more likely to act if there are cues to the seriousness of the situation from other bystanders. Once one person initiates action, others will follow.
> - The larger the number of strangers present who do nothing, the less likely an individual is to intervene. Each individual assumes that someone else will take the necessary action.
> - People fail to act if they perceive themselves incapable of doing anything to help. Conversely they are more likely to act if they feel they can do something useful to help.
> - People are less likely to act in ambiguous situations. For example, people are likely to ignore someone lying on the pavement if they think they may be drunk, rather than ill.

- People are more likely to take action if they have the opportunity to discuss the situation with other people first.
- Helping actions are influenced by the perceived 'deservedness' or culpability of the victim. This may relate to a 'just world' hypothesis in which people are presumed to get what they deserve in life.
- People who are facially, physically or behaviourally unattractive are less likely to receive sympathy or help.
- People are more likely to help if they are in a good mood!

Health care professionals are all trained to administer basic life support and are probably more likely to help in emergency situations. It is often puzzling why people do not immediately come to the rescue when someone collapses in a public place. But it is reassuring to know that, once you have initiated action, others are likely to follow and be supportive.

Non-verbal communication

Studies of patient satisfaction with health care have repeatedly shown that interpersonal aspects of care are central to patients' perceptions of quality of care. But it is not only what we do or say as professionals that matters, it is the manner in which we do it. Attitudes (Chapter 2) are evaluative responses that commonly involve approval and disapproval, usually expressed through non-verbal communication. If we disapprove of someone, or if we are nervous or annoyed, we show it in our facial expression, eye contact (or lack of it) and posture, and it is very hard to cover up our feelings or suppress these responses. We reveal a lot about ourselves through non-verbal communication. For example, we signal confidence or nervousness through our body and hand movements, facial expression, tone of voice and speed of delivery. Empathy, understanding, caring, pain and distress all involve communication, and non-verbal behaviours are the main ways of communicating caring.

Positive and negative attitudes such as pleasure or annoyance, approval or disgust, are revealed through non-verbal signals. Eye contact with a friendly smile normally conveys interest and a willingness to engage. People frequently use the avoidance of eye contact to signal that they have no wish to engage in social interaction. This may be why nurses become adept at walking through a ward without making eye contact. But while this prevents diversions, it can leave patients feeling ignored and frustrated.

A Dutch study (Caris-Verhallen *et al.* 1999) provided a detailed analysis of nurse–patient communication. The researchers measured characteristics of the nurse (age, gender, education level, years of employment, attitudes towards older people, job satisfaction), characteristics of their patients (age, gender, health status, time in care) and type of care environment (community or nursing home) and characteristics of the environment that might affect communication (time pressure, patients per shift, hours worked per week). During observations of care interactions, they measured the use of verbal and non-verbal communications.

The only nurse variable that affected communication with patients was educational level – nurses with a higher level of education engaged in less small talk and banter with patients, and more structured interaction. More worrying, higher level nurses engaged in less non-verbal communication (including eye contact), showed more irritation and dominance, and were independently observed to be less involved in patient care. This was to some extent ameliorated by positive attitudes towards older people and years of experience. Patient characteristics had little impact on verbal or non-verbal communication, although long-term residents received a much greater level of instrumental touch. Time pressures in residential care appeared to limit talk about lifestyle and emotions which, as the authors observed, is important to patient well-being.

It is very unfortunate if education really does reduce care and compassion and this is an important issue for educators to address. We acknowledge the time pressures on staff, but suggest that it is often possible to use time more selectively and effectively for the benefit of older patients, for example, while undertaking routine assessments, observations and tasks.

Interpersonal skills

Interpersonal skills are essential for people to be able to engage in all aspects of life. Communication is often treated as synonymous with the use of language. But we only have to find ourselves in a foreign country where we don't speak the language to discover how relatively easy it is to get by with the use of non-verbal communication. Much can be learned from observing mothers interact with pre-verbal babies, or by watching children who do not share a common language develop friendship through play. It would appear that interpersonal skills are normally present or learned from a very young age. Some of this learning is taught by adults and the child reprimanded for breaches of etiquette. But most is learned informally by modelling (Chapter 5).

Many of the rules of social engagement are implicit and difficult to learn through formal teaching. Children who find it difficult to learn by observation, for example those with learning difficulties or autism, are disadvantaged and socially excluded because of their poor interpersonal skills. The inability to communicate effectively can lead to frustration and inappropriate or challenging behaviours. The lowering of inhibitions, associated with alcohol misuse or serious mental health problems, can cause severe embarrassment or lead to violent attack. In all situations, poor social skills have the potential to lead to social isolation, which in turn contributes to mental health problems.

Key elements of interpersonal skills include:

- *Facial expression.* This indicates the emotional state of the individual, for example, joy, distress, fear are all normally discernible. Absence of facial expression as happens early in Parkinson's disease, may be interpreted as disinterest or may generate discomfort because the observer is unable to 'read' the individual's emotions. The presence of facial tics is disconcerting not just because they appear odd but because they can mask expression.
- *Reciprocity.* One of the earliest signs of language in children is the ability to take turns, as in a conversation. The small baby watches the mother's face intently while she talks, and then responds by mouthing similar sounds. In adult conversation, turn-taking signals interest and engagement, as opposed to self-absorption or disinterest.
- *Body posture and gesture.* These can signal a variety of intentions. For example, Caris-Verhallen *et al.* (1999) noted that leaning forward signals interest and engagement. A colleague recently needed to remind a student, who was preparing to interview older people, that sitting with arms folded did not signal empathy or interest.
- *Personal, social and public space.* It is normally perceived as uncomfortable or threatening when others get too close. Relatives and close friends are normally allowed closer than strangers. But it is important to recognize that personal space is largely determined by cultural rules of acceptability. Therefore people from other cultures may unwittingly breach social etiquette. Nurses are normally permitted to breach personal space in order to carry out necessary tasks, though it is common for older people with dementia to protest at being approached by 'strangers'. Similarly those under the influence of drugs or alcohol may 'misread' these approaches as a sexual advance or threat.
- *Eye contact.* Avoiding eye contact may be a result of uncertainty or low self-esteem, but may be interpreted as 'shifty'. Fixed eye contact is uncomfortable or threatening. Non-friendly eye contact is seen in many cultures and subcultures as a mark of disrespect, or act of aggression, which can provoke attack. Occasional eye contact, on the other hand, is usually acceptable and signals interest and engagement.

Many people who breach the rules of social etiquette are unaware they are doing this. People with Asperger syndrome have particular difficulties with communication and psychologists are working to develop innovative 'virtual reality' techniques to improve these (Parsons *et al.* 2000). They have also tried to develop programmes to assist with orientation into different cultures (Bhawuk and Brislin 2000). Care workers need to be able to identify reasons for, and respond appropriately to, inappropriate behaviours in order to avoid misunderstandings, conflict or injury.

Managing conflict

Conflict is an inevitable consequence of life. It is caused by competition for scarce resources, competing ideologies, and stereotypes and prejudice. Conflict can easily progress from feelings of threat to annoyance to aggression or violence. Violence by patients or their caregivers against care staff has increased substantially during the last decade. The most important way of avoiding conflict is to try to understand the perspective or point of view of the other party. If someone comes to a hospital or clinic, they are normally trying to communicate a need. When someone complains or gets annoyed it is usually because they feel that their needs have not been recognized or adequately responded to.

The natural response to a complaint or criticism is to defend one's position and offer an explanation. But a defensive response is usually interpreted as counter-attack and serves to intensify feelings of annoyance. It is necessary first to listen to the individual and acknowledge their needs. An apology for any annoyance or distress caused to an individual is useful in building or maintaining good interpersonal relationships. Patient services managers have recently become rather good at using this approach to deal with patient complaints.

Janice, in her new role as health care assistant, gave a patient some advice. The staff nurse told Janice off because it was for trained staff to deal with this. Janice believed that she was acting in the patient's best interest and responded defensively. This led to bad feeling between the two members of staff, each of whom saw themselves as the victim of the other's persecution.

This type of situation is easily resolved if one of the players stops defending their position and apologizes. The other, not wishing to be pushed into the role of persecutor by refusing to accept an apology, will normally respond in the role of rescuer by saying 'that's all right' or 'don't worry about it' or 'it wasn't really your fault'.

Janice acknowledged that she should have checked with the staff nurse and apologized. The staff nurse told Janice that she was only doing her best for the patient and to think no more about it.

Knowledge of these rules of engagement can help in all sorts of potentially confrontational situations. People with aggressive tendencies tend to expect and perceive hostility in others. When confronted with people who appear angry or upset, remember to act as rescuer and not as victim:

- Acknowledge, verbally, that you have seen that they are angry/upset. Look concerned.
- Ask them what they are angry/upset about. Look interested.
- Acknowledge their right to feel angry/upset in the situation as they perceive it (this is not the same as admitting responsibility). Look sympathetic.
- Try to negotiate a solution. Look sincere.
- The rules of reciprocity normally oblige the angry/upset party to listen to the reasons why you might have difficulty meeting their demands.

Rules of reciprocity and conventions of communication break down under the influence of alcohol or drugs, particularly when people are aroused because of fear or anxiety. In these situations, it is necessary to avoid any verbal or non-verbal behaviour, such as eye contact or dominant posture that might be interpreted, rightly or otherwise, as unsympathetic or confrontational. Similarly, touch can provoke attack if seen as an attempt to dominate or control. Hence, those working in situations where there is a high risk of attack, such as mental health units or accident and emergency departments, should receive special training in conflict avoidance and management. The following exercise was developed in response to students' complaints that they were frequently attacked or had objects thrown at them by older patients on general wards who were suffering from dementia.

The exercise is best undertaken in the skills laboratory and involves role play. The individual who will learn most is the one taking the part of the patient, so it is a good idea to take this role in turns. The parts are as follows.

Scene 1

- The patient in bed is a fiercely independent old person who has been admitted reluctantly from home. They have soiled the bed and are attempting to conceal it from the nurse by wrapping the faeces in a tissue.
- The 'nurse' locates the source of the smell and signals obviously to her colleague as s/he approaches the patient, saying loudly that they will need to clean them up; starts to tug at the bedclothes.
- The patient responds to the encounter and is then asked to report how it made them feel.

Scene 2

- Once the 'patient' has discussed how this made them feel, a similar scene is enacted using a much more sympathetic and discrete approach, starting with a conversation about how the patient feels about being in hospital and leading later to the issue of the soiled bed.

None of the students who took part in this exercise wanted to play the part of the 'nasty nurse', although all said that they had seen this type of incident in practice! The 'patients' instinctively clutched at the bedclothes, said that they felt humiliated and had a strong urge to hit the 'nasty nurse'. People with dementia who have previously experienced disrespectful treatment may subsequently react against the sight of a uniform. Attempts to gain their cooperation may be interpreted as further violations of their personal space or autonomy.

Adhering to culturally accepted rules of social etiquette by attempting to establish a relationship before engaging in close contact is particularly important in these circumstances. Violations are likely to have repercussions for future interactions with other care staff, no matter how nice. The skills of conflict avoidance and resolution are particularly important in mental health settings, where patients often lack emotional control. These problems led Cowin *et al.* (2003) to produce a research-based de-escalation kit, with computer disk and poster, free of charge.

Group interaction

Irving Janis, a psychologist famous for his work on stress, was prompted by a major international incident to investigate group decision-making in more depth. The incident was the American decision, in 1961, to support the unsuccessful invasion of Cuba in what became known as 'The Bay of Pigs' disaster. This prompted the Cuban missile crisis of 1962 and led the American president, Kennedy, to admit that a dreadful mistake had been made by his highly expert group of advisers. But how did this happen and why? Janis (1982) analysed the group processes involved and proposed that they had been victims of '**groupthink**'. Some of the main symptoms of groupthink are identified below.

* *Illusions of invulnerability*. Positions of power can lead people to believe that they cannot be proved wrong.
* *Collective rationalization*. Unrealistic assessments are supported by 'rational' arguments and used to convince other group members.
* *Belief in the inherent morality of the group*. This reflects the belief that the group is in the right and good must triumph.
* *Stereotypes of out-groups*. Outsiders are often automatically classified as 'bad guys' or enemies who must therefore be in the wrong.
* *Direct pressure on dissenters*. Dissenters are silenced and this discourages critical evaluation. Certain group members may take the initiative to reduce dissent by persuasion or coercion, and foster an illusion of unanimity. Silence is interpreted as support.

Groupthink leads to biased and often frankly wrong decisions that are not based on the best available evidence. It is wise to be aware of these effects when contributing to or developing a team charged with a specific task. Work on group or team composition suggests that groups which include a mixture of individuals with different skills and viewpoints are probably more effective in reaching an informed decision. 'Heterogeneous' groups are less likely to succumb to groupthink. Group size is an important consideration. It is rare for groups exceeding 12 to be effective, while a group of 5 or 6 people facilitates the active participation of each member. The chairperson plays an important and impartial role in encouraging each member to voice their opinions, and encourage the debate of any doubts.

These principles underpin developments in interprofessional learning and problem-based learning.

The potentially divisive nature of social groupings, in terms of inter-group discrimination and prejudice, was demonstrated by Tajfel (1982). Tajfel's work suggests that members of a social group generally work towards maximizing profits or rewards for members of their own group (the in-group), often at the expense of other groups (the out-group) (see also Chapter 2). Illustrations of this are to be found in battles between special-ities for scarce resources within health and social services. Within health care, examples of in-group/out-group conflict have been found in the rela-tionships between different professional groups, hospital and community, private and public services or between similar units in different localities. This can have a serious effect on multi-professional teamworking.

Anna had the opportunity to sit in on multi-professional case conferences held regularly to plan treatment and care for patients in an elderly care unit. It soon became clear that the group was not operating effectively. For example, the medical consultant persistently arrived late, put forward his point of view, and then left. Another group member always selected a higher chair than the others and tried to direct decisions. Eventually, a senior nurse broached this with other members and found that nobody was satisfied with the meetings or the quality of the decisions reached. Group members identified that the room was too small, the furniture inappropriate to facilitate sharing and decisions were not fully agreed and not implemented. As a result of this investigation, a larger and more comfortable meeting room was found and a set of ground rules agreed. These included all professionals dedicating time to attend, having a rotating chairperson, a short presentation by the lead professional, limited time for discussion, and an agreed plan of action with named persons responsible for implementation.

Multi-professional teamworking is generally recognized as central to good patient/client-centred care, but brings with it the potential for con-flict. Effective interprofessional teamwork depends on having an agreed goal. Observations of meetings at various levels in health care suggest that representatives of different professions and services are often good at voi-cing what they want to do, but not always clear about what they wish to achieve. Failure to agree a common goal leads to disputes, confusion and disillusionment. At this point weaker contributors normally give in to the ideas of stronger members, even though these are not necessarily the best. Sharing an agreed goal helps to keep group activity focused and reduces sources of disagreement. The ability to achieve this depends on effective leadership.

Leadership styles

Just as the rise of Hitler and the aftermath of Hitler's Germany stimulated Stanley Milgram's work on obedience, so it stimulated Kurt Lewin to study the issue of leadership. Lewin had escaped from Nazi Germany before the war and initiated a series of studies with colleagues in America into the effects of authoritarian, democratic and laissez-faire leadership styles. These styles of leadership are similar to the classification used to describe parenting styles (Chapter 3). Findings from these experiments revealed the following:

- *Democratic leadership* encourages participation, engenders a sense of ownership and commitment within the group and generally leads to higher morale, friendliness, cooperation and productivity. Democratic leaders facilitate change while recognizing resistance and seeking to work with dissenters.
- *Authoritarian leadership* is based upon coercion and is generally associated with lower morale among the group or workforce. It can be useful in order to achieve an important task quickly, but may place undue stress upon some members of the group. Authoritarian leaders order and direct change, but are likely to encounter covert, if not overt, resistance.

Most people prefer to work with strong but democratic leadership. Although psychological research has identified characteristics of good leaders, leadership also involves skills and techniques that do not come automatically. Therefore, management training is essential in the preparation of those who are appointed to take on leadership roles within health and social care services, particularly at a time of rapid change. One of the main challenges for leaders of these organizations is to break down barriers between different professional groups, promote interprofessional working and be prepared to work with representatives of patient and other voluntary organizations to ensure that services meet the needs of those they serve in the most efficient and effective way.

Summary of key points

- Persuasion can be enhanced by paying attention to particular features of the message sender, the nature of the message, characteristics of the target audience and immediacy of action or commitment to action.
- Obedience to authority figures and the desire to conform may occur without awareness, and can easily lead to unprofessional, unethical or undesirable practice.
- Helping and caring attitudes and responses are more easily elicited by those who are judged attractive or deserving.
- Non-verbal behaviour is an important source of communication in health care.

- Complaints and conflict may be diffused by listening to, understanding, responding appropriately to and acknowledging the other person's point of view.
- The creation of homogeneous groups, strong group identities and poorly determined goals can lead to inter-group conflict, poor decisions and poor interprofessional working.

Exercise

See after Chapter 10.

Further reading

Brehm, S.S., Kassin, S.M. and Fein, S. (2005) *Social Psychology*, 6th edn. Boston, MA: Houghton Mifflin.

Cowin, L., Davies, R., Estall, G., Fitzerald, M. and Hoot, S. (2003) De-escallating aggression and violence in the mental health setting, *International Journal of Mental Health Nursing*, 12(1): 64

Myers, D.G. (2002) *Social Psychology*, 7th edn. Maidenhead: McGraw-Hill.

Taylor, S.E., Peplau, L.A. and Sears, D.O. (2006) *Social Psychology*, 12th edn. London: Pearson.

STRESS AND COPING

- **What is meant by the term 'stress'?**
- **How can we understand stress and coping?**
- **What is the relationship between physiological and psychological responses to stress?**
- **Are there individual differences in responses to stress?**
- **What are the important characteristics of stressful situations?**
- **What do we mean by 'social support'?**
- **How does stress influence health and illness?**
- **How can professional carers help themselves and others to deal with stress?**

Introduction

It seems nowadays that everyone suffers from stress. Briner (1994) argued that in the late twentieth century, stress had become a modern myth, similar to demons and witches of the middle ages or 'nerves' in the 1950s. So what exactly does this mean? There are many common symptoms that could be indicative of stress:

- *Emotional*
  - Feeling upset and crying more than usual
  - Feeling irritable and behaving unreasonably
  - Losing your sense of humour
  - Unreasonable fears
- *Cognitive*
  - Feeling a failure
  - Worrying a lot
  - Difficulty in making decisions
  - Not wanting to be bothered
- *Behavioural*
  - Not eating *or* eating too much
  - Taking time off for minor illnesses
  - Using alcohol, tobacco or other substances to feel better or forget problems
  - Withdrawing from usual activities

- *Physiological*
  - Having difficulties sleeping
  - Indigestion or nausea
  - Panic attacks
  - Headaches and muscle tension

We all experience some of these symptoms some of the time but we are at risk of developing a stress-related illness if we experience quite a few of them a lot of the time. Stress can have important consequences for care professionals and their clients or patients. A common problem faced by nurses is to distinguish the symptoms of stress from those of mental or physical illnesses, since stress can worsen or mask the symptoms of disease. In health and social care staff, stress can lead to **'burnout'**. In both groups it can induce behaviours such as smoking that increase health risk. Therefore stress and coping are important concepts in health and social care.

Definitions of stress

There are many definitions of stress in the literature. This is because stress is not a fact, but a concept that depends on a theoretical explanation. One of the simplest and most commonly used definitions of stress reflects the notion of 'imbalance': 'Stress refers to an imbalance between a perceived demand and the perceived ability of the individual to respond to it' (McGrath 1970: 17).

Theories of stress assume that there is:

- a stressor that poses a demand, challenge or threat;
- an awareness or perception of the stressor;
- a response that includes emotional, physiological, cognitive and behavioural changes.

Some people find a situation stressful because it is unfamiliar and they don't know how to respond. Others hardly notice the same situation because it is well known to them and they respond without having to give it much thought.

When Anna started her degree course at university, she had little idea what was expected of her and felt very anxious. She envied third year students who seemed so confident. At that early stage of her training, it would have been easy to give up and work in a shop. But she stayed and by her second year had a much better idea of what was expected. By this time, she was enjoying the challenges of nursing. The things that had bothered her so much in her first year now seemed routine, and she felt much more relaxed and confident.

What is a stressor?

A stressor normally involves a change that has the potential to 'tax or exceed the adaptive resources of an individual or social system' (Lazarus 1966: 27) and is therefore seen as a threat to survival, quality of life or well-being. The threat may be physical, psychological, environmental or social. A physical threat involves a bodily change such as that caused by trauma, illness or age. A psychological threat is one that interrupts or prevents progress towards the achievement of an important goal (Monat and Lazarus 1991) or threatens self-esteem (Chapter 2). Environmental and social threats include hassles at work and at home, as well as life-changing events and losses. We explore these types of situation later in this chapter.

Stressors command attention and action, but not all stressors are bad for us. Dealing successfully with them enhances our self-esteem, develops our skills, prepares us to deal with future challenges and boosts our immune systems. But what is seen as a challenge by one person may be very stressful for another. The transactional model of stress and coping is the only theoretical model that takes full account of this.

The transactional model of stress and coping

The transactional model of stress was proposed by Richard Lazarus in the 1960s and later developed with Susan Folkman into the most widely accepted psychological theory of stress and coping. Previous models failed to explain why some individuals find certain situations stressful while others do not. For example, the behaviourist view assumed that there was a direct relationship between the situational demand (the stressor) and the emotional and behavioural stress response. But this is clearly not the case since people can respond quite differently to similar situations. Using a psychodynamic framework, stress-related emotions such as anxiety and depression might be attributed to poor attachment relationships in early life (Chapter 3), but this fails to recognize the stress-provoking character-istics of certain events or situations. Lazarus bridged the gap by proposing that 'cognitive appraisal' acts as a mediator between the situational demand and the individual response. This is summarized in Figure 8.1. The concepts contained in Figure 8.1 are considered in the following sections, starting with the appraisal and coping processes.

Cognitive appraisal

Appraisal is part of the process of perception by which the individual determines if the situation poses a threat or challenge, and decides what, if anything, to do about it. Appraisal is not necessarily a conscious pro-cess, since we respond automatically to a wide range of familiar situations. But Lazarus argued that differences in the ways individuals appraise an

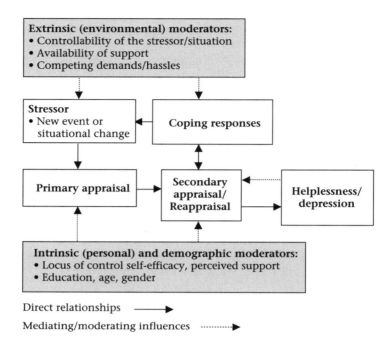

Direct relationships ———▶

Mediating/moderating influences ┈┈┈┈▶

Figure 8.1 Overview of relationships between stress, appraisal and coping (based on Lazarus and Folkman 1984)

event or situation help to explain differences in the ways they respond to it. For example, people who experience the same symptoms of illness can react in quite different ways.

- one person may view the symptoms as unimportant;
- another may view them as important but manageable;
- yet another may view the same symptoms as catastrophic.

Take the example of three people with arthritis:

- the first person has learned to ignore it and get on with life;
- the second has made some adaptations to their lifestyle and learned to manage it using a combination of prescribed medications, complementary therapies and exercise;
- the third finds the pain and limitation totally unacceptable and keeps going to the doctor in the hope of finding a cure, or may even decide that life is not worth living.

Each of these three people may be described as having different ways of appraising and coping with arthritis. A similar range of responses can apply in any type of situation, be it a medical condition, social problem, the task of caring for a family member, dealing with death and dying, or whatever.

Lazarus (1966) was the first theorist to identify thought processes (appraisals) as mediators between the situational demand or threat (the stressor) and the emotional and behavioural coping response. Lazarus and Averill (1972: 243) proposed a three-stage model of appraisal.

1 **Primary appraisal** is the initial response to a demand, situation or event, whereby the individual determines if it represents a threat. There are three possible outcomes to primary appraisal:
   - the situation is disregarded as irrelevant or unimportant
   - it is evaluated as a challenge likely to have a positive outcome if appropriate action is taken
   - it is identified as a potential threat to physical or mental well-being
2 **Secondary appraisal** refers to the appraisal of coping alternatives, during which the individual decides what, if anything, to do about the perceived threat. Very broadly, the behavioural choices available reflect the three dimensions of locus of control (Chapter 5) and include:
   - take personal action to deal with the situation (internal or personal control)
   - seek help from others to deal with the situation (external 'powerful other' control)
   - do nothing/ignore it/hope it will go away (external 'chance' control)
3 *Reappraisal* then takes place. This is where the individual reviews the outcome of their coping response and, where necessary, considers alternative options.

The outcome of primary appraisal is determined largely by previous experiences. Those who have previously dealt successfully with similar demands are more likely to perceive the situation as a challenge rather than a threat. Those who have no experience of similar situations, and have little information about what is happening, are likely to experience uncertainty and anxiety. Those who have had difficulties coping with similar previous situations, or perceive that they lack the resources to deal with it, are likely to perceive the situation as a threat and react with fear, anxiety or even a sense of hopelessness.

Secondary appraisal and reappraisal are likely to be influenced by the individual's knowledge about the controllability of the situation, their beliefs about their own responsibility, or that of others, for the actions necessary to achieve a successful outcome (their locus of control) and their confidence in using relevant practical and problem-solving skills (their sense of self-efficacy). If the individual has not encountered similar situations before, they are less likely to experience stress if they have information about the best way to deal with the situation or have help available to achieve a successful outcome. Care professionals can do much to assist people facing new or difficult situations by showing them the best ways to deal with them and supporting them until they feel confident.

When Mark was admitted to hospital for the first time, he was very anxious because he didn't know what to expect or what was expected of him. But he was given an information sheet telling him what he needed to take with him, what to expect and when visiting hours were. This did much to reduce his anxiety. The helpful manner in which he was greeted on the ward, shown round, introduced to other patients and informed about what would happen next was very reassuring. As a result, his level of stress following admission was quite low.

Coping

The outcome of the appraisal process is referred to as the coping response. Most people develop strategies for dealing with certain types of situation. A number of researchers agree that there are two contrasting types of coping strategy, though they have given them different names.

- Rosenstiel and Keefe (1983) refer to **active versus passive coping**. Active coping refers to taking direct action to deal with the problem. Passive coping refers to doing nothing or relying on others to deal with it for them.
- Roth and Cohen (1986) refer to *approach versus avoidant coping*. Approach coping refers to confronting reality and dealing with problems. Avoidance coping refers to ignoring the situation or avoiding the likely consequences.
- Folkman and Lazarus (1985) refer to **problem-focused coping** *versus* **emotion-focused coping**. Problem-focused coping is an active or approach strategy in which the individual actively seeks ways to mitigate or deal with a perceived threat. Emotion-focused coping is used to reduce the feeling of distress or fear associated with the perceived threat. This often involves avoiding having to think about or face up to it or deal with the demand or threat, or leaving it to others to deal with.

The best recognized of these definitions is that of Folkman and Lazarus, who drew on psychoanalytic theory to propose that emotion-focused coping (including the use of social support) is aimed primarily at managing feelings of anxiety, whereas problem-focused strategies are directed at dealing with the problem. Research findings from a variety of contexts suggest that active or problem-focused strategies are generally related to better psychological adjustment and health outcomes than passive emotion-focused strategies, provided the situation is potentially controllable and the individual has adequate coping resources available. By coping resources, we include personal skills, social supports and financial means. Avoiding thinking about or facing up to problems is generally associated with negative or poor outcomes.

Jo found it difficult to settle down to work after he left home. He eventually met up with Sasha who already had a small child, Lee, and moved in with her. Sasha's mother and father had rejected her when she became pregnant with Lee and life was lonely as a single mother. Sasha is now pregnant by Jo and they live on Sasha's social security benefits. Jo is a

> pleasant and caring young man who means well and likes having a ready-made family. But he has no idea about household management and operates by crisis management. They have recently spent a lot on new baby equipment and things to brighten up the flat. Jo knows the debts are mounting up, but hides the bills from Sasha to stop her from worrying.

Jo is using emotion-focused, avoidant coping strategies, trying to preserve an immediate sense of well-being by ignoring problems and avoiding the inevitable long-term consequences. Stress and coping is a dynamic process. The way people cope with one problem can affect future demands on their lives. For example, the more Jo ignores their financial problems, the more the problems mount up and the more difficult it becomes to find a solution.

The concepts of problem-focused and emotion-focused coping are widely applied in stress research as a convenient classification. However, Folkman and Lazarus (1985, 2003) actually described a range of common coping strategies which, apart from the last two, cannot automatically be labelled as problem-focused or emotion-focused. They include:

- *confrontational coping*: aggressive efforts to alter the situation which suggests some degree of hostility that could lead to labelling as a 'difficult' client or patient (Chapter 2);
- *distancing*: cognitive efforts to detach oneself and to minimize the significance of the situation;
- *seeking social support*: efforts to seek informational and emotional support as well as practical help;
- *escape-avoidance*: wishful thinking and behavioural efforts to escape or avoid the problem;
- *problem solving*: deliberate problem-focused efforts to alter the situation, coupled with an analytic approach to solving the problem.

Generally speaking, dealing with a problem by acknowledging it and trying to resolve it is better than ignoring it, but the outcome depends on whether or not the situation is within the control of the individual and those (if any) who provide support. A mismatch between the type of stressor and the coping strategy used can actually induce stress (Park *et al.* 2001). For example, Merritt *et al.* (2004) presented experimental data to suggest that those who put a lot of effort into coping without the financial means or social resources to achieve success, may be at greater risk of stress-induced cardiovascular disease.

Review of the transactional model of stress

The Lazarus and Folkman approach to stress and coping has become popular because it addresses cognitive and behavioural components of coping.

It was adapted for nursing by Benner and Wrubel (1989), who provided a detailed analysis of the relationship between stress, coping and caring in different contexts. It is now the main theory of stress and coping in health psychology, reflecting the current emphasis on social cognition. However, below there are a number of issues that we will consider in more depth.

- The transactional model initially gave little consideration to the nature of the stressor. More recently, Folkman and colleagues (Park *et al.* 2001) have focused on the importance of controllability (see later in this chapter).
- Folkman and Lazarus (1985) originally included social support within the concept of emotion-focused coping. However, recent analyses confirm that social support needs to be treated as a separate dimension of coping (Chesney *et al.* 2006).
- It may be unwise to treat social support as a single entity. Different types of social support (informational, emotional and practical) serve different functions and are associated with different outcomes, some positive, some negative. They therefore deserve to be treated separately.
- Some emotion-focused coping strategies, such as smoking and drinking, help to relieve anxiety, but pose significant risks to long term health and can contribute to stress-related illness. Therefore the short and long term outcomes of stress may be different.

In the following sections, we explore these issues in greater depth, starting with the relationship between stress and illness.

Stress and stress-related illness (psychoneuroimmunology)

Stress is a physical as well as a psychological phenomenon. For example we experience anxiety as both a physical and a mental state and it is sometimes difficult to distinguish the symptoms of anxiety (e.g. heart racing, nausea, muscle pain) from those of physical illness. Furthermore, stress really can make us ill. Therefore it is important to have some understanding of the physiology of stress.

When faced with a sudden or new demand or threat, there is an immediate arousal of the autonomic nervous system (alarm response, Selye 1956) and release of adrenaline and endorphins. This prepares the body for action and was described by Cannon in the early twentieth century as the 'fight or flight' response. It causes the release of glucose stored in the liver in readiness for muscular activity; increases cardiovascular activity as indicated by increases in heart rate and blood pressure; increases the viscosity of the blood, re-routing of blood from the digestive organs and skin to the brain and muscles; increases the rate and depth of breathing and widens the pupils of the eyes. If the individual is unable to address the demand or threat using their usual coping strategies (the timescale is variable), corticoids are released into the bloodstream while coping attempts continue. Corticosteroids provide energy for adaptive reactions and stimulate the body's natural defence systems (Selye 1956 termed this physiological response the stage of resistance). Gradually over time, these resistance mechanisms decline in strength and stress-related illness may occur (Selye termed this the stage of exhaustion). Selye described how, finally, resistance to stress declines rapidly, resulting in a state of collapse or even death, particularly in those whose immune system is compromised. Below, we have illustrated this process, linking the psychological coping tasks with physiological responses.

When Mark was diagnosed as having Type 2 diabetes, he was initially quite shocked. He immediately experienced physical sensations (heart racing, sweating). His first thoughts were of the threats to his health, his lifestyle and sense of identity. Over the next few weeks, he learned to develop the knowledge and skills to deal with his diabetes with support from Janice. He also needed to adapt his diet, cut down on his drinking and change other aspects of lifestyle. All of this took time, during which corticoids were released and Mark oscillated between optimism and frustration.

Long-term outcomes
If Mark finds effective ways of controlling the diabetes and adapting to his changed circumstances, his sense of well-being will be restored and **homeostasis** re-established.

OR

If Mark is unable to find effective ways of coping with his life or his diabetes, he may experience a state of helplessness and hopelessness (chronic anxiety and depression). His diabetes may become uncontrolled, partly due to his behaviour and partly due to the onset of Selye's stage of exhaustion. He will be at increased risk of other stress-related illnesses. If faced with a life-threatening illness, his body systems are more prone to collapse and death could occur.

Long-term exposure to stress appears to lead to changes in the homeostatic mechanisms that regulate heart rate and blood pressure, leading to hypertension, cardiovascular disease and other stress-related illnesses. Recent research has focused on the role of the immune system, which is influenced by the endocrine system and release of corticoids. Through this mechanism, stress has been shown to affect a number of important aspects of health, including:

- rate of wound healing;
- susceptibility to infectious disease;
- development and progression of cancer;
- development and progression of autoimmune diseases;
- progression of HIV infection (Kiecolt-Glaser *et al.* 2002).

Kiecolt-Glaser and her colleagues have identified that immune function and stress-related illness might be influenced by the following mechanisms:

- physiological changes in the endocrine system, including the release of pituitary and adrenal hormones which affect the immune system in multiple ways;
- the effects of stress-related behaviours, including tobacco, alcohol and drug use, poor nutrition (e.g. comfort eating) and insufficient exercise;
- disruption of sleep pattern;
- anxiety and depression appear to be directly related to changes in immune response.

We have illustrated some of these associations in Figure 8.2.

Optimum functioning of the immune system is particularly important in babies whose immune function is yet to be fully developed, people with immune deficiency or other diseases where the immune system is compromised, and older people whose immune function has declined naturally with age (Kiecolt-Glaser *et al.* 2002). Therefore, stress reduction and management is particularly important in the care of these groups.

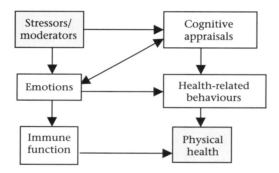

Figure 8.2 Predicted relationships between stress and physical health

Positive versus negative effects of stress

It is not uncommon to find stress referred to as potentially positive. Indeed, some laboratory experiments designed to test the effects of stress show that exposing people to demands such as mental arithmetic actually enhances immune function (e.g. see Peters *et al.* 1999). The reason is quite simple. Effortful coping strategies associated with overcoming challenge have been shown to be associated with positive emotions and enhanced immune function. In contrast, it is the sudden intense, or prolonged or repeated exposure to uncontrollable stressors, particularly in the presence of concurrent stressors and/or absence of adequate support that causes chronic anxiety and/or depression and compromises immune function. We give examples of the relationships between stress, immune function and stress-related illness in the following sections.

Mediators and moderators of stress and stress-related illness

Although we have previously argued that stress is determined by an individual's appraisal of events or situations, there are certain properties of events and situations that lead them to be appraised by the majority of people as stressful. The most important property is controllability, by which we refer to the extent to which it is humanly possible to determine or influence the outcome of an event or situation.

Perceived controllability

The concept of control has become increasingly important in research into stress and coping. Control refers to the achievement of important goals. It is affected by the achievability of desired goals and the availability of the resources (knowledge, skills, support, money) necessary to accomplish them. Not all situations are controllable, although most have some aspects that can be controlled, depending on the individual's willingness to compromise or shift their desired goals (see Chapter 3 on adult development). However, it is important to note that stress is associated with *perceived control* (the extent to which the individual *believes* the situation to be controllable) and not actual control.

Uncontrollability

This refers to situations where goals are unattainable or outcomes unlikely to be affected by human intervention, much the same as in learned helplessness (Chapter 5). In these situations, problem-focused coping strategies are of little use and stress may increase as a result of failure. A number of researchers have used certain chronic or terminal illnesses, experienced as either patient or caregiver, as examples of uncontrollable stressors because they are incurable and surrounded by a high degree of uncertainty, or the certainty of death. In such situations, it has been suggested that emotion-focused coping strategies may be more adaptive (Park *et al*. 2001). Faced with a life-limiting illness, it makes sense to focus on short-term or alternative goals that are achievable, such as recording one's life story or finishing a painting. But researchers have found that the denial or avoidance of reality, when used as a form of self-protection, is reported as consistently ineffective at alleviating distress (Wiebe and Korbel 2003). This may be because it as a barrier to communication and the giving and receiving of emotional support.

Sanders-Dewey *et al*. (2001) examined the use of coping strategies in individuals with Parkinson's disease and their caregivers. They found that emotion-focused coping strategies were associated with increased psychological distress for both patients and caregivers. Interestingly, they

> found that the use of problem-focused coping by the patient was
> associated with a higher level of distress in the caregiver. This may be
> because attempts by patients to manage their own condition conflict
> with caregivers' instincts to care and protect.

Perceived control and emotions

Positive emotions are generally associated with working towards achieving
desired goals and successfully addressing challenges. The experience of
gaining personal mastery over new or difficult situations leads to increased
self-confidence and self-esteem. For a long time psychologists have recognized personal mastery as an important source of personal satisfaction and
motivation (Walker 2001). As noted in Chapter 6, it appears that our cognitive processes normally have a positive bias towards perceptions of control
and optimism. Perhaps this helps to explain why most of us feel fairly
positive most of the time, even when faced with adversity.

Perceived uncontrollability leads to learned helplessness (Chapter 5),
which is an important cause of stress-related mental and physical illness. It
has cognitive and behavioural dimensions:

- perceived uncertainty: 'I don't understand what is happening';
- perceived unpredictability: 'I don't know what is going to happen';
- perceived uncontrollability: 'I don't know what to do' or 'there is nothing that can be done'.

Perceived uncertainty and unpredictability may be due to lack of effective
knowledge or skills, but may equally be caused by lack of adequate information on which to act successfully. They are associated with feelings of anxiety. Knowledge deficits may be reduced or eliminated by the provision of
appropriate   information   and   education   (informational   support).
Sometimes, uncertainty and perceived lack of control can be due to lack of
self-confidence and may respond to the provision of encouragement or
emotional support. The belief that there is nothing that can be done reflects
a state of hopelessness and may be associated with feelings of depression.

Because humans are social beings, there are two sources available to
achieve control: personal action or help from others. Figure 8.3 demonstrates the hypothetical relationship between perceived control, perceived
support and emotional state.

The following scenario illustrates and analyses what happens when
someone develops a persistent symptom or illness, in this case pain.

> Janice has developed back pain. With reference to Figure 8.3, the
> following analysis illustrates the relationship between Janice's control beliefs
> and her emotional outcomes, given different levels of personal control
> (self-management) and/or social support in the form of medical help.

- *High control, low support.* Janice successfully treats the pain without help using a combination of tablets and exercise. This strengthens her sense of self-efficacy and internal locus of control with respect to back pain.
- *Low control, high support.* Janice cannot relieve the pain herself, so she seeks advice from an osteopath who treats it successfully. She has no personal control over the pain, but is confident that she can depend on him to relieve it if it happens again. This reinforces external (powerful other) locus of control.
- *High control, high support.* As well as treating the pain, the osteopath gives Janice exercises to deal with future episodes of back pain. Janice now has confidence in two alternative sources of control (internal and external powerful other).
- *Uncertain control, uncertain support.* The backache fails to respond completely to treatment and the pain fluctuates so Janice searches for other sources of relief. In the meantime, she feels helpless and very anxious. This is typical of patients waiting for treatment and strengthens external (chance) locus of control.
- *Low control, low support.* If nothing Janice or anyone else does has any effect, she is left feeling hopeless and depressed.

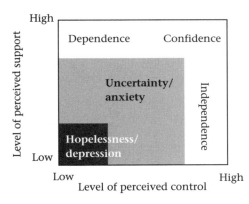

Figure 8.3 Interaction between control and support (Walker 2001)

The above analysis illustrates the relationship between perceived control, perceived support and emotional outcomes.

Ross and Mirowsky (1989: 214) conducted a large-scale American telephone survey. They asked people about their level of psychological distress, using a measure called the Center for Epidemiological Studies Depression Scale (CES-D) which includes items related to depression and anxiety. They asked some structured questions about the degree of

> control and level of support informants had in their lives. Their findings
> reflect exactly the pattern of response predicted in Figure 8.3.

Both theory and research support the prediction that perceived control
and perceived support complement each other in achieving desired outcomes and determining emotional response. Therefore, social support is an
important determinant of mental and physical health.

Uncontrollability and physical health

Learned helplessness (Chapter 5) is commonly used as a model for depression in stress research. For example, a learned helplessness experiment was
used to identify uncontrollability as a cause of gastric ulceration (Overmier
and Murison 2000). But it is now known that gastric ulceration is caused by
Helicobacter pylori infection. What the findings may actually suggest is
that a state of helplessness creates physiological and immune changes that
allow this type of pathogen to proliferate.

A number of researchers wishing to research the effects on immune function of chronic persistent (uncontrollable) stress have studied the caregivers
of older people with dementia. These are people who have been identified
as at particular risk of health problems including cardiovascular disease,
certain cancers, Type 2 diabetes, periodontal disease, arthritis, frailty and
decline (Kiecolt-Glaser *et al.* 2002).

> Vedhara *et al.* (2002) studied the caregivers of dementia patients and
> found that T-cell proliferation was impaired, NK cell numbers and activity
> were reduced, and there were elevations in herpes virus antibody titres
> (which explain increased susceptibility to shingles). A longitudinal study
> by Kiecolt-Glaser *et al.* (2003) indicated that health problems in this
> group are also mediated by the release of IL–6, a proinflammatory
> cytokine. Garand *et al.* (2002) demonstrated that a home-based
> intervention programme designed to improve coping strategies resulted
> in an immediate improvement in T-cell function among dementia
> caregivers.
>
> *Note: T-cells and NK (natural killer) cells are protective. Proinflammatory
> cytokines make disease worse. For a detailed but readable explanation, see
> Ader et al. (1995).*

There are many reasons why caregiving in this situation is so stressful.
These include the constant need for attention and caring demands, the
unpredictability and uncontrollability of the dementia sufferer's behaviour,
and the loss of emotional and practical support from the individual who

now requires help. These give rise to mixed feelings of anxiety, fear, guilt, shame, anger, loneliness, depression, similar to responses to bereavement loss (Chapter 6). Many caregivers are themselves approaching old age, so these stressors arise at a time when immune function is already somewhat compromised, meaning that they are particularly at risk of stress-related illness.

Gaining or promoting control

In controllable situations, the use of problem-focused coping strategies is associated with better outcomes since these are directed at resolving the problem. To ignore or avoid a demand or threat that requires direct action is not adaptive. For example, when faced with the appearance of a breast lump, ignoring it is likely to lead to a poor outcome. If the individual does not have the knowledge, skill or resources to deal effectively with a situation that is potentially controllable, it makes sense to seek expert help.

Situations such as chronic illness are often viewed as uncontrollable and can lead people to feel helpless. But a readjustment of goals or review of resources can give back some sense of control.

When Ted went to live with Janice and Mark, they recognized that he needed to retain some independence and feel useful in spite of his limitations (he has chronic heart disease). His real love had been growing vegetables in his garden, so they bought him a large greenhouse where he could grow tomatoes and strawberries. This gave him something to do and made him feel a useful member of the family. It gave him back a sense of control over his life and something to aim for.

It is clear that social support can be used to promote personal control or compensate for self care deficits in a variety of situations and is therefore an important mediator of stress.

Social support

Most of us live in families or other communities and form relationships with other people in a variety of different contexts. When faced with problems, we often share these with others and give and receive emotional comfort as well as practical advice and help. This is what we commonly refer to as 'social support'. There is now a large body of research that has identified social support as an important determinant of stress-related outcomes, including mental and physical illness. There are a number of different types of social support. Some have positive effects on health, while others can have negative effects.

- *Informational support.* This refers to the giving or receiving of information or advice that supports problem-focused coping and has been shown to have a positive effect on health outcomes. The advice given by a grandmother to a new mother about child care is one example. The information sheet given to a patient is another. Health and social care professionals and self-help groups are important sources of informational support with respect to health, illness and social problems (Chapter 9).
- *Emotional support.* Cobb (1976) described this as information that leads individuals to feel cared for, loved and valued. Emotional support provides reassurance and encouragement. It facilitates the individual's sense of self-confidence and self-esteem and is associated with positive health. It can be linked to secure attachment relationships (Chapter 3).
- *Instrumental support.* This refers to the giving of practical help to deal with problems, including financial support. It is essential at the beginning and often the end of the lifespan or where people are unable to look after themselves. It is beneficial so long as the help provided is essential and does not take over from tasks the individual could and should do for themselves. Practical help beyond this leads to dependence (see Chapter 10 on chronic pain).
- *Social affiliation/social network.* Social affiliation refers to a sense of belonging. It usually involves a system of mutual obligations and reciprocal informational, emotional and instrumental social support. A social network of family and friends normally provides this. Self-help groups can also provide it. Reciprocity is an important component of successful social networks.

People who are socially isolated seem to be more at risk of developing mental as well as physical health problems, leading to a vicious cycle of deprivation and stress.

Janssen *et al.* (2002) reviewed studies of stress, coping and attachment in people with an intellectual disability (*sic*). They reported evidence that intellectually disabled people were more vulnerable to stress and use less effective coping strategies. Studies of attachment indicated that people with intellectual disability are at risk of developing insecure or disorganized attachment. This may put them at risk for developing challenging behaviours, particularly when faced with stressful situations or life change.

Social support and health outcomes

Sephton *et al.* (2001) reported growing evidence of links between social support, stress, emotional state, endocrine and immune function. Social support has been shown to mediate the relationship between stressors and immune function. Emotional support appears to be the most important dimension responsible for this effect (Uchino *et al.* 1996). This explains why loss of a loved one is so often associated with physical illness. Bereavement loss not only has a direct emotional effect on the immune system, but it can deprive the individual of the person who previously provided the emotional support they now urgently need (see Carman 1997). Support groups offer important sources of all types of support, tailored to meet the needs of a particular group of people.

> Andersen *et al.* (2004) set up a clinical trial to see if a support group for women following surgery for breast cancer had any impact on their health and well-being. In total, 227 women attended one session a week for four months, completing questionnaires and giving blood samples before and after. Compared to a control group who received usual care, they showed significant improvements in perceived social support, less anxiety, better dietary habits, smoking reduction and stable or increased T-cell proliferation compared to T-cell decline in the control group.

Emotional support is essential for children in early life, which is why Bowlby (1969) identified attachment relationships as important (Chapter 3). Secure attachments have been shown to act as a buffer against stress (Fox and Card 1999). In addition, these early relationships may provide a template for future relationships. The lack of secure attachments reduces close social affiliations and networks in the long term, leaving people more susceptible to mental and physical stress-related illnesses throughout their lives.

Negative aspects of social support

Early research into social support tried to measure availability in terms of quantity. People were asked about other members of their household, whether they had neighbours and relatives living nearby and how many close friends they had. This proved to be of little value in understanding the relationship of social support to stress-related illness because a social network can have negative as well as positive influences. On the positive side, Hobfoll (1988) suggested that people with close social networks have people around them who recognize when they are under stress or are ill, and persuade them to consult a doctor, take a holiday or other appropriate form of coping action. He also proposed that effort put into maintaining a social network acts as a kind of insurance policy in case help is needed in the future.

On the negative side, a person's social network can provide a source of peer group pressure to engage in unhealthy lifestyles and influence whether or not they come into contact with possible disease-causing factors, as in the case of sexually transmitted diseases and HIV. Relationships that involve conflict or seek to undermine the individual can have deleterious effects on physical and mental health. There are also surprising negative effects from well-intentioned supportive actions.

> Ross and Mirowsky (1989) identified from their survey that, contrary to their predictions, the more people used talking to others as a strategy for coping with stressful situations, the more depressed they tended to be.

This suggests that talking aimed at grumbling or eliciting sympathy (gripe sessions) is not beneficial, probably because it is not problem-focused. Equally, too much instrumental support (practical help) has also been shown to lead to negative health outcomes because it can create passivity and dependence (see the example of chronic pain in Chapter 10). This suggests that control and support need to be considered together, in conjunction with the demands of the stressor. For example, support groups work well if they encourage and facilitate personal control, but not if they encourage people to focus on the awfulness of their situations.

The spiritual dimension of support

Spiritual support can offer a lifeline for those who feel helpless or hopeless including:

- those with depression;
- those unable to find meaning or purpose in their lives;
- those who lack an established network of social support;
- those faced with uncontrollable situations such as financial ruin, homelessness, relationship breakdown, abuse, terminal, chronic or life-threatening illness or other losses.

Spiritual or religious beliefs have been shown to be associated with increased psychological well-being and better health (Koenig and Cohen 2002). Spiritual support implies a special form of emotional support. It does not necessarily require formal religious affiliation, although participation in organized religion can provide additional sources of informational, emotional and instrumental support.

> Sephton et al. (2001) studied the impact of spiritual belief on immune function in women with stage IV metastatic breast carcinoma. They found that higher expression of spiritual belief was associated with higher levels of white blood cells, lymphocyte count, helper T-cells, cytotoxic T-cells and NK cells. Attendance at religious meetings was associated with higher lymphocyte count and immunity against infection.

There are a number of ways of explaining possible relationships between spirituality and health. In so doing, it is necessary to separate out spiritual faith from religious affiliation and religious activity. In western societies, belief is often separate from religious affiliation. Having a spiritual faith provides existential meaning and coherence (Levin 2003; see also Chapters 2 and 3). Activities, such as praying or reading religious texts, provide effortful coping strategies. Attendance at religious meetings provides access to a supportive social network that provides reassurance and help in times of need.

There is, however, some potential for psychological harm in those who expect protection in exchange for religious activity or affiliation. People are sometimes heard to say 'What have I done to deserve this' or 'Why is God punishing me like this?'. As with social support, the individual balance of positive and negative effects makes it more difficult to study the benefits of spirituality with any degree of certainty.

Other mediators and moderators of appraisal and coping

Demographic influences

Those who lack coping resources such as knowledge, skills, social support networks or money, are clearly disadvantaged when appraising and coping with many of life's demands. This explains why stress responses are likely to differ according to such variables as age, gender, education and social class, and provides an important link with sociology. As people grow older, they have a wider range of cognitive strategies they can draw on to compensate for declining physical strength. Younger people often perceive less danger while some actively seek out the challenge of dangerous activities, particularly in response to peer group pressure, thereby exposing themselves to increased health risks. Men and women are often exposed to different types of challenge or danger during their lifetimes, acquire different skills, and demonstrate different ways of coping, and may therefore respond differently. For example, it appears that women are more likely than men to seek and provide social support (see Matthews *et al.* 1999).

The 'Whitehall studies' (Griffin *et al.* 2002) were set up nearly four decades ago to explore stress over a long period of time in people of all grades working in the British Civil Service, from top administrators to those in the lowest paid jobs, including those facing the public in social benefits offices. Some of the findings are summarized below.

- A greater proportion of women than men were classed as depressed or anxious.
- Younger women and men were more likely to be depressed than working people who were older.
- Women reporting low control at home had over twice the risk of depression than women reporting high control, even after controlling for marital status, number of children and caregiving status.

- Low home control increased men's risk of depression.
- Men who were caregivers consistently had a significantly higher risk of depression and anxiety.

Mirowsky and Ross (2003) explained gender differences in psychological distress (anxiety and depression) by the degree of control women have over their lives in comparison to men, including the division of responsibility and labour within the home. Their work showed that in contrast to women, marriage seems particularly important for the mental health of men, probably because of the quality and security of the supportive relationship provided for men within a marital relationship.

People of different levels of educational attainment and job experience are likely to vary in the knowledge and skills they bring to different types of situation. Those with strong social networks of family and friends are more likely to have people available to provide advice and reassurance, compared to those who are socially isolated. Those who can afford to pay for assistance when they need it are clearly advantaged over those with no financial resources. All of these variables are likely to interact to determine the outcome. But it is certain that those with limited knowledge and skills, and who are socially isolated and poor, are least likely to cope successfully with the demands and challenges of life. This immediately places illiterate and homeless ex-prisoners at the top of the list of those at risk of mental and physical stress-related health problems.

Individual differences

It has long been recognized that many diseases associated with stress, including heart disease, are influenced by family history. Genetic susceptibility is likely to be an important factor (Marsland *et al.* 2002). However, some of this influence may be accounted for by family patterns of coping behaviour, passed on during childhood socialization.

Psychologists have also been interested to identify if there are any stable differences in personality or coping style that could account for differences in susceptibility to stress and stress-related illness. Early attempts to identify a stress-prone personality type generally met with failure. In the 1970s, Friedman and Rosenman (1974) proposed a 'Type A' behaviour pattern or 'coronary prone personality' that consisted of sense of time urgency, competitiveness and aggressiveness. In the 1980s, Temoshok (1987) proposed a Type C behaviour pattern (passivity, compliance and suppression of anger) which was identified as being associated with cancer proneness or poor survival rates. More recently, researchers have investigated the 'Big 5' personality characteristics (Chapter 2) as potential mediators of stress responses with little success. Research findings tend to prove inconsistent, largely because of the interaction between the individual's appraisals, their behaviour pattern and the demands of the situation. There is currently little evidence to support an association between these personality types and health outcomes.

Hardy personality

Kobasa (1979) identified certain 'hardy' personality characteristics as predictors of health, longevity and protection from stress-related illness. According to Kobasa, hardiness consists of three dimensions:

- *commitment*: active involvement in life activities;
- *control*: a belief in autonomy and the ability to influence life events
- *challenge*: a belief that change is normal and growth-enhancing.

These dimensions appear to reflect a combination of internal locus of control, optimism and sense of coherence (Antonovsky 1985). Several studies have confirmed that hardiness is associated with enhanced immune function (Dolbier *et al.* 2001). Nicholas (1993) found that those scoring high on hardy characteristics were more likely to engage in good self care behaviours and were therefore less susceptible to illness caused by smoking, alcohol, poor diet or lack of exercise. It has been suggested that they may be associated with greater job satisfaction and lower incidence of burnout for those working in caring professions. However, much is likely to depend on the extent to which the working environment supports those with these characteristics. For example, workers with 'hardy' personality characteristics may be more likely to become frustrated and disillusioned when faced with lack of autonomy, adequate resources and managerial barriers in the workplace.

Optimism, pessimism and negative affectivity

Researchers have investigated optimism and pessimism as traits likely to be associated with responses to stress. A number of studies suggest that optimists have better psychological adjustment and immune responses to stressful life events than pessimists.

Brissette *et al.* (2002) suggested that optimists use more effective coping strategies and have more supportive social networks and this is why optimists are usually found to be less prone to stress (though it is difficult to distinguish between cause and effect.) Cohen *et al.* (1999) compared the immune responses of optimists and pessimists to acute and chronic stressors. They found that optimists had better immune function following acute stress, whereas pessimists showed no effect. But in situations of persistent high stress, optimists showed more immune depression than pessimists.

Optimists may be more optimistic because they are better at dealing with situations and gain most positive feedback. Their success enables them to view demands as challenges and put more effort into achieving mastery. However, when faced with uncontrollable stressors, optimists experience a stronger sense of helplessness and failure, whereas pessimists get what they expect. Although optimism and pessimism are somewhat stable over time, they reflect expectations that can change in the light of experience.

Negative affectivity refers to a disposition to experience aversive mood states, including anger, contempt, disgust, guilt, fear and nervousness, which are often present in anxiety and depression. Some researchers are using this as a marker for stress and studying its relationship to stress-related symptoms. One of the main problems, however, is to identify if these feelings represent cause or effect. For example, they may represent a particular sensitivity to external demands, or a mood disposition that regulates responses in all or particular types of situation, or they may generate behaviours that create stress (Spector *et al.* 2000). The matter is unresolved and illustrates some of the complexities involved in stress research.

Hostility

The concept of suppressed hostility or anger has generated a lot of research in the field of hypertension and cardiovascular disease. It is based on the notion that the inability to express frustration and anger leads to pent up feelings that raise blood pressure. Hostility and anger are also associated with depression, and particularly with increased depression and health risk in men. Kivimäki *et al.* (2003) suggest that this is because anger is associated with the failure to gain control, and may also reflect a lower ability to benefit from social support. These issues led Bishop *et al.* (2005) to develop and test a programme of psychosocial skills training for men undergoing coronary artery bypass graft surgery, with encouraging outcomes in terms of lowering depression and blood pressure reactivity.

Locus of control

Locus of control (Chapter 5) refers to an individual's beliefs about who or what is responsible for what happens to them – self, others or chance. It is important to note that locus of control refers to patterns of belief that may be different in different situations and are amenable to change over time. As was seen earlier in this chapter, control beliefs may guide the individual's use of coping strategies. For example, external chance locus of control is more likely to be associated with emotion-focused coping strategies and inaction. Because of the interaction between the person and the situation, there are no clear evidence-based links between locus of control, stress and health.

Sense of coherence

Antonovsky (1985) proposed 'sense of coherence' as a key predictor of long-term mental and physical health. It means seeing the world as rational, predictable, controllable and meaningful. It includes the belief that daily activities give pleasure and anticipating that life in future will be full of meaning and purpose (Bowling 2004). Sense of coherence has been shown to be associated with successful ageing and with a range of positive health consequences including immune function and pain tolerance. Stressful life events, illnesses or losses disrupt an individual's biographical coherence (Chapters 2 and 3) and narrative therapy may offer a way of strengthening sense of coherence (Chapter 6).

Review of individual differences as mediators of stress

There is no doubt that different people have unique outlooks on life and develop different responses to certain types of situation throughout their lives, starting in childhood. There is little evidence that these remain fixed throughout the lifespan or that they apply across all situations (with the possible exception of those with severe depression). Attempts to measure the effects of personality types on stress-related outcomes have generally met with failure, largely because of the complex interactions between all of the personal and situational variables. It is nevertheless helpful for care professionals to focus on the fit between the individual's beliefs and the demands of the situation they are facing, and to try, where possible, to help to reduce discrepancies.

Stress in different contexts

Illness and hospitalization

When people are ill, their immune systems are often compromised or under strain. It is therefore particularly important to help them find ways of reducing uncertainty and unpredictability, enhance personal control, and provide appropriate informational, emotional and instrumental support. Information-giving and patient education are essential to reduce uncertainty and unpredictability, and increase controllability in health care settings. Even when problems seem overwhelming, health care professionals can help patients to identify aspects of their situation that they can control. For example, when someone has developed a chronic illness or disability, they need time to mourn their loss of health and identify short-term achievable goals.

Janice encountered Mike, aged 32, in the outpatient department. He had recently had bilateral hip replacements, necessitated by a congenital bone deformity. Although the operations were successful, he complained of pain 'everywhere' and appeared depressed. Mike explained he had always been very fit, but after his hip operations he watched old ladies getting up and going home while he could hardly move. This made him feel helpless and demoralized. At this visit, the pain consultant suggested a short-term goal of improving his physical fitness. In addition to helping him mobilize, exercise would help him to regain cardiovascular fitness and increase the circulation of endorphins to help reduce the pain. At his three month appointment, Mike reported that the pain was now controllable and he was feeling optimistic. At the end of six months, his business was flourishing and his partner was expecting their baby.

Patient education and self-management programmes aimed at increasing self-efficacy and personal control is essential to the management of chronic illness (Chapter 9).

Lund and Tamm (2001) conducted a qualitative study in Sweden into the process of adjustment in older people who had been ill and undergone rehabilitation, but remained disabled. They found that initial care focused on physical rehabilitation and involved interaction with health care professionals. Following this, participants reported a period in which they struggled to come to terms with what had happened and find new meaning in their lives. As time progressed, they had to negotiate changes in interpersonal relationships and deal with stigmatizing attitudes in their daily lives. Lund and Tamm commented that although professionals in Sweden claimed rehabilitation took a holistic approach, participants received little help or support in dealing with these psychosocial aspects of change.

People's goals change as their lives and their health changes and care professionals have an important role to play in helping with this process of adaptation (Chapters 9 and 10).

Life events

Holmes and Rahe (1967) developed a measure of life events called the Social Readjustment Rating Scale (SRRS). It consisted of 43 common positive and negative life-changing events, ranked in order of importance. Marriage was given an arbitrary score of 50. Loss of a spouse was presumed to be most stressful and was given a score of 100. The SRRS proved a popular tool because it was simple and easy to use. But it is now seriously out of date and fails to take account of the many cultural changes that affect perceptions of stress.

Some evidence has supported a link between life events and subsequent illness, but generally the correlation (statistical measure of association) has been low and the results disappointing. An important reason may be because the SRRS fails to distinguish between events that are controllable and those that are uncontrollable. In addition, the notion of a direct association between life events and stress-related illness overlooks the fact that many stress-related illnesses are caused by maladaptive coping responses, such as smoking, drinking excess alcohol or comfort eating. Life events can never predict an individual's emotional or physical response because this is mediated by their appraisal process. For example, the death of a spouse is scored highest and for most people events involving loss, such as death, trauma or job loss, also involve loss of control over one's life and loss of support. But such assumptions are not always correct. When a nurse sympathized over the recent death of her husband, one older woman responded with total lack of remorse saying: 'Well you needn't be [sorry], because I wasn't'. It is therefore helpful to assess how patients have experienced these life changes, find out how they are coping with them and what support they need.

Daily hassles

People who have had relatively little exposure to major life events may nevertheless be susceptible to the development of stress-related illness. 'Daily hassles' refers to the accumulation of minor annoying things like missing the bus, being late for work or spilling the coffee. A considerable volume of research suggests that daily hassles are indeed associated with depression.

People who are disadvantaged through poverty, illness or disability are likely to experience a much greater number of what Hewison (1997) observed to be cumulative hassles and recurrent crises. These include negotiating with benefits agencies and hospital systems while attempting to deal with financial and various other losses and relationship problems (Walker *et al.* 1999). A good way of finding out the sorts of hassles that patients experience is to listen to their accounts of health care, observe reactions during episodes of care or read qualitative research reports of patient experiences of care. Many of the hassles experienced while in hospital, such a noise at night, can easily be reduced and stress diminished, leading to improvements in patient satisfaction and health.

Traumatic events and post-traumatic stress disorder

We reviewed post-traumatic stress disorder (PTSD) and its management in Chapter 6. In the context of stress, it may be seen as a response to a single catastrophic uncontrollable event, which is associated with high uncertainty and unpredictability and therefore high physiological arousal and anxiety. It may be viewed as exposure to a stressor that results in total loss of control. The individual is rendered totally helpless as all supportive resources and effective coping responses are comprehensively removed or inaccessible. A review of the neurophysiology of PTSD was provided by VanItallie (2002). Responses include hypersensitivity of sympathetic nervous system responses to trauma-related cues, giving rise to panic attacks. This also suggests that people with PTSD may be more susceptible to stress-related cardiovascular disease in the longer term. For successful treatments, see Chapter 6.

Organizational stress and burnout

Much of our life is spent at work and the working environment has proved an interesting source of research into stress and stress-related illness. It used to be thought that stress was a result of work pressure and was therefore associated with the high-flying executive or senior management. But findings from the **Whitehall studies** indicate that this is not the case.

Theories of organizational stress tested as part of these studies include the 'demand-control-support' and 'effort-reward imbalance' models. Findings show that effort-reward imbalance (people do not get what they feel they deserve) and low job control are related to the incidence of coronary heart disease (Marmot *et al.* 1999). Family life, social support and leisure activities are important buffers against the effects of work-related stress. Stansfield (1999) observed that since social support plays an important role in preventing physical and psychological morbidity, interventions to improve social cohesion at work are important.

A few years ago, Mark was working as a regional sales representative for a firm selling office supplies and working from home. But he had become increasingly anxious and depressed and was eventually signed off sick with 'depression'. He received help from a counsellor. A brief initial analysis revealed that his stress was probably job-related. His pay depended on sales and he invested a high level of effort for relatively little return. He felt he had little control over the management of his work schedule and was swamped with paperwork. He had no colleague or supervisor support since the office base was 50 miles away. High effort and low reward, plus high demand, low job control and low job support equals high stress. Mark resigned from the job and his depression lifted almost immediately. He obtained a more autonomous job as a groundsman, working with a team of others. The rewards were less, but so were the demands, and Mark felt well supported.

The caring services are subject to financial constraints and targets that expose employees at all levels to high levels of demand, but with varying degrees of job control and support. Stress is increased when staff have personal, financial or health problems, or lack adequate emotional support outside work. The problem of burnout has long been recognized among the caring professions (Maslach *et al.* 2001). This is where stress leads to low job satisfaction, poor performance and a lack of ability to empathize with patients as staff are no longer able to cope with the emotional demands of caring. Support groups for staff are an increasingly popular method of supporting professional carers. These need careful facilitation to provide emotional and problem-solving support and avoid negativity.

The reduction and management of stress

In terms of stress reduction, prevention is better than cure. A review of stress management practices (Cooper and Cartright 1997) indicates that those focused on the individual offer only temporary improvement. Elkin and Rosch (1990) offered the following management strategies to reduce work-based stress:

- review the task, the work environment and work schedules and redesign where necessary;
- encourage participative management;
- include the employee in career development;
- analyse work roles and establish goals;
- provide social support and feedback;
- build cohesive teams;
- establish fair employment policies;
- share the rewards.

There are actions that individuals can take to protect their own well-being at study and at work (see Palmer *et al.* 2003). These include developing the skills of prioritizing, time management, seeking help when necessary and assertiveness (to stand up for one's needs where necessary). If stress-related problems are caused by relationship problems or the failure to come to terms with past events, counselling may be helpful. A counsellor can also help the individual to review their goals and help them to focus on achievable aims. For those with more severe anxiety or depression, cognitive behaviour therapy (CBT) uses psychological principles to improve the ability of the individual to be able to confront and deal successfully with life stresses (Chapter 6).

Health and social care professionals can do much to reduce stress for patients and clients, including keeping them adequately informed, assessing their needs and negotiating realistic goals, identifying appropriate coping resources, providing appropriate advice and offering suitable referrals for support, as necessary. The first aim of stress management should be to help the individual assess the number, nature and controllability of the stressors they face, help them identify if their goals are realistic and if they are using effective ways of coping to achieve their goals.

Listening to people's problems is important, but does not imply an obligation to solve their problems for them (Chapter 6). The act of offering a sympathetic ear is an important part of the caring process. Asking if the individual would like further help and, if so, identifying appropriate sources of support are the next steps.

Caring for a child with a life-threatening or terminal illness is one of the most stressful and distressing situations imaginable. Although parents receive professional support, it is not always well structured. Sahler *et al.* (2005) tested the effects of eight sessions of cognitive-behavioural problem-solving skills training to see if this would help. Compared to usual care, mothers receiving this therapy reported improved problem-solving skills and decreased negative affect, some of which were sustained at three-month follow-up. In these types of situation, people gain not only from the content of the programme, but from respite and from the additional support of those attending and running the programme. It might be more helpful if such programmes provided opportunities to continue to meet on a regular basis in order to review strategies and

> maintain support as the demands of caring accumulate or change over time.

In the next chapter we also review how cognitive behavioural principles help to reduce stress for people with chronic illnesses or disabilities.

Summary of key points

- Stress involves an interaction between a stressor, the perceived ability of the individual to achieve a desired outcome, and the individual's coping response.
- Effective coping strategies are those that enhance sense of control and immune function. These include problem-focused, active and effortful coping when used in controllable situations.
- Supports that protect against stress include informational support (advice, information and guidance), emotional support (loving, caring) and spiritual support.
- Anxiety, depression and anger are natural emotional responses to stress.
- Physiological and immune responses to stress are closely associated with positive and negative emotional consequences of stress.
- Traumatic and other major life events (particularly those involving loss), daily hassles (particularly when associated with poverty and deprivation), illness and hospitalization, and organization in the workplace are all important sources of stress and stress-related illness.

Exercise

See after Chapter 10.

Further reading

Cameron, L.D. and Leventhal, H. (eds) (2003) *The Self-regulation of Health and Illness Behaviour*. London: Routledge

Marmot, M. and Wilkinson, R.G. (eds) (1999) *Social Determinants of Health*. Oxford: Oxford University Press.

Mirowsky, J. and Ross, C.E. (2003) *Social Causes of Psychological Distress*, 2nd edn. New York: Aldine de Gruyter.

Palmer, S., Cooper, C.L. and Thomas, K. (2003) *Creating a Balance: Managing Stress*. London: British Library Publishing.

Sarafino, E.P. (2006) *Health Psychology: Biopsychosocial Interactions*, 5th edn. Hoboken, NJ: Wiley.

Walker, J. (2001) *Control and the Psychology of Health*. Buckingham, Open University Press, Chapter 8.

PSYCHOLOGY APPLIED TO HEALTH AND ILLNESS

- **What do we mean by the terms health and illness?**
- **How can we promote health for people who are well and those who are ill?**
- **What are the main reasons why people choose not to take health advice?**
- **Why is it difficult to predict with any certainty whether or not people will change their behaviour, even when they want to?**
- **How can we motivate and help people to change their lifestyles?**
- **Why is it important to identify key individual goals when planning self-management strategies?**
- **What resources are available to help and support people with chronic illnesses?**

Introduction

This chapter focuses on the application of psychology to the promotion of health, and the prevention and management of ill health. To a health professional, the concepts of both mental and physical illness are usually defined by a set of symptoms which are either present or absent. But the concepts of health and illness reflect subjective beliefs and experiences and need to be understood from the perspective of each individual person. Psychologists have drawn on certain common aspects of belief and experience to build theories that can help to guide assessment, interventions and evaluation.

The theories used to explain health-related beliefs and predict health-related behaviours are termed 'social cognition' (or social cognitive) theories. Social cognition combines theoretical positions from cognitive science, social and behavioural learning and social psychology to identify factors likely to influence health-related behaviours and behaviour change. These enable health care professionals to assess the likelihood that an individual will engage in or change health-related behaviours and identify barriers to health action. They also guide the development of programmes likely to promote health and well-being in health and illness. Although illustrated for use within physical and mental health, some of the models are applicable to all types of behaviour and may be useful in the field of social care. Those working with children and people with learning difficulties or cognitive deficits will need to be selective or adapt the models to take account of the developmental and learning needs of their client group (Chapter 3).

Social cognition models presented in the context of **primary prevention** and **secondary prevention** of disease are related to the behaviours of patients and professionals. The principles of **tertiary prevention** and rehabilitation focus on self-management and include ways of measuring and evaluating health outcomes in practice. We start by considering the meaning of health and illness.

Defining health, illness and disease

We touched on some issues related to health as a multi-dimensional concept in Chapter 1. The most widely cited definition of health was provided by the World Health Organization (WHO) (1946): 'health is a state of complete physical, mental and social well-being, not merely the absence of disease or infirmity'. It has since officially remained unchanged, although it is now emphasized that health is a dynamic and not a static state. It is helpful to distinguish between illness and disease. Eisenberg (1977) suggested that patients experience illness, while doctors diagnose and treat disease. Similarly, Blaxter (1990) defined disease as a biological or clinically identified abnormality, and illness as the subjective experience of symptoms. Therefore, she argued, it is possible to have an illness without a disease, and a disease without feeling ill.

> Mark has hypertension, which is a disease associated with high blood pressure. It is an important cause of heart disease, stroke and kidney failure and places Mark at high risk of further health problems. But hypertension often remains symptom free until the late stages and is therefore an example of disease without illness. This makes it difficult for Mark to perceive it as a problem.

It is often difficult to define someone as either healthy or ill because these are relative concepts. Most people take their health for granted unless or until they become ill or perceive themselves at risk of ill health – often as they get older. It is interesting that older people often rate themselves as healthy in spite of diagnosed disease or disorder (Grimby and Wiklund 1994). Medical diagnoses themselves are not static but change as medical technologies improve and attitudes change. Mental health provides many examples of how medical explanations and treatments have changed over time. Diagnosis of mental illness is based on symptom classification, which is subject to cultural changes in attitude as well as knowledge. For example, homosexuality is no longer classified as a mental illness, while bulimia nervosa was not recognized as a mental health disorder until the 1970s. Mental health classifications sometimes respond to political demands. Drapeto-mania (the tendency of slaves to run away from their masters) in nineteenth-century America, and dissidence in twentieth-century USSR are examples of politically convenient 'mental illnesses'. The classification of 'personality disorder' might be seen by some as a political response to the management of asocial behaviour. A useful account of some of these issues is provided by the WHO (2001).

It is important to note that the definitions of illness and disease used here are based on the assumptions of western biomedical science. Alternative explanations are to be found outside western medicine, including the east-ern traditions that inform some complementary therapies. Cross-cultural and lay explanations of physical and mental health vary widely and it is essential to take account of these understandings when working with people from different cultural backgrounds. An exploration of these issues is to be found within the sociology of health and illness, which provides an important contextual background to the psychology of health and illness.

We commence this chapter by focusing on the psychology of health promotion and education in relation to preventable diseases, including cardiovascular disease and diabetes.

Promoting health and preventing ill health

When considering how to apply psychology to health, it is important to distinguish between three distinct types of activity (WHO 2001, based on definitions by Leavey and Clark in 1965):

- *primary prevention*: the avoidance of disease;
- *secondary prevention*: early detection and treatment to arrest a disease pro-cess already initiated;
- *tertiary prevention*: rehabilitation and symptom management to restore the individual to their previous level of function or maximize their remaining capacities.

Each of these is associated with a particular set of actions. We commence by examining psychology in relation to primary and secondary prevention, starting with a focus on the aims, and the assessment and evaluation of outcomes.

Assessing health outcomes: primary and secondary prevention

Primary prevention

Important causes of mortality and morbidity in western populations include heart disease, stroke and cancers (DoH 1999). Primary prevention therefore needs to focus on risk factors such as smoking, diet and exercise. The aim of primary prevention is to keep people well and prevent illness, but the epidemiological outcomes in terms of disease reduction may not be observable for many years. Other than conducting a large-scale study of the same cohort or group of people over a long time period, it is rarely possible to study the outcomes of a health promotion programme in terms of disease prevention. While it is desirable to gain objective information about behaviour change, this is not always feasible. Therefore psychologists often rely on self-reported changes in health-related risk behaviours. Of course, people are not always entirely honest, particularly when they want to present themselves in a good light (Chapter 7). Therefore, it is a good idea to include at least one objective measure if one is available. The systematic process of identifying suitable outcomes is illustrated in Table 9.1 in relation to cardiovascular disease.

The same principles can be applied to other diseases where there are known risks factors.

Table 9.1 Illustration of outcome assessment in primary prevention

Priority health problem	Modifiable risk factors include	Risk behaviours	Behaviour change required	Examples of self-report outcome measures	Examples of objective outcome tests
Cardio-vascular disease	Inhalation of tobacco smoke

Lack of exercise

High cholesterol | Smoking

Sedentary lifestyle

Saturated fat consumption | Stop smoking

Brisk 30 min walk 3 times a week

Cut down on fatty foods | Reduction in cigarettes smoked

Increase in reported exercise

Reduction in fatty foods | Salivary nicotine metabolites

Treadmill tolerance

Blood cholesterol |

Secondary prevention

Early detection involves attending screening tests for conditions such as cervical and breast cancer, diabetes, hypertension and hyperlidipaemia (blood cholesterol); self-examination for breast and testicular cancer, and melanoma; and seeking medical assessment or advice at an early stage of the disease process. Psychologists are interested in factors that promote these courses of action. Outcome measures include medical attendance and self-report of self-monitoring activity, as appropriate.

Tertiary prevention

From a psychological perspective, the main concerns are adherence to medical regimes and rehabilitative actions that promote quality of life and focus on outcomes that measure this. Prevention involves behaviour change. The models considered in this chapter are designed to identify key factors likely to predict behaviour change, so that health promotion and education programmes can focus more closely on these.

Social cognition

Social cognition is concerned with how individuals make sense of social situations (Conner and Norman 1995). Social cognition theories focus on the thoughts or beliefs that lead to health-related behaviours or behaviour change in particular social contexts. They are based on the assumption that changes in beliefs and attitudes precede changes in behaviour, as illustrated in Figure 9.1. (It is an assumption rejected by behaviourists who argue in favour of a direct relationship between external cues and behaviour, see Chapter 5.) The 'cues' in Figure 9.1 refer to such things as health messages, media images, health advice, illness symptoms, family and peer influence, each of which needs to be understood within the social and cultural context of the individual or group of individuals concerned. The following models are both based on social cognition principles

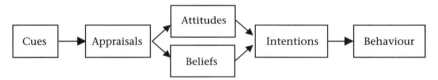

Figure 9.1 Causal assumptions associated with social cognition theories

The health belief model (HBM)

The health belief model (HBM) is what is termed in behavioural psychology an 'expectancy-value' model. This means that it assumes that action is based on the individual's evaluation of the likely outcome for them of a particular behaviour or behaviour change. The HBM was originally developed by Hochbaum in the 1950s, at a time when tuberculosis was an important health problem. He interviewed people to find out why so many people failed to attend for chest X-ray screening, and developed the health belief model from his findings (Rosenstock 1974a). The HBM was reported by Rosenstock (1974b), reviewed by Becker and Maiman (1975), modified by Janz and Becker (1984) and extended by Rosenstock *et al.* (1988). It has proved a popular and durable model within health education. The components are shown in Figure 9.2.

Applying the HBM to dietary change, it is predicted that we are more likely to make a change to a healthier diet if we:

- believe that failure to change increases our risk of getting a disease that could have serious consequences for us (referred to as perceived vulnerability and perceived severity, or in combination as perceived threat);
- believe that the benefits of making the change outweigh the barriers to change (referred to as benefits versus barriers or cost–benefit analysis); the barriers include psychological barriers, such as perceived lack of ability to achieve the change (perceived self-efficacy, Chapter 5);

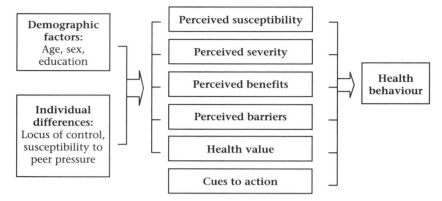

Figure 9.2 The health belief model (adapted from Rosenstock 1974b; Rosenstock *et al.* 1988)

- value our health sufficiently to be motivated to make the effort to change (health value);
- are prompted to change by external cues, such as health messages, advice, information, or the development of symptoms (cues to action).

The model predicts that we are more likely to take action to protect ourselves if we believe ourselves to be at risk from a disease that could have severe consequences. These beliefs are influenced by demographic factors, such as educational level, gender and age, as well as knowledge and experience. But even if we perceive ourselves to be vulnerable, we still need to see that the benefits of action will outweigh the difficulties involved in making a change.

> Before Jo moved in with Sasha, Anna was very concerned about his diet because he lived on pizza and other convenience foods, and refused to eat fresh fruit or vegetables. Anna used the health belief model to assess the likelihood that he would change his diet. Jo did not believe that his diet placed him at risk. He identified a range of barriers including his food preferences, lack of time to buy and prepare food, inability to cook and peer group pressure to eat pizza. He was aware of health messages (cues) in the media, but did not feel that they were relevant to him. He believed that heart disease was a disease of older people and took his own health for granted. Anna concluded that it was unlikely he would change to a healthy diet in his present situation. Fortunately, these beliefs changed when he moved in with Sasha and took on more responsibilities.

Review of the HBM

The HBM was developed from interviews about screening attendance and this explains its focus on disease prevention. Screening attendance is part of secondary prevention (early detection of disease) and involves a single action aimed at protection. The model has also been used to predict the likelihood that people will take medication once they become ill. It is legitimate in these contexts to claim a causal link between health beliefs and health behaviour. However, the HBM has since been applied to a range of lifestyle activities such as smoking, eating, drinking, exercise and sexual activity. These behaviours are clearly related to health from a public health perspective, but not necessarily in the minds of people at the time they engage in them (Galvin 1992). People smoke, eat, drink and engage in sexual activity because they give pleasure or have other reinforcing effects (Chapter 5). Therefore, the HBM may be less relevant in explaining these health-related behaviours and behaviour change.

Tests of the model indicate that the most important reasons for failure to change lifestyle behaviours are perceived vulnerability and barriers to implementation (Sheeran and Abraham 1996). Those who believe themselves vulnerable to adverse consequences are more likely to take notice of health promotion campaigns. But barriers can prevent change even when motivation is high and intentions to change strong. Many of the barriers involve social pressures that are unforeseen at the time of making a commitment to act or change. Therefore, if the HBM is to be a useful aid to patient assessment, it is essential to encourage the individual to think through all possible environmental, social and psychological barriers likely to interfere with their ability to make specific changes.

The theory of planned behaviour (TPB)

The theory of planned behaviour (TPB) (Ajzen 1991) was designed by social psychologists to explain any behaviour, including buying a car, choosing a shirt or smoking a particular brand of cigarette. The original theory was called the theory of reasoned action (TRA, Ajzen and Fishbein 1980). Later, an additional variable 'perceived behavioural control' (similar to self-efficacy) was added to increase the power of the theory to predict behaviour and the theory was renamed the TPB. The TPB (see Figure 9.3), is currently the most popular and most widely used social cognition model in health psychology.

The TPB is based on the assumption that people's behaviour is based on rational decisions. According to the theory, the intention to behave in a certain way, or make a change, is determined by three factors.

1 *Attitude towards the behaviour* reflects a value judgement made by the individual about whether or not the action or change is a good thing. It is based on an evaluation of the desirability of the outcome of the proposed action.
2 *The subjective norm* refers to individual beliefs about what others who are important to them think they should do, together with their motivation to comply with their wishes.
3 *Perceived behavioural control* refers to an assessment of the degree of control the individual perceives him or herself to have over the particular course of action. It is based on an appraisal about whether or not they

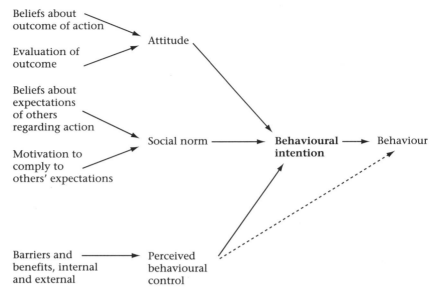

Figure 9.3   The theory of planned behaviour (adapted from Ajzen 1991)

have the necessary skills, abilities and resources to achieve the behaviour. It is similar to Bandura's concept of self-efficacy (Chapter 5), but takes account of available resources, such as money, social support and opportunity.

Janice has had an invitation to attend for a mammogram and is deciding whether or not to attend.

Attitude. Janice believes that attending for screening will have positive benefits. If it proves negative, it will reassure her. If it proves positive it will enable her to receive early treatment for breast cancer and this will improve the outcome for her.

Subjective or social norm. Janice believes that her family would wish her to attend for screening. Her friends all attend and expect her to do the same.

Perceived behavioural control. It is quite easy for Janice to attend for screening as the unit comes to her workplace. She will need to change the appointment to fit in with her shift at work, but the contact details make it easy for her to do this. She knows about the procedure and is not frightened about what will happen.

In this situation, the model predicts that Janice will attend for a mammogram unless there is an unforeseen obstacle, such as illness or the car breaking down. However, the analysis is more difficult when applied to lifestyle behaviour, such as smoking, drinking, eating or exercise, where external influences are greater and change more difficult to put into action.

> Mark was advised by the cardiologist to walk for at least 20 minutes per day, but has so far failed to do this. He believes that exercise would do him good (positive attitude). Janice and Anna want him to do this (subjective norm). He knows that he could easily do it if he wanted to (perceived behavioural control) because he has the ability and the resources (equipment, environment) to do it. Therefore he really intends to it. But somehow, he keeps putting it off until tomorrow when the weather is better, or he has more time.

The TPB fails to identify why Mark has not so far implemented his good intention. Research with the TPB indicates that the model is reasonably good at predicting intentions (Ajzen 1991) but less good at predicting actual behaviour. A recent meta-analysis (synthesis of research findings) suggests that the TPB accounts for about 39 per cent of the variance for intention and 27 per cent of the variance for behaviour (Armitage and Conner 2001). These percentages are estimates of the explanatory power of the model. The most important variable is perceived behavioural control, which in many instances is shown to have a direct influence on behaviour as well as intention. But the longer the gap between expressing intentions and taking action, the less likely it is that the action will take place. Therefore an immediate demonstration of commitment is desirable. Once again, unforeseen barriers are probably important in preventing people from carrying out their good intentions. Some authors have recommended combining the TPB with the HBM to strengthen their ability to predict health behaviours (e.g. Maddux 1993). This allows for the identification of psychological and social barriers likely to reduce self-efficacy at the point of action.

Critique of social cognition models

The HBM and TPB have provided the basis for a lot of health psychology practice and research in relation to primary and secondary prevention. The TPB has proved to be the most popular model because of its versatility in explaining a wide range of behaviours. But although reasonably good at predicting intentions, it has proved modest in predicting actual behaviour. There are a number of practical reasons to consider.

Unlike behaviourist learning theory (Chapter 5), social cognition models assume that health-related behaviours are based upon rational processes of reasoning and deliberation. This is reasonable when applied to the decision to engage in a one-off action like attending for screening. But most lifestyle behaviours that influence long-term health outcomes, such as eating, drinking and smoking, are *habits*. Habits are, by definition, things that we do routinely and without thinking (using the language of behaviourism, these behaviours are under stimulus control, Chapter 5). They are therefore hard to change even when we want to do so.

Hunt and Martin (1988) provided a useful analysis of lifestyle behaviour change. They suggested that daily life needs some kind of interruption to bring an existing habit or lifestyle into conscious focus, so that it can be changed. An example might be meeting a new partner who eats a healthy diet (as in the case of Jo and Sasha), or moving to a new area with a new set of friends. They also suggest that new behaviours, such as taking up exercise, are unlikely to be maintained until they have become habits and take place without having to think too hard about them.

Social cognition models do not distinguish between different types of behaviour change. For example, smoking, drinking and substance use are behaviours that need to stop. Therefore, some other activity needs to be introduced to compensate for the time spent engaged in these activities. Exercise involves the introduction of a new behaviour that needs to displace some other activity or routine. Dietary change involves substitution, which is not so difficult provided it is evaluated as the same or more desirable. Mark might not want to exercise because he sees this as less attractive than relaxing in front of the television, particularly in winter when the weather is bad. Perhaps he might have more success in summer, or needs a friend to join him? Behaviour change requires careful analysis in relation to the individual's lifestyle, goals and desires, as well as their health needs.

Many health-related behaviours are actually coping strategies used for dealing with stress (Chapter 8). Smoking, comfort eating and drinking alcohol are good examples. These will be difficult to change while the individual is under stress, so it is a good idea to help people identify and address sources of stress when developing an action plan.

Little attention is given in the literature to age-related differences, though it is generally recognized that people take their health more seriously as they get older. A small unpublished student project, which compared healthy people aged 18 to 28 with those aged 55 to 65, found that the TPB was a fairly good predictor of exercise in the older age group, but failed completely to predict exercise in the younger group. Additional information indicated that the older group exercised primarily for health reasons, while those who were younger did so primarily because it was a social recreational activity.

A final important criticism of all social cognition models is their lack of emphasis on the immediate and often unforeseen social cues, particularly in the younger age groups.

Coleman and Ingham (1999) interviewed young people about their use of contraception. They found that first sexual experiences were usually

> unplanned and protection not used. They observed that the association of a condom with disease prevention could actually inhibit use, since wearing a condom, or asking a partner to use one might imply a lack of trust. Coleman and Ingham discussed this in relation to the need for enhanced communication skills in young people. Ingham (1993) also observed that when the lights are low, the alcohol flowing, and passions rising, good intentions are inclined to be forgotten.

Finally, some of the tools used to measure health beliefs have limited validity. For example, the HBM measure developed by Champion (1984) to predict breast self-examination, and cited in Conner and Norman (1995) as an example of instrument development, omits the most important barrier of all – fear of finding a lump! This clearly reduces the power of the model to predict behaviour, though the problem is with the measure and not the model. It is really important to involve participants in the development of measures to ensure that all relevant issues are covered.

In spite of relatively modest success with predicting change for health habits, these models are widely used to help focus health education and promotion programmes on important aspects of beliefs and skills. The HBM and TPB are both theories of decision-making. Next we consider a theory of motivation which should be considered as complementary to these.

Stages of change (transtheoretical) model

Prochaska and Diclemente (1983) recognized that another important determinant of health-related behaviour change, particularly in relation to smoking cessation, was the individual's motivational state – their readiness to make a change. They argued that interventions will be more successful if tailored to the individual's state of readiness to change. It is fairly logical to assume that those who are not aware of the need to change need information. Those who know about the risks need persuading to want to change. Those wanting to change need an action plan. Those who have changed need a strategy to maintain change. Prochaska and DiClemente produced the 'stages of change' model (also called the transtheoretical model or TTM) in order to classify people according to the following stages in the change process:

- *pre-contemplation*: the individual is not considering change in the near future, and may not even recognize the need for change;
- *contemplation*: the individual has recognized a need to change and is starting to think about possible ways to achieve this;
- *action planning*: the individual is planning how to make the change;
- *implementation*: the individual is in the process of trying to change;
- *maintenance*: the individual has made the change and is trying hard not to relapse.

A useful review of the model and its application, based on research by their own research team, is provided by Prochaska and Norcross (2001). The model has been applied to most health risk behaviours and is widely used in the field of smoking and 'addictions'. The process of ensuring that people receive interventions appropriate to their stage of change should, in theory, improve the outcomes of health promotion and education programmes.

Below, we illustrate how the stages of change model could be used as a framework, in conjunction with social cognition models of decision-making, to address important issues in achieving behaviour change.

- *Pre-contemplation*. At this stage, health promotion is important to draw attention to the need to change and to encourage a set of shared values that will lead people to want to consider changing their behaviour. The media plays an important role in highlighting health issues and raising awareness. Personal advice from health professionals and physiological feedback on personal fitness are important cues to change. The perceived health threat components of the HBM and the attitudes component of the TPB are useful aids in identifying individual beliefs and attitudes that need to be addressed at this stage.
- *Contemplation*. If the individual is thinking about change, the cost–benefit analysis component of the HBM may help to assess potential barriers that might deter them. It is also helpful to use the subjective norm component of the TPB to assess social influences on the individual's intention to change. Health education needs to focus on reinforcing the need for change and helping the individual to set up an action plan.
- *Action planning and implementation*. The perceived behavioural control element of the TPB, and barriers component of the HBM, are likely to be particularly important in developing and implementing a sustainable plan of action. In the example given previously, Mark wanted to change and intended to change, but did not feel sufficiently in control of the barriers to make and maintain the change. Health education can be used to ensure that the individual has the skills to make the change and to recognize and identify ways of overcoming potential barriers.
- *Maintenance*. Maintaining a change in behaviour is often more difficult than making the initial change. For example, relapse rates for those quitting smoking and drinking are high. Health education programmes need to encourage individuals to identify the factors most likely to tempt them to relapse and to plan how to deal with these situations. Social support is particularly important at this stage (see the buddy system in the smoke stop programme in Chapter 4).

Critique of the stages of change model

The stages of change model is intuitively attractive, extremely popular among clinicians and researchers, and widely used as a basis for planning health promotion interventions. However, Riemsma *et al.* (2003) reviewed research from a wide range of sources (not just the original research team) and found little evidence that programmes based on the stage model are more effective than other approaches. He did suggest this could be due to problems with the rigour of patient assessment. Now over 20 years old, considerable controversy surrounds the model. Those interested in robust academic debate should read the editorial by West (2005) together with commentaries on the following pages (including one by an even more vociferous opponent, Sutton) and followed by a reply from Prochaska (2006). West argued, in the context of smoking, that 'the problems with the model are so serious that it has held back advances in the field of health promotion and, despite its intuitive appeal to many practitioners, it should be discarded' (West 2005: 1036). His reasons are incorporated into the summary below.

- The model is descriptive, but not predictive. It is possible to classify people, but this gives little indication of their future progress.
- There is actually no evidence that people progress smoothly through a series of 'stages'. (This argument applies equally to other stage models of development and change, Chapters 3 and 6.)
- The model assumes that people make conscious and stable plans – many do not (see critique of HBM and TPB).
- People may not respond honestly to an assessment of their stage of change (particularly when engaging in a stigmatized behaviour such as smoking or other substance use).
- To label someone as a 'precontemplator' when they have no intention to change is not helpful.
- The model allows health promoters, educators and researchers to claim success for an intervention just because people have moved from one stage to the next, even if no behavioural change has actually taken place.
- The model has become so popular that it has inhibited the development of better models. This argument applies to many models and measures commonly used in psychology. You will find an alternative model in the later section on self-regulation.

It is interesting to note that much of this debate takes place in the context of smoking cessation. The reader needs to bear in mind that smoking may be conceptualized as an addiction, or a health habit, or self-medication against anxiety and stress (Chapter 8). Different conceptualizations lead to different therapeutic approaches and need to be considered against a background of powerful vested interests, including the tobacco industry and the manufacturers of nicotine replacements, which can determine the research agenda. Reviews of the stages of change model in relation to other lifestyle behaviours, such as exercise, offer conflicting evidence of efficacy. The following example, based on Hunt and Martin (1988), offers some insights into why the model might fail to predict change.

Take the example of Jo's dietary preference for living on pizza. It is clear that prior to meeting Sasha he had no intention at all of making a change. However, after moving in with Sasha, his dietary behaviour changed completely – but with no intention or effort at all on his part. No social cognition model predicts change in the context of chaotic lifestyles or unpredictable life changes.

In spite of his criticisms, West suggested that it is important to assess both decision-making and motivation. Accordingly, we suggest that if the stages of change model is to be used, this should happen in conjunction with social cognition models such as the HBM and TPB, as illustrated previously (see also Courneya *et al.* 2000). Hodgins (2005) has argued that it might be helpful to outline the stages of change to patients or clients and invite them to make their own judgements about where they fit. This fits with our own recommendation that practitioners work with clients and patients as partners to ensure that any course of action fits in with their personal goals and the resources they have to achieve these, as in the self-regulation model reviewed below.

Self-regulatory theory: the importance of having a goal

Self-regulation implies that people have, or can develop, autonomy, self-control, self-direction and self-discipline (Purdie and McCrindle 2002). The assumption is that all behaviours are motivated by the desire to achieve goals that are personally important (Gollwitzer and Oettingen 2000). The notion of the self-regulatory system has its origins in systems theory (from which also come the concepts of control and homeostasis, see Chapter 8). Self-regulation depends on feedback through which the individual can appraise and adjust their performance. The amount of effort put into achieving a goal is likely to depend on its desirability and achievability.

Bandura (2005) argued that if health is to be seen as a goal, health promotion targeted at changing lifestyle habits is the best way to achieve it. One problem is that many individuals and some groups enjoy their unhealthy lifestyles and do not share the same goals as health professionals. Another is that when considering a lifestyle change, people often face competing or conflicting desires (Taylor and Gollwitzer 1995). For example, in our scenario, Mark wishes to stay healthy but also enjoys eating unhealthy snacks. Taylor and Gollwitzer (1995) also identified the tendency for people to be unrealistically optimistic in their beliefs about their ability to achieve their goals, but poor at anticipating the amount of effort required to overcome habits, social pressures and likely distractions. These issues led Gollwitzer and Oettingen (2000) to argue that behaviour change requires a goal implementation strategy and not just a goal-directed intention, as proposed in the TPB.

When Mark developed angina, he needed a plan to avoid the temptation of buying crisps and chocolate. He enjoyed the daily chat with the newsagent from whom he bought chocolate bars and who had become a good friend. So he planned to share his problem with his friend and engage his help in buying chewing gum and nuts instead. Meanwhile, he and Janice worked out a lunchtime diet that would satisfy his hunger as

> well as his dietary needs. This new strategy worked very well. Mark lost weight and started to feel better.

Bandura highlighted that 'health promotion and risk reduction programs are often structured in ways that are costly, cumbersome and minimally effective' (2000: 316). He reasoned that it is impossible to achieve success if the individual has a goal without a plan to achieve it; or if they have a plan without a clearly identified goal. According to Bandura, self-regulated change does not rely on willpower but on having a comprehensive plan. The self-regulatory model does not exclude the models previously discussed, since these may be helpful in assessing readiness for change and identifying potential barriers and resources that need to be incorporated into the implementation plan. Bandura, like Prochaska, identified the importance of identifying readiness to change but identified three different *levels* of readiness (not stages), based on the concept of self-efficacy (Chapter 5).

- *Level 1*: these are people with a high sense of efficacy and positive expectations for achieving behaviour change who need minimal guidance.
- *Level 2*: these individuals have self-doubts about their efficacy and the likely benefits of their efforts. They make half-hearted attempts and are quick to give up when they run into difficulties. They need individual support and guidance which may be provided by telephone or via the internet (see Bandura 2000).
- *Level 3*: they believe that their health habits are beyond their personal control, effort futile, and are highly sceptical of the need to change. They need a great deal of personal guidance in a progressive structured programme (Bandura 2005).

Bandura (2000) drew on behavioural principles to recommend that the individuals at Levels 1 and 2 need to identify short-term attainable sub-goals to motivate and guide their efforts. The type of programme he recommends is quite similar to the one outlined by Marks *et al.* (2005, see Chapter 5) and incorporates a range of activities to improve health.

Critique of Bandura's self-regulation model

Bandura's concept of self-regulation builds on his concept of self-efficacy. By self-efficacy, Bandura means the belief that one is able to exercise control over one's behaviours and habits. The weakness of Bandura's levels appears to be that they still focus too closely on personal control over health-related behaviour change. A real danger for health professionals is to assume that health is an important goal for everyone. Practitioners need to understand and acknowledge the competing goals faced by people who generally struggle to balance their desire to remain healthy with their desires to engage in enjoyable and sociable, but risky or unhealthy, activities. Practitioners and researchers need to focus carefully (as did Marks, see Chapter 5) on the ability to manage social contexts where there is likely to be strong peer pressure to continue to engage in unhealthy behaviours in spite of the best intentions. Where individuals are struggling to address competing demands, help with sorting these out might well take priority (see Chapter 8). One way of helping people to identify these issues is through the motivational interview.

The motivational interview

Didactic (instructional) approaches to health education, and those based on persuasion, often fail to work for reasons we have considered (see also Chapter 7). Motivational interviewing (Miller and Rollnick 2002) is a technique that was developed for use in the field of addiction and is now being used to motivate change in other health settings (Britt *et al.* 2004). It starts with a narrative approach in which the patient is encouraged to talk about their interpretation of their problems and worries in the context of their everyday lives and highlight key areas of concern. The clinician then steers them towards their own recognition of the need to change, and encourages them to identify achievable goals and develop a plan for achieving these. This promotes concordance (see below) and can lead people from the stage of precontemplation to action planning and implementation in a relatively short time. This technique has demonstrated success in a variety of settings (Rubak *et al.* 2005), including changing perceptions of drug-related harm and reducing drug consumption in young people (McCambridge and Strang 2004).

Medical help-seeking

The outcome of many illnesses depends on early detection. In order to seek medical help, it is first necessary for people to recognize that there is something wrong with them. Then it is essential that they seek help as soon as possible. Cancer and myocardial infarction (MI) are good examples of how delay in medical help-seeking can affect the outcome.

Grunfeld *et al.* (2003) surveyed well women about their beliefs and intentions to seek help for breast cancer symptoms, using the theory of planned behaviour. Older women were more likely to express the intention to seek help than younger women. The inability to recognize breast cancer symptoms predicted delay in all age groups. For women aged 35–54, lack of perceived behavioural control (not knowing what to expect or what to do) was found to be an important predictor of the intention not to seek help. In women aged over 65 years, beliefs about the disabling or disfiguring consequences of having breast cancer were important.

Findings such as these have important implications for health promotion and education. People need clear information about what to look for and when to seek help, but they also need information about outcomes. Based on their study, Grunfeld *et al* suggest that providing information about cosmetic outcomes may be particularly important for older women whose friends or relatives might have received surgery at a time when aesthetic outcomes were poor.

In the case of MI (myocardial infarction) or stroke, delay to the commencement of thrombolytic (clot-busting) intervention can have serious adverse consequences. Yet people often delay calling for help for several hours. Older people may be less likely to summon help because symptoms are less typical or severe. Women may be more likely to delay than men if they view MI as a disease of men, but other than this there is little evidence that delay is due to lack of knowledge. An important reason for delay is likely to be found in the social processes of help-seeking. A German interview study of post-MI patients (Kentsch *et al.* 2002) found that key factors associated with delay included not wanting to bother anybody and waiting to ask others for advice.

> When Mark first experienced an attack of angina, he wondered if he might be having a heart attack and was very frightened. It was late afternoon and he was at work. He managed to convince himself that it was probably indigestion and made an excuse to leave early, knowing that Janice would be home. It was Janice who phoned for the ambulance. Fortunately, tests revealed it to be an angina attack and his symptoms responded to treatment. But had it been an MI, his delay could have been fatal.

This scenario is fairly typical. People commonly seek the help, advice and reassurance from others when they feel ill and it is often a family member or friend who prompts help-seeking. This confirms that those who are socially isolated are at greater risk (see Chapter 8 on social support). People are particularly inclined to delay seeking medical help for mental health problems. Christiana *et al.* (2000) conducted an international survey of members of patient advocate groups suffering from anxiety disorders and found a median delay of eight years. Older people were more likely to seek help earlier. An important reason for delay may be the stigma associated with mental illness (Chapter 2).

Tertiary prevention: managing illness

Disease management in western traditions depends primarily on taking prescribed medicines. For some illnesses, such as infection, this involves a short course of antibiotics (which many people fail to complete). In the case of chronic illnesses, it can mean a lifetime taking a range of drugs in addition to other demands such as dietary restrictions and self-monitoring. There is strong evidence that people find it really difficult to stick to these treatment schedules in spite of the potential consequences.

Compliance with, adherence to, or concordance with, medical advice?

Compliance is the term traditionally used to describe acting in accordance with the doctor's instructions. Non-compliance is costly for patients in terms of their health; for professionals in terms of the frustrations and help-lessness caused; and to health services because of increased demands and wastage.

Compliance has been extensively studied in relation to diabetes. In addition to control over glycaemia (blood sugar), control over blood pressure and lipidaemia (blood fats) is needed to reduce long-term adverse health outcomes. Therefore medication and diet are essential aspects of diabetes management. A Canadian study (Toth *et al.* 2003) identified that only 10 per cent of their sample met guidelines for glycaemic control. But non-compliance was not restricted to patients. The researchers identified that only 22 per cent of diabetic patients had been prescribed aspirin in line with clinical practice guidelines.

Donovan and Blake (1992) argued that non-compliance by patients is often a process of reasoned decision-making, based on a cost–benefit analysis of treatment – many drugs have unpleasant side-effects which are perceived to be worse than the original symptoms. The HBM predicts that people will only put up with these barriers if the disease is sufficiently severe to warrant it, as in cancer treatment. However, it is important to note that compliance itself can have unfortunate or even lethal consequences. For example, some people continue to take medication in the face of adverse drug reactions, just because they were told to do so by the doctor (see external 'powerful other' locus of control, Chapter 5).

Fogarty (1997) suggested that non-compliance can be a reaction against loss of freedom. Talk to any group of patients and you will find some who just don't like taking tablets. Many people nowadays want to know *why* they need treatment and what to expect from it, rather than blindly following the doctor's instructions. The authoritarian and paternalistic attitude suggested by the term 'compliance' is now generally seen as unacceptable and was replaced by the term adherence. Adherence is intended to entail the doctor and patient reaching an agreement about an appropriate course of treatment, but it still implies that the main agenda is set by the doctor. Therefore, compliance and adherence both imply varying degrees of coercion, placing the patient in a passive role and discouraging personal control. These issues led Anderson and Funnell (2000) to claim that compliance and adherence are dysfunctional concepts.

More recently, the term 'concordance' has been encouraged within health care. Concordance implies a shared understanding between health care professional and patient about the nature of the illness, and its treatment and management. The intention is to involve patients as partners in order to ensure that their needs are met.

> Sanz (2003) identified that when dealing with children with chronic diseases, concordance is required between three partners: doctor, parent and child. Sanz pointed out that the medical consultation frequently involves a two-way conversation between the doctor and parent, while the children play a passive role. On the other hand, children with asthma or diabetes are expected to play an active role in the management of their disease. This requires the child to play an important part in establishing and agreeing goals and action plans. It also requires that they fully understand the implications of what they are required to do and why.

Partnership involves give and take. Patients need to understand the reasons for and advantages of adhering to a particular course of action. Professionals need to understand the barriers likely to make this difficult. Through partnership, a plan of action or, if necessary, a compromise may then be worked out. In reality, time constraints, the need to use evidence-based treatments and an unequal power relationship between doctor and patient can mean that coercion is implicit (Ferner 2003). Unequal power relationships are particularly problematic when the patient is someone with a learning difficulty or a child. However, educational programmes can be developed to overcome this.

> Igoe (1988, 1991) developed an education programme to improve children's involvement in their own health and health care. In one study, children were asked to draw the medical consultation. They depicted a large doctor, medium-sized mummy and, to one side, a small child, reflecting the interpersonal situation as they saw it. They then received training in what to expect in a medical consultation about themselves, and preparation in how to ask questions. After the programme, their drawings indicated a much more equal relationship between the three partners, as illustrated by the size and position of the three players.

Adherence by health professionals

Discussions about adherence usually refer to patients' beliefs and behaviours. However, those of staff are of equal importance to health outcomes. Ley (1997) catalogued activities in which health care professionals had been shown not to comply with standard protocols and procedures. These included observing rules about the administration of drugs, giving adequate patient information, attending professional updates and adhering to infection control procedures. Hospital-acquired infection, in particular, is extremely costly in terms of financial cost and human suffering. One of the most effective ways of reducing this is by effective hand washing and antiseptic gel use, yet compliance by health care professionals still appears poor. It is possible to apply the TPB to analyse this issue.

- Do staff believe that failure to cleanse their hands could have important consequences?
- Do staff believe that others who matter believe that they should cleanse their hands and how motivated are they to comply with that wish?
- Do staff feel able to engage in adequate hand-cleansing? What are the barriers?

Knowledge about the method and frequency of hand washing is clearly important, but education alone is not sufficient. Time is limited and seeing senior staff members cut corners leads others to do the same. But peer pressure can also be used as a force for change.

> A paediatrician told Anna how bacteria had been eliminated from a neonatal unit. Spot hand cultures were taken from staff. These showed that certain members of staff had unacceptable concentrations of bacterial growth. The infection control staff fed back the results to the unit without publicly naming names. People became aware that the eyes of others might be on them as potential culprits. A short time later, when cultures were taken, the results were all clear.

Understanding chronic illness

In this section, we focus attention on psychological issues in chronic illnesses – those that by definition are not amenable to cure. Psychologists in the 1980s found that there are five key questions that people normally want answered when they become ill (Leventhal and Nerenz 1982; Lau and Hartman 1983).

1 *Identity*: what is the name of the disease I have?
2 *Consequences*: what will happen to me?
3 *Time line*: what is the duration of the illness?
4 *Causes*: why has this happened to me?
5 *Cure*: what can be done about it?

The Illness Perception Questionnaire (IPQ, Weinman *et al.* 1996) was designed to assess people's understanding of their illness, based on these dimensions. Copies of the long and short versions are available on the internet (see end of chapter) for use in research and clinical practice. It has also been adapted for children. Asking about people's understanding of their illness will inform the sort of information the individual needs and can identify misconceptions. It seems a paradox that some patients express relief when given a potentially life-threatening diagnosis such as cancer or multiple sclerosis, but it can be very stressful and worrying to be uncertain about what is wrong. A diagnosis validates the illness and reason for help-seeking, and achieving a diagnosis is often an important goal for patients.

Aim of chronic disease management

The aim of chronic disease management is to improve quality of life and help patients or clients to attain achievable goals (see Bandura's self-regulatory model). These are very subjective, so assessment needs to include the individual's hopes, fears, expectations and aims. It is surprising how variable these can be and often not at all what nurses or other professionals expect.

> Anna spent an afternoon observing the assessment process in the pain clinic. All of the patients had chronic back pain. The first patient focused only on getting rid of the pain. The second wanted to understand the cause of the pain. The third was concerned that she would end up in a wheelchair. The fourth wanted to be able to walk further so that she could meet her friends in the local café.

Different professionals are trained to focus on different aspects of chronic illness: doctors on symptoms, physiotherapists on physical function, occupational therapists on role function, psychologists on emotional well-being and maladaptive behaviours, and so on. The danger is that each assesses their domain in isolation from the others. This can lead to fragmentation or conflict and meanwhile no one really address the patient's personal goals. This is why there is an urgent need for interprofessional working in partnership with patients who have a chronic disease.

Assessing outcomes in chronic disease

In the context of an ageing population, the Department of Health (DoH) (2000) refers to the importance of 'adding life to years', by which they mean improving quality of life. The same applies to all people with a chronic disorder. In order to achieve this, it is necessary to focus on each of the following dimensions.

- Illness-specific symptom management (e.g. pain, breathing, nausea, anxiety).
- Functional ability (e.g. mobility, self-care, ability to carry out normal roles).
- Anxiety and depression (see relationship to stress, Chapter 8).
- Quality of life. The WHO has identified key domains of quality of life, based on interviews worldwide, and incorporated these into the WHO

quality of life measure (WHOQOL: see Skevington *et al.* 1999; O'Connell *et al.* 2003) (see Figure 9.4).

Domain I	Domain III	Domain V
• Pain and discomfort • Energy and fatigue • Sexual activity • Sleep and rest • Sensory functions	• Mobility • Activities of daily living • Dependence on medication or treatment • Dependence on non-medicinal substances • Communication capacity • Working capacity	• Physical safety and security • Home environment • Work satisfaction • Financial resources • Health and social care: availability and quality • Opportunities for acquiring new information and skills • Participation and opportunities for recreation/leisure • Activities • Physical environments

Domain II	Domain IV	Domain VI
• Positive feelings • Thinking, learning, memory and concentration • Self-esteem • Body image and appearance • Negative feelings	• Personal relationships • Practical social support • Activities as provider/supporter	• Spirituality, religion and personal beliefs

Figure 9.4   WHO indicators of quality of life (Skevington *et al.* 1999)

In order to evaluate the outcomes of disease management programmes, it is necessary to have valid and reliable measures. A useful introduction to the measurement of health outcomes, together with comprehensive reviews of a range of health measures, is given by Bowling (2004). The following are generic measures (they apply to all chronic diseases). They are used mainly for research, but can also be used by clinicians to audit the outcomes of treatment programmes. Examples include:

- *psychological well-being*: Hospital Anxiety and Depression Scale (HADS);
- *life satisfaction and meaning*: Sense of Coherence scale (SOC);
- *general health status*: the Short-Form-36 Health Survey Questionnaire (SF36); Euroquol EQ–5D*;
- *Multidimensional quality of life*: WHOQOL.*

* Starred items are available on the internet, see end of chapter.

The general health status questionnaires referred to are used to compare the cost-effectiveness of disease management programmes. Bowling illustrates a range of disease-specific measures (including mental illness) in common use and her book is useful for interpreting research outcomes.

A recent innovation has been the introduction of patient-determined outcome measurement. Rather than being presented with a list of pre-determined symptoms and problems, this allows the patient to select those most relevant to their personal needs and is much more in keeping with the self-regulatory model. An example of a simple but valid and reliable tool is the MYMOP (Measure Yourself Medical Outcomes Profile – Paterson 1996) which is also available on the internet. This allows patients to select and rate important symptoms, activities and well-being.

After Ted developed chronic heart disease, he was fortunate to join a pilot self-management group. As part of the evaluation, he completed the MYMOP2 questionnaire (Paterson 2003). Before the programme began, he identified his worst symptom as breathlessness, which he scored 5/6, his difficult activity as gardening (6/6) and his well-being as 4/6 (NB high scores are negative). As a more objective measure, he was asked to record the number of visits to the doctor during the last month. One month after the programme finished, he was sent a follow-up questionnaire. This time, he rated his breathlessness as 4/6; his gardening ability as 4/6 and his well-being as 2/6. He had enjoyed the programme, learned new techniques and felt much less anxious about his condition. As a result, he felt less breathless and more confident to spend time pottering in the garden and greenhouse. The evaluation team was pleased to note that most participants reported less frequent visits to their doctor's surgery after the programme. This enabled them to calculate that the cost of putting on the programme was more than balanced by savings to health care.

Simple tools like this make it easy for health care professionals to establish whether or not interventions such as this are meeting patients' needs. In the next section, we consider the principles of self-management.

Self-management in chronic illness

Self-management implies making lifestyle changes, which we addressed earlier in this chapter. Making changes when also having to cope with a diagnosis of chronic disease and all its consequences and losses can be difficult. Patients who have a chronic or disabling health problem are often informed by doctors that they will have to learn to live with it, but are rarely told how. As the DoH (2002: 1) pointed out, the options are to suffer and do nothing; just take the medicine; or take charge and be an active self-manager. Drawing on the self-regulatory model and principles of motivational interviewing discussed earlier in this chapter, it is important to develop a goal-directed plan for how to achieve successful self-management. Some of the important issues faced by people with a chronic disease include (from Miller 1992):

- maintaining sense of the 'normal' in terms of daily routines and lifestyle;
- gaining knowledge and skills for symptom management;
- making decisions about treatment;
- using effective coping strategies;

- complying with essential medical regimes;
- dealing with stigma associated with the disorder;
- adjusting to altered social relationships;
- coming to terms with losses associated with the illness;
- maintaining hope;
- maintaining occupation or work.

Self-management programmes are designed to address these issues. Patients come together to learn ways of controlling their symptoms and regain control over their lives, with support. Programmes are based principally on cognitive-behavioural principles such as those listed below.

- Bandura's social learning theory (Chapter 5) supports the need to learn technical skills, such as the use of inhalers or giving of injections. Modelling and instruction are used to increase self-efficacy in these tasks.
- Behaviourist principles (Chapter 5) support the need to identify and reduce avoidance and risk behaviours, and build in treats to reward adherence.
- Beck's cognitive theory (Chapter 6) supports the need for positive thinking – focusing on what can be achieved, rather than on what can't be done. Hassles and losses need, where appropriate, to be identified and addressed.
- Self-regulatory theory supports the need to identify short-term achievable goals as well as longer-term realistic goals to maintain hope.
- Peer support is an important component of informational and emotional support (Chapter 8).

Self-management and cognitive behavioural programmes have been successfully used to manage rheumatoid arthritis, asthma, diabetes and a variety of other chronic conditions.

An early example of a successful self-management programme was designed by Thomas Creer to treat childhood asthma (Creer *et al.* 1992). As part of the programme, children were taught to understand their condition and their symptoms, use their inhalers correctly, monitor their own symptoms and learn to recognize early signs of an attack. This enabled them to use their inhaler to prevent or reduce an attack. The children rehearsed these skills for implementation at home and at school. The evaluation of the programme identified that the child's locus of control shifted from external to internal, meaning that they felt more control over their lives. However, the researchers noted that parents felt some loss of their parental role, which clearly would need to be addressed.

Asthma self-management programmes have also been developed for adults (see Kotses and Harver 1998). An evaluation by Muntner *et al.* (2001) identified that those who declined to participate in their programme had less knowledge about what to do in the event of an attack and less knowledge about the correct use of inhalers. This confirms that those with the greatest need for knowledge and skill are those least likely to attend a self-management programme. It is also worth noting that autonomy and control are not valued equally by all people, therefore self-management programmes may not appeal to everyone.

The Expert Patient Programme

In 1989, a team led by Kate Lorig reported on the long-term outcomes of a self-management programme to help people deal with rheumatoid arthritis (Lorig and Holman 1989). The Arthritis Self Management Course (ASMC) demonstrated sustained decreases in pain and depression, increase in perceived self-efficacy and decrease in visits to the doctor (Lorig *et al*. 1993). Self-management reduces costs because it addresses patients' own needs. At a time when the costs of supporting people with chronic diseases have rapidly increased, the DoH (2006) advocates this model of care for people with all types of chronic disease and disorder as part of what they term the Expert Patient Programme. The DoH recognizes that the main aims of self-management are to preserve and promote health and well-being *in spite of* chronic disease. Specifically, the aims are to:

• improve self-efficacy and personal control;
• improve effective symptom management;
• improve activity and function;
• reduce demands on health services in terms of consultations and admissions.

These programmes have now been established throughout the United Kingdom (see web address at the end of the chapter). The title 'expert patient' has proved controversial and most certainly does not imply, as some appear to have feared, an 'unappealing stereotype of the dissatisfied, middle-class consumer' (Shaw and Baker 2004: 723). This unfortunate phrase suggests that the empowerment of patients is seen as challenging to certain professionals who are used to holding on to medical knowledge as a source of power.

There are important differences between the Expert Patient Programme and other self-management programmes. While self-management programmes focus on groups with specific diseases or disorders, the Expert Patient Programme is generic, designed to address needs common to all people living with a chronic health problem, including mental health problems such as depression. While self-management programmes are normally run by health professionals, the Expert Patient Programme offers a structured programme facilitated by lay people who have undergone special training. Increasingly these are people who have a chronic health problem themselves, denoting the importance of self-help and peer teaching.

Peer teaching

Peer teaching forms an important part of the Expert Patient Programme. In some schools, it has been used as part of health education for quite a while, informed by Vygotsky's principles of developmental learning (Chapter 3). Additional principles are included in the research example outlined below.

> Campbell and MacPhail (2002) explored peer teaching in the context of HIV prevention among young people in Africa. They identified that traditional didactic methods of health education seek to change the views and attitudes of single individuals. By contrast, peer education promotes dialogue and argument between peers as they ask one another questions, exchange anecdotes and comment on one another's experiences and points of view. This provides a forum where peers can weigh up the pros and cons of a range of coping possibilities, using their own terminology and taking account of their own priorities.

Self-management group programmes that involve lay teachers or facilitators are becoming increasingly popular. Lay people often find it easier to learn from people who, like themselves, have had to learn to cope with a similar illness.

> Von Korff *et al.* (1998) conducted a randomized controlled trial to compare the effectiveness of usual care with four sessions of group problem-solving for people with back pain, led by trained lay people. The purpose of the programme was to reduce patients' worries, encourage self-care and increase activity levels. Participants in the problem-solving programme reported significantly less worry about back pain and more confidence in self-care. Half of the participants showed a 50 per cent or greater reduction in disability scores at six months, compared with 33 per cent among the usual care controls.

The DoH (2006) recommended an expansion in user-led self-management programmes, provided by patients and patient organizations in partnership with health and social care professionals. Self-help groups provide another valuable ongoing source of emotional and informational support to those who need it. Perhaps the last word on this should go to Nadine Johnson (2004: 30), the wife of Peter, who developed cancer of the larynx in 1997 and who, as a result, became a facilitator with the Expert Patient Programme.

> Nadine tells of how fellow members at a branch of the National Association of Laryngectomy Clubs passed on 'A wealth of essential, practical tips that you don't learn about in hospital and, to my mind, help to complete the circle of care. Peter learned that in his condition coughing up blood was not necessarily a sign of lung cancer. To a

seasoned laryngectomee, this could be a sign of a comparatively innocuous chest infection or dryness of the chest. The differences are mammoth when you live constantly with the fear of a relapse.'

Summary of key points

- Health and illness are subjective experiences that need to be understood in their social and cultural context.
- Social cognition models, including the HBM, the TPB and the stages of change model, can be used to assess patient needs and inform health-promoting activities.
- Motivational interviewing can be an effective way of promoting change and concordance.
- Health outcome measures, including quality of life, are important components in the evaluation of health-promoting interventions.
- Self-management is based on the principle of self-regulation and involves partnership between health care professionals and service users to promote expert patients.

Exercise

See after Chapter 10.

Further reading

DoH (Department of Health) (2002) *Self-management of Long-term Health Conditions: A Handbook for People with Chronic Disease*, www.expertpatients.nhs.uk/.

Marks, D.F., Murray, M., Evans, B.E., Willig, C., Woodall, C. and Sykes, C.M. (2006) *Health Psychology: Theory, Research and Practice*, 2nd edn. London: Sage.

Norman, P., Abraham, C. and Conner, M. (eds) (2000) *Understanding and Changing Health Behaviour: From Health Beliefs to Self-regulation*. Amsterdam: Harwood.

Ogden, J. (2004) *Health Psychology: A Textbook*, 3rd edn. Maidenhead: Open University Press.

Rutter, D. and Quine, L. (eds) (2002) *Changing Health Behaviour*. Buckingham: Open University Press.

Useful websites

EUROQOL: www.euroqol.org/

Illness Perception Questionnaire: www.uib.no/ipq/

Measure Yourself Medical Outcomes Profile (MYMOP): www.hsrc.ac.uk/mymop/

WHOQOL: www.who.int/substance_abuse/research_tools/whoqolbref/en/

PSYCHOLOGY OF PAIN

- **How are responses to pain learned?**
- **Why is the gate control theory of pain essential to our understanding of pain?**
- **What do we mean by placebo and why is it an important part of pain treatment?**
- **What are the differences between acute and chronic pain and why are these important for assessment and management?**
- **How does psychology inform the assessment and management of pain?**
- **How can we apply psychological principles to help manage complex pain problems?**

Introduction

This chapter seeks to address some of the challenges faced by professionals when advising and caring for people who have pain. We explore some important influences on pain perception and behaviours in response to acute and chronic pain and examine how this knowledge can be used to improve pain assessment and management. Our analysis draws on many of the psychological principles already covered in previous chapters. Therefore you will find that we often refer back to these for you to follow up in more detail. The examples used in this chapter are presented as if they were people and patients encountered by Anna and Janice. In fact, all are based closely on real observations and pseudonyms are used to protect confidentiality. We start by examining what is meant by pain.

Perceiving and expressing pain

Pain is a subjective emotional and physical experience which we feel as real in ourselves but can only interpret in others through their 'pain behaviours'. Like illness behaviours (Chapter 5), these include verbal complaints and self-report, non-verbal expressions and other behavioural reactions such as crying or limping, each of which is strongly affected by a diverse range of social, cultural and contextual influences. We are frequently reminded that 'pain is what the patient says it is', but this requires that we listen to what they say. When someone reports pain or complains about pain, it is important not to view it in isolation from the circumstances in which it occurs.

> Ellen was aged 84 and had trigeminal neuralgia (continuous intense facial pain) for 50 years. During that time, she had raised a daughter, run a successful dancing school and enjoyed retirement with her husband. But her husband and daughter had both died during the previous year. Now, she complained that the painkillers were useless, she could no longer bear the pain and wanted to die.

The pathology underlying Ellen's pain had remained unchanged in 50 years, but the pain had only recently become unbearable. It was her circumstances and emotional state that had changed. In this situation, any attempt to treat Ellen's pain without addressing her grief was unlikely to be of benefit. The same pain clearly can have different meanings for the same person at different points in time. It is therefore no surprise that it has different meanings for different people. Some people minimize pain while others express pain out of all proportion to its apparent cause. Professional judgements about pain are inevitably influenced by these different responses and also by the way they expect people to respond to a particular sort of pain. The following example illustrates how easy it is to draw the wrong conclusion about the 'severity' of someone's pain.

> Arthur was aged 82 and awaiting leg amputation because of severe peripheral vascular disease. He rated his leg pain as 'excruciating', but said he was not concerned about this as he had had it for a long time and knew what it was. His overwhelming concern was with a slight 'niggling' pain in his lower abdomen. Six years ago, he had surgery for bladder cancer and he was very afraid it might signal a recurrence.

Arthur illustrates how a mild pain is capable of causing more suffering than an excruciating pain. Pain assessment must take account of this and a good theory of pain must account for these types of anomaly.

Gate control theory of pain

Prior to the 1960s, it was supposed that there was some kind of direct relationship between the extent of tissue damage or injury and the intensity of the pain felt. Ronald Melzack, a Canadian psychologist, working with Patrick Wall, a London neuroscientist, radically changed this view with the publication of their gate control theory of pain (Melzack and Wall 1965). Gate theory explains a number of mechanisms by which pain signals are modulated between leaving the site of tissue damage and reaching the cerebral cortex.

Pain signals travel along fast and slow ascending pain transmission fibres from the site of tissue damage to the dorsal horn of the spinal cord where they enter a 'junction' (ganglion).

> When Lee started walking, he fell over and banged his knee. He felt a sharp blow, but didn't start to cry until a few moments later when a dull intense throb set in.

The timing of Lee's pain illustrates the effects of pain transmission along fast and slow pain fibres from the site of tissue damage. But when the pain signals reach the dorsal horn of the spinal cord, they may be modulated by competing ascending signals from touch fibres.

> When Lee bumped his knee, Sasha rubbed the area until he stopped crying.

Rubbing is effective in reducing pain because it stimulates the touch fibres to override the pain signal and effectively 'close the gate'. The effect of 'counterstimulation' led to the development of transcutaneous electrical nerve stimulation (TENS) for the management of pain (we refer to this later).

Also in the dorsal horn, the ascending pain signal is modulated by descending signals from the brain. The 'gate' is a metaphor for all these processes of modulation. It actually consists of various neurotransmitters and inhibitors which are released in the dorsal horn and either allow the full force of the pain to be transmitted to the brain (gate open), or prevent or limit the pain transmitted to the brain (gate closed). Research since the 1960s has identified a range of neurotransmitters that contribute to the 'pain gate' mechanism, including endorphins. Endorphins are the body's own (endogenous) pain-relieving substances, similar to opioids such as morphine, and opiates such as heroin. Table 10.1 identifies the main factors associated with the opening and closing of the pain gate.

Negative emotions indicative of suffering are largely responsible for the operation of the pain gate, just as they influence immune function (Chapter 8). Therefore stress plays an important role in the perception of pain.

Table 10.1 Factors associated with the opening and closing of the pain gate

	Factors that open the gate	*Factors that close the gate*
Physical	Extent of injury	Medication Counterstimulation
Emotional	Fear/anxiety Depression	Confidence/relaxation Optimism
Cognitive/behavioural	Focusing on the pain Having nothing to do Sense of helplessness/ hopelessness	Focused distraction/ active involvement Perceived control Perceived emotional support

Pain as a stressor

Pain is an unpleasant experience and is usually associated with injury or disease, which adds to stress (Chapter 8). Stressors directly associated with pain include:

- *Perceived uncertainty* about the nature of the painful condition and its potential consequences (Chapter 9). Questions patients are often afraid to ask include:
  - Have I picked up an infection?
  - Is it cancer?
- *Perceived unpredictability* about if and when the pain is likely to get worse, how long it will last and what the long outcome is likely to be, for example:
  - Will I end up in a wheelchair?
- *Perceived uncontrollability* if treatments and coping strategies are found to be ineffective:
  - Nothing I or anyone else does gets rid of this pain.

These appraisals cause anxiety, fear or depression, which in turn open the pain gate. Pre-existing or co-existing stressors, such as disability or loss, increase stress even more (Walker *et al.* 2006) and can make the pain unbearable. This helps to explain why responses to pain vary so much. But individual differences in pain perception and response are also caused by differences in experiences of pain throughout life.

Learning to perceive and express pain

Pain in babies

Pain is felt from an early stage of development. This presents particular problems for the care of premature, low birthweight and sick babies who are exposed to considerable pain and stress due to invasive monitoring and life-saving procedures. These include needle stick, suctioning and surgery. The long-term effects are not yet known, but may include hypersensitivity to pain and stress (Grunau *et al.* 2006). Good practice dictates that every attempt should be made to minimize the number of painful or stressful procedures wherever possible. Stress-reducing therapies before, during and afterwards include the use of pacifiers (non-nutritive sucking) and soothing music. As soon as is feasible, parental talking, singing, gentle stroking and cuddling should be encouraged (Halimaa 2003). Pre-emptive analgesia given in advance of invasive interventions is recommended although the long-term effects of opiates on the developing child are largely unknown.

Learning how to cope with pain

Decades of research indicate there is no such thing as a 'pain-prone' personality. But socialization is an important determinant of the ways people respond to and deal with pain and also accounts for cultural differences in pain behaviours.

> After he started walking, Lee fell over frequently but rarely injured himself, so Sasha became less concerned. When she heard a thud, she would call out 'you're all right'. Usually, the cry would stop immediately. If it didn't, she would run to find out what was wrong.

Why did Lee cry in the first scene but not in similar circumstances in the second? The answer lies in the process of modulation by descending signals from the brain. Lee gradually learned that pain did not automatically signal harm. This allowed his attention to be quickly diverted away from the pain. The combination of 'perceived low threat' and distraction was sufficient to 'close the gate' on his pain. Contrast this with Lee's friend, Jack.

> When Jack started walking, his mother was very afraid that he might hurt himself. She ran to check each time she heard a bump. She was upset and cuddled him whenever he cried.

Because of his mother's reactions Jack became afraid of hurting himself, leaving the gate wide open whenever he injured himself. Children such as Jack are often very nervous on admission to hospital, as are their mothers. On the other hand, when Jack went to play with Lee, he learned that falling over was not taken seriously and he did not cry so much. These age and often gender-related experiences shape adult responses to pain.

Alison and Clare, both aged 14, experienced premenstrual pain. Each month, Alison's mother encouraged her to go to school as usual, while Clare's mother allowed her to stay at home. Alison soon learned to control the pain with exercise and distraction whereas Clare relied on rest and painkillers. Clare also found that she could avoid demanding situations at school if she complained of pain. Thus Clare learned to use avoidance pain coping strategies, while Alison learned approach strategies (Chapter 8).

There is some evidence in the literature to suggest gender differences in pain, but these are also likely to be influenced by differences in pain experience. Musculoskeletal injuries are more common in boys, but boys are less experienced than girls at dealing with internal pains. Therefore it is likely that boys and girls grow up to respond differently to different types of pain.

Placebo and nocebo responses

The placebo response refers to an improvement in pain due to a placebo or 'dummy' treatment that confers no specific therapeutic benefit. It is caused by having a positive expectation about the effect of treatment. The opposite of placebo is nocebo:

- the placebo closes the pain gate and reduces pain;
- the nocebo opens the pain gate and makes the pain worse.

The placebo response to pain is mediated by the release of endorphins that 'close the gate' (Hoffman *et al.* 2005). The size of response depends on the level and type of expectation.

Anna could not understand why some people in hospital claimed their painkillers did not work as well as the same sort they took at home. She learned that changes in the size, shape or colour, caused by change of brand, can eliminate the placebo effect. One patient, when given an infusion of saline, reported that it had relieved her pain. Her colleagues claimed that this demonstrated the pain was not real. Anna was able to explain that the patient's belief in the infusion had led to the release of endorphins that were strong enough to provide significant pain relief.

Did you know?

- The placebo was shown to be mediated by endorphins because naloxone (the antidote to morphine) eliminates the effect (Benedetti *et al.* 2005).

- Because of this, placebo analgesia can induce respiratory depression in the same way as morphine (Benedetti 2006).
- A placebo can affect only the site at which the individual expects to gain pain relief (Benedetti *et al.* 1999).
- The placebo response is capable of producing a large effect. In an experimental study by Benedetti *et al.* (2005) the application of a placebo cream caused a mean reduction in reported pain of between 46 and 57 per cent, compared to 'no treatment'.
- Placebo responses are not confined to pain. A placebo intervention in patients with Parkinson's disease triggers the release of dopamine, while serotonin is implicated in the placebo response for patients with depression (Benedetti *et al.* 2005). Placebo effects have also been found to influence blood pressure, asthma, social phobia, hot flushes and many other problems.
- The placebo effect may be diminished in people with Alzheimer's disease because expectations are not so strong (Benedetti *et al.* 2006).

A significant proportion of the effect of many medications and treatments is likely to be due to placebo. It seems that the placebo harnesses the body's own healing mechanisms. This is why Gracely (2000) observed that health professionals should seek to use their gifts of empathy to promote natural healing responses in their patients. These qualities of caring may help to explain the success of many complementary therapies.

Psychological principles of pain assessment

Pain assessment is an important way of establishing the therapeutic relationship. Assessment is designed to elicit important information about the holistic needs of the patient. But as has already been demonstrated, to focus exclusively on pain is totally inadequate.

Diana was aged 75 and had rheumatoid arthritis for many years. The community nurse was asked to visit because she persistently complained of uncontrollable pain. The nurse assessed the intensity and location of the pain, together with the extent to which the pain limited Diana's ability to care for herself. As a result of this assessment, she made various recommendations for pain-relieving measures and home aids to facilitate independence. But following this, Diana continued to complain of uncontrollable pain. What the nurse had missed was the overwhelming sense of loss and guilt felt by Diana at having recently placed her learning disabled daughter in a care home.

Basic pain assessment should include the following:

- Measure and record pain over time:
  - Is it getting better or worse? It should never be used to compare one patient's pain with that of another.
- Monitor the impact of pain on the individual, as appropriate to the cause and duration of pain:
  - Physiological effects: blood pressure or signs of shock (acute pain).
  - Emotional effects: feelings about the pain, events surrounding the pain and their impact on well-being, quality of life and lifestyle (Chapter 9).
  - Functional effects: mobility, ability to perform self-care and other physical and role function tasks.
- The extent to which interventions have improved pain and well-being, for example, comfort measures, heat, exercise, analgesia.
- The extent to which interventions have given rise to unwanted side-effects, for example, indigestion, nausea or vomiting, constipation.
- If the pain is not well controlled or is getting worse, listen to, agree and record the patient's key concerns, goals and expectations.

In this way, pain assessment can be linked more directly to the type of intervention that is most appropriate to the patient, the problem and the situation (see Hodgins 2002). It may range from the giving of analgesia or a laxative, or requesting aids to independence, to inviting the chaplain to visit.

Measuring and recording pain

Key issues covered next include:

- what to measure;
- how to measure it – any measure must be shown to be valid and reliable and suited to the needs of the individual;
- when to measure it.

Location of the pain

- The location should be recorded on a body chart (see Brief Pain Inventory, below) – patients who are able may do this for themselves, but many confuse left with right and need help.
- If there is more than one site or cause, these should be assessed and recorded separately.
- Children, and many adults, particularly those with cognitive deficits, have difficulty locating pain. Children often use the term 'headache' to refer to any sort of pain, including tummy ache or sore throat. It is important to ask people to show you exactly where the pain is.

Severity or intensity of the pain

The most common measures of pain intensity used with adults are as follows.

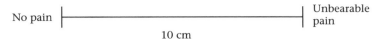

Figure 10.1   Visual Analogue Scale (VAS)

Visual Analogue Scale (VAS). The VAS usually consists of a 10 centimetre line that reflects the distance between 'No Pain and 'Worst Pain Ever (or imaginable)' (see Figure 10.1). Many patients report that it is hard to know what the worst pain would feel like and find it easier to relate to the term 'unbearable'. The validity of the VAS score is reported to be improved if administered vertically (Stephenson and Herman 2000). The pain score is measured from the 'no pain' end with the aid of a ruler. This form of measurement is normally considered most sensitive for research purposes. However, some find it conceptually difficult and it excludes those with poor eyesight. If it is used, always make sure patients are wearing clean spectacles, if they have them, and check they can read the writing at each end of the VAS.

Numerical Rating Scale (NRS). The NRS is normally a number from 0 to 10. This has the advantage of verbal administration, but is problematic for those with hearing deficits.

Verbal Rating Scale (VRS). The VRS is the easiest pain measurement scale to use in practice. It is reported as most appropriate for use with older people and can be used with those with all but severe levels of cognitive deficit (Ferrell *et al.* 1995; Closs *et al.* 2004). It consists of a series of words that reflect the intensity of the pain. It can be administered either verbally or visually and recorded as a number. It is increasingly common to find the use in practice of a four-point scale (0 no pain to 3 severe pain). However, this can lead to a 'ceiling effect', which means that it fails to differentiate between severe and extremely severe pain. A six-point scale (0–5) is generally more acceptable to patients and more sensitive to change. Examples include the Present Pain Intensity scale (PPI, Melzack 2005) and the Evaluative scale of the McGill Pain Questionnaire (MPQ, Melzack 2005) which measures bearability.

	PPI	**MPQ Evaluative scale**
0	No pain	No pain
1	Mild	Annoying
2	Discomforting	Troublesome
3	Distressing	Miserable
4	Horrible	Intense
5	Excruciating	Unbearable

Selection of 'miserable, intense or unbearable' from the evaluative scale provides an indicator of psychological distress, as do the words 'frightening' and 'punishing, cruel and vicious', taken from the affective scale of the MPQ. People who use these words are generally not coping well with their pain and need additional support.

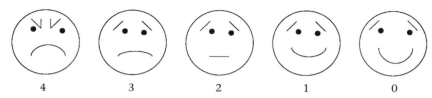

Figure 10.2   Happy/sad faces scale

Pictorial scales

Happy/sad faces scales are available for use with children and those with a moderate to severe cognitive deficit. An example is given in Figure 10.2. It is important to note that pain may be indistinguishable from other sources of distress when using this measure.

Measure of pain relief

Similar scales can be used to measure relief from pain, ranging from no relief to total relief. It is important to identify how long the relief lasted, and if there were any adverse effects of treatment, such as nausea, indigestion, tiredness, loss of concentration or difficulty maintaining balance.

Temporal pattern of pain

It is necessary to measure and monitor changes in the location and intensity of each pain over time. In hospitalized patients, routine assessment may take place four-hourly, or more frequently if the pain is not under control. However, there is little point in asking someone who has chronic pain, or is visited at home, what their pain is like 'right now'. Instead, using a VRS or NRS, ask the following:

- During the last day (or week or month), how would you rate your pain when it was at its worst?
- During the last day (or week or month), how would you rate your pain when it was at its least troublesome?

You can use this information to find out what influenced these changes. Patients living at home may be asked to keep a diary of pain and surrounding events for a short period, to identify 'trigger' factors (see below).

Sensory description of pain

Not all pain feels the same and variations in description can help with diagnosis. Yet people find it very difficult to find the right words to describe their pain. The MPQ describes ten separate sensory and miscellaneous dimensions which include: 'throbbing, shooting, stabbing, sharp, gnawing, burning, stinging, aching, penetrating'. The MPQ is rarely used in clinical practice, but similar words are included in the Brief Pain Inventory (see below) and may be useful for diagnostic purposes.

Pain triggers and contextual factors

Having assessed the pattern of pain, it is important to investigate what influences it for better or worse. This can help to identify interventions to promote comfort and relief. For example, people who have arthritis typically have worse pain and stiffness in the mornings and may need analgesia to help them to get moving. The gate control theory emphasizes the importance of assessing concurrent stressors, which can range from worry about the care of a pet, through concerns about the longer term implications of the painful condition, to recent loss of a partner or spouse. The following incident highlights the potential impact of patients' concerns and the importance of assessing these.

Brenda mentioned a pain, which she rated as 'mild', to the practice nurse at a routine visit. Fortunately, the nurse noticed her high level of anxiety and took time to elicit her concerns. It transpired that her friend had died of breast cancer. When Brenda developed a persistent unilateral (one-sided) pain across her back, painkillers had no effect at all. She had become convinced that she, too, might have the disease. The nurse arranged for the doctor to give her a detailed examination at which he excluded cancer and diagnosed post-herpetic neuralgia – Brenda lived alone and probably never spotted the shingles rash on her back. The next time she attended the surgery, Brenda reported that the pain was still there, just the same, but now she hardly noticed it. She described her life as 'transformed' by the care she received at her last visit.

This incident serves as another reminder of the significance of the patient's concerns.

Pain coping strategies

These include all of the pain-relieving or comfort measures that people use to help control their own pain and are often more effective than analgesia. People who have a chronic or persistent pain often find the pain gets worse on admission to hospital because they no longer have access to their favoured strategies. These include: having comfortable pillows, mattresses and chairs; doing housework, getting meals, moving around at night and making a cup of tea; exercises, music, hot water bottles, favourite rubs, sprays, over-the-counter medications and complementary therapies. Even if they have no medical validity, these strategies promote perceived control (Chapter 8), which in turn helps to close the pain gate.

Global assessment of chronic pain

The Brief Pain Inventory (BPI, Cleeland 1991) encompasses most of the aspects discussed above and is freely available on the internet at the time of writing. The long form is more comprehensive and has been adopted for use in many pain clinics. The short form (two pages) focuses on the pain location, intensity (worst, least), relief obtained and interference with activities. This would provide a very helpful tool for assessing persistent pain in hospital settings. There are cultural differences in pain expression, and in some situations assessment may be undertaken using a language that is not the patient's own, or using a translator. Therefore, Lasch (2000: 19) has identified a series of questions that might be helpful. We have adapted these for general purposes.

- What do you call your pain? How do you describe it?
- Why do you think you have this pain?
- Do you have any fears about your pain? If so, what do you fear?
- What are the chief problems that your pain causes for you?
- What kind of treatment do you think you should receive?
- What are the most important results that you hope to receive from the treatment?
- What remedies have you tried to help you with your pain?

Pain assessment in those unable to communicate

Babies and those with severe cognitive deficits who are unable to communicate pain present a serious challenge, since pain must be deduced from non-verbal and behavioural expressions. These include a combination of the following.

- Signs of current or former physical trauma or disease normally associated with pain.
- Physiological responses indicative of stress (Chapter 8).
- Vocalizations: grunting, whimpering, crying.
- Facial expression, grimacing, signs of tension, fear.
- Body language: rocking, guarding, agitation.
- Behaviour change: loss of appetite, bouts of confusion or aggression.

A number of observational tools have been developed, based on these types of observation, but all require 'knowing the person'. The following may be helpful, depending on the client group.

Babies and young children

For a review of available approaches to assessment and management, see American Academy of Pediatrics (2006). Scales include the Bernese Pain Scale for Neonates (Cignacco et al. 2004).

Older people with dementia

There are a number of observational tools. A systematic review by Zwakhalen (2006) identified two valid and reliable tools, of which the DOLOPLUS2 scale is most easy to use (freely available on the internet at the time of writing).

People with severe learning difficulties

There is little literature on this topic and no valid and reliable tool tested for this group. The literature focuses on behavioural signs (see above), which depend on intimate knowledge of the client's usual behavioural pattern. A review of assessment and management challenges is offered by Jones (2003). As people with severe learning difficulties live longer, they can expect to experience similar chronic pain problems as the general population. Carers should remember to look out for signs of common causes of pain in otherwise healthy individuals. For example, head-banging might suggest toothache; doubling up and rocking could indicate constipation; stiffness in older people may indicate arthritis.

The aim of pain management

Having assessed pain and its impact, it is essential that all members of the multidisciplinary team share a common aim for pain management, bearing in mind that it is not always possible to relieve pain entirely. Don Berwick, a leader in the field of health care improvement, proposed that the primary aim should be to 'eliminate or reduce human suffering'. Physical pain (nociception) and suffering are not the same (see Bendelow 2006). Suffering implies distress. Pain does not always cause distress, as illustrated by Lee's falls, but distress can leave the pain gate wide open. As illustrated by Ellen, it is not unusual for someone who has suffered a bereavement or other distressing event to find that a bearable pain has become intolerable. Based on these observations, a group of nurses attending a pain workshop proposed that a suitable aim might be: 'No individual should ever have more pain than they are willing or able to bear'.

Promoting coping

Understanding, sympathy, comfort, security, reassurance, confidence and someone to listen are rated highly as ways of promoting coping.

The following responses were received from older people to the question, 'What do you think that nurses can do to help people in pain?'

- Be someone you can rely on – gives you a feeling of security.
- Give them confidence and be truthful.
- A sympathetic ear – though not soft as people must cope.
- The worst thing is uncaring and unkindness.

Lack of time is no excuse:
- She [the district nurse] gave me the assurance that she had the time, even though she did not really (Walker 1994).

Martin was partially sighted, had poor health and had attended hospital

> many times. He expressed much dissatisfaction with various episodes of care, but reported a very positive memory of attending an accident and emergency department with acute urinary retention. The doctor greeted him by observing, 'You poor thing, you must be in agony.' He observed, 'She was wonderful.'
>
> (Walker *et al.* 1998)

Acts of kindness and compassion or merely acknowledging pain can help to close the gate on pain and leave a lasting positive memory for the patient. Acts of unkindness and lack of compassion open the pain gate and also store up a lasting sense of fear for future occasions. These principles apply to all types of pain.

Types of pain

Different types of pain pose different demands and therefore require different approaches to coping and management. From a psychological perspective, it is helpful to distinguish between the following.

Acute pain

This refers to pain associated with a single episode of tissue damage due to injury, trauma or surgery, which is normally expected to resolve upon healing.

Chronic cancer pain

Pain due to the invasion of cancer cells or effects of cancer treatment. It is chronic in the sense that it is continuing and often progressive, but it is usually bounded in duration by the limited life-expectancy of the patient. However, cancer patients often experience acute episodes that need to be treated as acute pain and may develop persistent pains that are not directly caused by the cancer.

Chronic or persistent benign pain

Pain associated with a known disease process such as arthritis, or unknown pathology where malignant causes (red flags) have been excluded. It may be continuous, as in the case of neuropathic pain, or intermittent as in the case of migraine or angina. Barring spontaneous resolution or new technologies, it may last for the remainder of the individual's life, no matter how young they are.

'Neuropathic' pain is an important cause of chronic and cancer pain. It is so named because damaged nerves continue to transmit pain signals spontaneously and continuously, even long after disease or trauma. Examples include trapped nerves (as in carpal tunnel syndrome); accidental mechanical damage due to trauma, vibration injury or surgery; toxic nerve damage due to chemotherapy; post-herpetic (shingles) and other neuralgias (see the example of Ellen); arthritis, metabolic nerve damage including diabetic neuropathy; and phantom pain in which pain continues to feel as though it comes from an amputated limb or other body part. Although tricyclic antidepressants, opioids and anticonvulsant drugs can provide modest relief, there is no cure for neuropathic pain. Therefore psychological management is fundamental to pain control.

Psychological issues in acute pain

Pain and acute trauma

> Mark read an account in the newspaper of a farmer whose arm was severed in farm machinery but felt no pain until he got to hospital. Anna had recently been on placement in accident and emergency and made a similar observation, but was not sure how to explain it.

Beecher (1959) reported similar observations among soldiers injured on the battlefield during World War II. He explained it in terms of their relief at escaping from the front line. It is more likely, based on recent research, that intense focus on escape or task completion leads to the release of endorphins that close the pain gate (Wall 1999). Not all people experience this to the same degree, giving rise to wide variations in pain following comparable injuries.

Post-operative and post-trauma pain

Interventions that help to control acute pain include:

- emotional support, so that the person in pain feels secure and cared for;
- regular assessment of pain, along with emotional state and key concerns, combined with adequate frequency and strength of analgesia;
- information aimed at reducing uncertainty and anxiety about pain and promoting sense of control;
- timely advice and reminders about using appropriate coping strategies and comfort measures;
- patient-controlled analgesia (PCA) and/or adequate and reliable offering and giving of analgesia.

Acute pain, if uncontrolled, can lead to chronic pain (for mechanisms, see Carr and Goudas 1999).

Anxiety, information and pain

It has been recognized since the 1950s that anxiety increases pain. In the 1970s, Hayward (1994) showed that pre-operative information-giving reduced post-operative anxiety and pain. At about the same time, Langer went further by demonstrating that the type of information is important.

> Langer et al. (1975) compared two groups of surgical patients. One was given standard procedural information about what would happen during surgery; the other group was taught how to use imagery to control their anxiety following surgery. Langer observed that procedural information raised anxiety in the immediate term and had no effect on post-operative anxiety or pain. In contrast, information about how to use imagery lowered levels of post-operative anxiety and need for pain relief.

Information about what sensations to expect post-operatively and how to deal with these, including when and how to ask for help, are important aspects of pre-operative information-giving. McCann and Kain (2001) provide a useful review of pre-operative anxiety management in children, for whom similar principles apply.

Patient-controlled analgesia (PCA)

During the 1960s and 1970s, psychology experiments demonstrated that the belief they could terminate a painful stimulus enabled people to tolerate more pain. These studies were instrumental in piloting and introducing PCA into clinical practice. A meta-analysis of research findings (Hudcova et al. 2005) found that, in general, PCA leads to better pain control and patient satisfaction. PCA, within defined limits, has been shown to be effective in children and adolescents (Berde et al. 1991) provided they are able to understand the concept (Chapter 3). Not all patients are capable of or want to control their own analgesia (see locus of control, Chapter 5). In order to make effective use of PCA, patients require good preparation and continuing support from staff. Therefore PCA should not be seen as a time-saving option. The duration of PCA should be linked to assessment of the pain and analgesia consumption. Its removal should be a matter of negotiation between staff and patient, though we are aware that this often fails to happen. If the patient is still in severe pain, it is unethical to reduce or withdraw analgesia without full medical examination, since it may indicate the presence of infection or the onset of neuropathic pain.

> Diane was the mother of two children with severe learning difficulties who also required a lot of physical care. She had carpal tunnel syndrome (trapped nerves) in both wrists and opted for surgery to her right (dominant) hand. Post-operatively, her complaints about pain in her right shoulder were dismissed: 'Your operation was on your hand, not your shoulder.' Following discharge, the pain in her arm and shoulder became unbearable. After several months, she was referred to the pain clinic where she was diagnosed as having a form of neuropathic pain caused by the surgical nerve damage. Sue was most angry about the response to her pain in hospital. As someone who gave her life to caring for others, she felt she deserved better.

Techniques and strategies that help to control pain are reviewed towards the end of this chapter.

Psychological issues in terminal illness

Pain is not an inevitable consequence of cancer or terminal illness, though pain control was one of the reasons that Dame Cicely Saunders started the modern hospice movement. Symptom management and particularly pain control is one of the most common reasons for referral to specialist palliative care. However, people diagnosed with terminal illnesses may be cared for in general or specialist hospital wards, hospices or at home. Therefore all nurses need to understand the principles. According to the World Health Organization (WHO) working parties for adults and children (Sepúlveda *et al.* 2002), palliative care starts at an early stage and aims to achieve the following:

- relief from pain and other distressing symptoms;
- integrate psychological and spiritual aspects of patient care (adults), evaluate and alleviate physical, psychological and social distress (children);
- offer support to help patients live as actively as possible until death;
- offer support to help the family cope during the patient's illness and in their own bereavement;
- enhance quality of life.

Using the BPI, Twycross *et al.* (1996) demonstrated that most cancer patients have pain from more than one source. It is important to assess all of these and negotiate which needs most urgent attention. Wherever possible, early intervention should facilitate self-management (Chapter 9). Numerous support networks exist, and self-help information is available on the internet (see end of chapter). Cancer patients should be helped and encouraged to maintain their desired lifestyle or substitute other enjoyable activities for as long as they can, in order to stimulate the release of endorphins and provide distraction from pain. People with cancer and their caregivers face considerable threat and loss and may need help to deal with anticipatory grief (Chapter 6) or depression (Williams and Payne 2003).

The analgesic ladder (WHO 2007) should act as a guide to analgesia, starting at a level appropriate to the severity of the pain experienced. PCA can be used effectively by many patients, including children, provided they are adequately prepared. From a psychological perspective:

- There is no reason whatsoever to ration the use of morphine or opiate analgesia for patients who have a terminal illness, unless or until the patient decides that the side-effects outweigh the benefits.
- It is important to assess patients' attitudes towards strong analgesia and address misapprehensions. Risk of addiction is unlikely and irrelevant in this group of patients.
- People often weigh the benefits of treatment against the adverse effects. Assessment and management of medication side-effects and other symptoms should take place alongside the assessment and management of pain, in order to facilitate optimal use of analgesia.

There is good evidence that patients themselves appear reluctant to complain of pain or take adequate analgesia to control the pain, no matter how advanced their disease.

> Coward and Wilkie (2000) reported on narrative interviews with 20 patients who had metastatic bone cancer. Although pain interfered with work, social activities and relationships, most participants preferred not to tell others, including health care providers, about their pain. More than half did not take pain medications in accordance with their prescription.

Refusal to take medication can cause considerable distress for all concerned.

> Wendy, in her 50s, was in the late stages of cancer and being nursed at home by her husband and daughters. Her family did not want her to have morphine because they believed that signalled 'the end', and Wendy refused to have it. Her pain became so bad that she screamed when the nurses tried to move her. They found this very distressing and blamed the family. At her funeral, the family and the nurses were unable to look at or speak to each other.

The problem here is that the focus of the nurses' attention was on the pain, rather than on the emotional needs of the patient and her family. This probably caused them to miss issues that left the pain gate open. Furthermore, the nurses appear to have adopted a didactic or authoritarian approach to pain management which has been shown not to be effective (Schumacher 2002). A shared problem-solving approach involving dialogue between nursing staff, the family and Wendy was more likely to have achieved mutual agreement about the problems and possible solutions.

As it was, Wendy's death involved immense suffering which left the family and the nurses with very distressing memories to resolve. Contrast this with a positive scenario:

> Anna accompanied the palliative care nurse to visit a family whose daughter Susy, aged 9, had an inoperable tumour in her spine. The palliative care nurse had taught Susy and her family how to use PCA to control pain (with an anti-emetic to control nausea). This enabled Susy to use her wheelchair and maintain a range of activities, with advice and support from the social worker, occupational therapist and school teacher. She spent short periods in the local children's hospice for review of symptom management and respite, but died peacefully at home. All the staff mentioned supported the family at the funeral and it was agreed that the palliative care nurse would continue to provide supportive contact during their bereavement.

Psychological issues in chronic or persistent benign pain

Chronic pain is often defined as pain that has lasted for at least three months, although some persistent pain may need to be treated as potentially chronic prior to this. Others define it as pain that has persisted beyond the healing time needed for recovery from injury or tissue damage (Chapman *et al.* 1999), although some conditions, such as arthritis and cancer, involve persistent tissue damage. Chronic pain is so-named because there is no known medical cure.

Nurses and other health care professionals increasingly encounter hospital patients who have acute exacerbations of chronic pain, or chronic pain in addition to the acute condition they are being treated for. It is inappropriate to treat chronic benign pain as if it was acute pain, using the analgesic ladder, because continued use eventually reduces its effectiveness (this is termed tolerance). Similarly, medical interventions such as nerve blocks offer only short-term solutions to a long-term problem. The emphasis needs to be on self-management (Chapter 9) and the development of effective problem-solving coping strategies which aim to reduce suffering (not just pain) and improve quality of life.

Those with chronic pain have a choice of pain management programmes delivered by pain clinics, the Expert Patient Programme (Chapter 9), local self-help groups such as those run by Action on Pain, and internet support from sites such as Dipex (see information at end of chapter). Evidence from systematic reviews of the effectiveness of multi-professional pain management programmes is currently lacking due to methodological problems (Thomsen *et al.* 2001). However, a community-based nurse-led programme (Lefort *et al.* 1998), based on Lorig's arthritis self-management course (Chapter 9), demonstrated improvements in important aspects of quality of life including pain, dependency, self-efficacy, vitality, role functioning and life satisfaction.

Coming to terms with chronic pain

Chronic pain often starts out as acute pain (see example of Diane). Persistent pain leads people to a search for a diagnosis and a cure (Chapter 9). A lot of people with chronic pain, including those with back pain and low abdominal pain, have no verifiable diagnostic signs, often because it is caused by soft tissue injury or disease. To make matters worse, a number of studies have demonstrated that patients without a confirmed diagnosis or whose condition fails to respond to treatment are stigmatized by medical and nursing staff (Walker *et al.* 1999; Higgins 2005; Holloway *et al.* in press; see also the unpopular patient, Chapter 2). Some people spend years searching for a 'magic bullet' cure. Doctors are often reluctant to remove hope and offer one treatment or consultation after another, but this just maintains false hope and prevents effective coping. Pain management depends on developing a goal-directed approach that promotes quality of life *in spite of pain*.

Managing the transition from acute to chronic pain is currently a major challenge for clinicians who view the inability to cure as defeat. Some important factors that affect successful pain adjustment are discussed below. Helpful overviews of current psychological issues in the management of chronic pain, including back pain, can be found in Eccleston (2001) and Main and Williams (2002).

Ways of improving quality of life for those who have chronic pain

Understand the patient's real needs

- Patients sometimes complain of physical pain, rather than admit to feelings of anxiety, helplessness or loss. It is important to assess the circumstances that surround the pain including those that have suddenly made the pain worse, as in the case of Ellen.
- Where appropriate, ask the patient why they sought help at this particular time.
- Ask about the individual's chief concerns and how they are coping with life.
- Clarify their understanding of the causes and consequences of their pain and options available to help them cope with it.

Opioid analgesia and NSAIDs

The use of opioids in chronic benign pain is contentious. The pharmaceutical industry is keen to encourage their use, while one of the main aims of pain management programmes is to reduce their use. The regular use of opioids inevitably causes constipation, which some people regard as worse than the original pain. Non-steroidal anti-inflammatory drugs (NSAIDs) are quite effective in controlling pain from arthritis and other conditions, but long-term use can lead to gastric side-effects (including haemorrhage) and increased risk of heart disease. Overall, these are important reasons for hospital admission in elderly people. Alternative helpful interventions include:

- encouraging and supporting as many other ways of coping with pain or controlling the pain as possible, including the use of complementary therapies;
- giving information about the local pain clinic, self-help group or self-management programme (see suggestions at the end of this chapter).

Hospital admissions

Chronic pain often gets worse on admission to hospital because the patient loses access to their usual pain coping strategies and is under stress because of illness. People who have chronic pain can find themselves avoided or ignored because staff don't understand their needs.

- Provide opportunities for patients to maintain their coping strategies while in hospital.
- Patients may need an increase in analgesia while in hospital, but need to understand that this is not a long-term solution.
- There should be a discharge plan to help patients reduce analgesia and develop other coping strategies on discharge (see above).

Ensure that advice is evidence-based and patients understand potential adverse reactions

Some people adhere to treatment regimes and recommendations in spite of adverse reactions, mostly because explanations about potential side-effects were not given. Yet some medical interventions have recently been found to be ineffective or even damaging.

Janice and Mark had a friend, Ray, who had suffered from back pain for the last ten years. When his back initially seized up for no apparent reason, he was advised (incorrectly) to take bed rest. When the pain persisted, he tried various medications, treatments and complementary therapies to no avail. He was unable to return to work and eventually lost his job. He spent more and more time lying down for fear that pain on movement indicated further harm to his back. He kept returning to his doctor in the hope of finding a cure.

The advice to take bed rest was routine until quite recently. But research into its outcomes led Waddell (1992: 544) to describe it as 'the most damaging treatment ever devised for backache and a potent cause of iatrogenic [medically induced] disability'. Bed rest leads to loss of muscle strength, encourages passive coping (Chapter 8) and seriously reduces cardiovascular fitness.

- Professionals need to ensure that the advice and information is evidence-based and suited to the type of pain experienced.
- Patients taking medication over a long period of time need to be made

aware of the potential side-effects and ways of overcoming or avoiding these wherever possible.
- Increasing activity and exercise are important components of all pain management programmes.

Reduce fear-avoidance

Patients avoid movements that cause pain for fear that they are causing themselves damage. Explanations that focus on degenerative disease are particularly unhelpful (people believe that their body is wearing out). Researchers have suggested that 'fear-avoidance' is the main cause of disability in people with chronic pain (Vlaeyen and Linton 2000), and have developed behavioural programmes to reduce them (Boersma *et al.* 2000; see Chapter 5). Fears need to be identified and addressed at an early stage. All pain management programmes emphasize that chronic pain is no longer associated with tissue damage, and focus on ways of increasing exercise and activity levels which also increase the circulation of endorphins. Once activities have become severely restricted, a programme of 'paced' exercise, such as walking, is required (starting very gently from a baseline well within pain tolerance and increasing very slowly). Patience and perseverance are needed to improve function in the long term.

- Before giving advice, find out the patient's beliefs (Chapter 4).
- Professionals should emphasize that chronic pain does not signal damage is occurring.
- Explanations for pain that focus on damage, wear and tear or degeneration should be avoided since they induce fear and hopelessness (Eccleston 2001). A lot of musculoskeletal pain is caused by muscle spasm.
- Optimistic advice on improving fitness, no matter how modest, is helpful – there is always some part of the body that will benefit from exercise.

Catastrophizing

Catastrophizing refers to the belief that things are awful and can only get worse (Janssen *et al.* 2002; see negative affectivity, Chapter 6). It remains unclear if this is due to having a pessimistic disposition (Sullivan *et al.* 2001) or to the impact of loss (Walker *et al.* 2006). But when dealing with patients who have a negative outlook, it is worth making time to listen to their stories because they usually present reasonable explanations for their distress, some of which are amenable to change.

- It is helpful to listen to the reasons for negative attitudes (see Chapter 6) and offer recommendations or referrals for further support (on discharge if necessary).
- It is a good idea to explain the gate control theory of pain so that patients understand the link between emotions and pain (and this does not imply that the pain is 'in the mind').
- If a patient seems depressed or admits to feeling depressed they need to be referred for proper assessment (Chapter 6).

Practical help with daily living

As was identified in Chapter 8, instrumental support can encourage passive coping and it has been shown that having an attentive spouse or partner, the sort who takes over roles or activities from the person in pain, is associated with greater levels of pain behaviours and depression in those with chronic pain (Walker and Sofaer 1998; Thieme *et al.* 2005). Help is often given with the best of intentions – it is very hard to see a loved one struggle. Professionals need to work with family members as well as the patient to encourage self-care, exercise and other activities.

Another potential negative influence arises if state disability benefits are withdrawn once the individual is judged fit to work. It is difficult for those with a history of chronic pain to obtain work and the threat of loss of income limits improvement and encourages passivity. It is advisable to ask the patient to identify such potential barriers and ask them how they think they might be able to overcome these, or negotiate how it is possible to work within these constraints.

Co-existing stressors and stress-related disorders

We have dealt with most of these aspects already. But it is worth noting that there is a relatively high incidence of post-traumatic stress disorder (PTSD) in people with chronic pain and it often goes unrecognised. If someone has experienced a traumatic injury or incident, check for symptoms of PTSD (see Chapter 6). If appropriate, advise them to ask their doctor for a referral to a psychologist who specializes in the treatment of PTSD.

Evidence-based therapies for acute and chronic pain

Most of the following techniques are helpful for all types of pain, provided the patient has adequate preparation.

Transcutaneous electrical nerve stimulation (TENS)

TENS is based on the principle of counter-stimulation (see gate control theory). It consists of a battery-operated device that delivers a small variable electrical current to the region of the pain via adhesive pads. Because it is operated by the patient, it serves the additional purpose of promoting personal control (Chapters 5 and 8). TENS has been shown to be effective in improving pain control in labour (van der Spank *et al.* 2000) and in chronic pain due to known pathologies such as knee pain (Osiri *et al.* 2000). Reviews of its effect on other chronic pains, including back pain, have proved inconclusive (Carroll *et al.* 2006). This may be because of the complexity of the psychosocial issues associated with chronic pain. But TENS is non-invasive and worth a trial.

Relaxation and imagery

Relaxation is intended to counter anxiety (Chapter 5) and reduce muscle tension which contributes to muscle spasm and pain. The most common approach, taught in antenatal classes, is progressive muscle relaxation (PMR), pioneered by Jacobson in the 1920s, in which the individual tenses and then relaxes each muscle group in turn until a complete state of relaxation is achieved. Imagery helps to maintain relaxation by diverting the mind from other concerns and promoting calmness.

In their systematic review of relaxation for acute and chronic pain, Kwekkeboom and Gretarsdottir (2006) found only 15 published studies that focused solely on the effect of relaxation on pain. Interventions ranged from a single session for acute pain to several months in the case of chronic pain. Relaxation was compared with various control interventions including 'usual treatment' and massage. Of the 13 studies in which patients used relaxation repeatedly over a period of time, 8 demonstrated pain relief, whereas one-off use (for acute pain) showed no effect. The authors suggested that frequent practice of relaxation over several weeks or months is required to achieve positive outcomes.

When faced with a patient in acute pain, the instruction to 'relax' is potentially unhelpful since it can trigger a stress response in individuals who have no prior training and find relaxing difficult to achieve.

Mindfulness meditation

Unlike other forms of mental imagery where the individual is encouraged to focus attention away from the body, mindfulness meditation is based on a Buddhist tradition that encourages the individual to focus on the reality of the present moment, without allowing the intrusion of thoughts about or emotional reactions to the situation (Kabat-Zinn *et al.* 1985). It has recently regained popularity as 'mindfulness-based stress reduction' (MBSR) (Baer 2003; Grossman *et al.* 2004). This has been shown to be effective in assisting in the self-management of chronic pain, cancer pain and a variety of other medical conditions.

Acupuncture

Acupuncture involves the subcutaneous insertion of fine needles that are believed to stimulate the release of endorphins. There are two different types of acupuncture: Chinese acupuncture where needles are inserted in distal meridian points, such as the ear; and western acupuncture where needles are inserted close to the site of the pain, with or without additional electrical stimulation. Some evidence has been presented for the effectiveness of acupuncture in the treatment of musculoskeletal pain (Ezzo *et al.* 2000) and cancer pain (Lee *et al.* 2005). But many of the studies have been of poor quality and much of the effect may be due to placebo. Anecdotal information from patients attending a pain clinic suggests that even where acupuncture does not relieve pain it can promote relaxation and sleep for a limited period.

Cognitive behaviour therapy (CBT)

There is good evidence that CBT (Chapter 6) is effective in helping to promote the self-management of chronic pain (Vlaeyen and Morley 2005), though these authors identify the need for further research to match people and problems to particular aspects of treatment.

> Morley *et al.* (1999) reported a systematic review and meta-analysis of CBT compared to control treatments and no treatment for chronic pain (an update is awaited at the time of writing). Compared to waiting list control, CBT was associated with a moderate level of improvement on all measures. Compared to alternative active treatments, CBT produced significant improvements in pain experience, cognitive coping and appraisal (positive coping measures), and reduced behavioural expression of pain. It did not show a reduction in depression, cognitive appraisals of coping or social role functioning. In spite of this, the authors concluded that CBT was an effective treatment for the management of chronic pain.

As we have argued, different people have different needs and therapeutic goals. Therefore, it is important that outcomes for people with chronic pain are judged according to their own priorities (Chapter 9). Pain research has yet to address these important issues.

Case study: Pam

This in-depth case study is based on an encounter that took place in an outpatient clinic and involves multiple problems of the kind that makes care professionals feel helpless. We use it to illustrate how a person-centred approach, rather than a pain-centred approach, can help all concerned. It incorporates principles of motivational interviewing (Chapter 9) which are transferable to many other situations.

> The nurse met Pam and Rob in the corridor after they had attended for a consultation with the pain consultant. Pam was in tears and her husband looked angry.

Non-verbal signs of anger and distress suggested that neither Pam nor Rob felt their needs had been addressed as a result of their consultation (Chapter 7). The nurse took them to a private room and asked them to tell their story.

Rob spoke while Pam sat with her head in her hands and cried. He explained that Pam had extremely poor circulation. Pam held out her blue hands as he explained that the fingers on her left hand had already been part amputated and those on her right hand caused excruciating pain most of the time. They had come to the clinic to seek relief from the pain, but the doctor told them he was unable to provide treatment until Pam gave up smoking. Rob expressed the view that everyone in health care was anti-smoking, but that it was unreasonable to expect Pam to succeed in view of her problems.

The treatment considered was sympathectomy. This involves cutting the sympathetic nerve supply to the arms to increase the circulation to the hands. But smoking would negate this because nicotine constricts the peripheral blood vessels. The doctor had probably explained this, but neither Pam nor Rob had either heard or understood it (Chapter 4). They had interpreted the advice to stop smoking as an instruction, but the doctor had not offered an action plan to help them (Chapter 9).

The nurse explained why it was necessary to stop smoking. She sympathized and commented that since the doctor was himself a heavy smoker he would appreciate these difficulties.

The psychology of persuasion suggests that health advice is better received if it appears unbiased (Chapter 7). Rob felt Pam was being stigmatized for lack of willpower (Chapter 2). But it was becoming clear that Pam was under a lot of stress due to her illness and possibly other issues (Chapter 8), leading to a sense of helplessness and hopelessness, which in turn increased the pain. The nurse decided to adopt a motivational interview style (Chapter 9), starting by inviting Pam and Rob to tell their story.

Rob explained that he and Pam, aged 42, had been married for over 20 years. About 10 years ago, Pam had developed a drink problem which became so bad that he left her.

Alcohol is often used as self-medication to reduce pain and help people to forget traumatic experiences. It is a form of emotion-focused coping (Chapter 8). A little later, it might be helpful to find out the reasons for her drinking, as it might contribute to her current emotional state.

Her circulation gradually got worse and then, two years ago, Pam had a stroke that left her with a slight right-sided weakness (she was left-handed) and slow in formulating speech. This, Rob explained, was why Pam did not like talking to people. Rob returned home to look after her on the promise that she would give up drinking, which she did.

Rob paused at this point while both he and the nurse shared admiration for Pam. Alcoholism in women is stigmatized (Chapter 2), and there is a tendency to focus on the addiction, rather than the success of stopping.

Rob explained how he cared for Pam. He took her breakfast in bed, helped her dress and undress, did all the housework and cooking. He was self-employed and went home at lunchtime to get her a midday meal.

The literature on chronic pain suggests that instrumental support (practical help) can reduce personal control and lead to dependence (Chapter 8 and this chapter). By this time, Pam had gained confidence to join in the conversation and it was obvious that speech therapy was no longer needed. The nurse asked Pam to describe her typical day.

Pam described how she watched television all day. But she could identify only one programme that she enjoyed and this was something she and Rob watched together in the evening.

Pam appeared to have little positive reinforcement in her life (Chapter 5), other than Rob's company and smoking. The nurse asked about her life prior to the pain.

Pam described how she had spent her early life in a children's home. She had then married Rob and had one child who was born with a severe mental and physical handicap and died at the age of 6. They had no other children. After the death of their son, Pam became withdrawn and started drinking. It became clear that she had not come to terms with this and had a very low opinion of herself.

It was important that Pam chose to present this aspect of her biography. She appears to have had little opportunity to develop a secure attachment relationship during her childhood, which might have left her vulnerable to low self-esteem, depression and substance abuse (Chapter 6). Since marrying Rob, she had experienced a series of serious losses, uncontrollable life events and hassles associated with the death of their son and her subsequent illness (Chapter 8). Although Rob appears to be a good source of emotional support, she may fear that Rob will leave again. This highlights the importance of keeping him involved in her pain management.

It was necessary to clarify Pam's main goal (Chapter 9), which was to obtain relief from pain. So the nurse focused next on assessing the pain. What was it like? When was it worst? Could she find any ways of gaining relief? Was she ever pain-free?

> Pam likened the pain to a constant toothache in her hands. She took a high dose of sustained release morphine and was on an antidepressant, which also helped pain and sleep.

The nurse then focused on the pattern of Pam's pain.

> Rob observed that Pam usually awoke free of pain and the pain commenced after she had her first cigarette. Pam nodded agreement.

The identification of pain as an immediate negative consequence of smoking (Chapter 5) validated the doctor's advice and provided an important incentive to quit. As a check, the nurse asked Pam to keep a pain diary for a week, in which she would record her levels of pain intensity at regular intervals, together with what she was doing immediately before and after. This 'functional analysis' (Chapter 5) would provide important feedback on factors that influenced pain, including smoking. As a start, the nurse suggested a simple technique to reduce the desire to smoke, based on Marks's smoke-stop programme (Chapter 5). Pam's personal message to be read out before smoking each cigarette read:

> This cigarette will cause me a lot of pain.
> This cigarette is making me ill.
> I don't want to smoke this cigarette.

Smoking serves a number of important functions (Chapter 5) and it was necessary to compensate for these if Pam were to cut down. In Pam's case it appeared to calm her feelings of anxiety, gave her something to do, and she enjoyed it. Pam and Rob were encouraged to think about alternative enjoyable ways of filling her time, focusing on things that Pam could do, rather than what she could not do. It was emphasized that active involvement leads to the release of endorphins that help to alleviate pain. It was important to find activities that kept Rob involved.

> Pam agreed that she could prepare sandwiches for their lunch, instead of Rob getting them. Rob would continue to come home at lunchtime to provide company and help to break up the day.

Stress management is an important part of smoking cessation, pain and depression management programmes so the nurse asked if Pam would consider attending a CBT programme (Chapter 6). Pam rejected this. Rob explained that she was embarrassed because people stared at her hands and she found it difficult to speak to strangers. So the nurse enquired about relaxation techniques to help her control her anxiety.

> Pam had learned yoga years ago and found it beneficial. She was willing to try relaxation exercises at home and Rob agreed to support this.
>
> It was important to find means of distraction from the pain, and the nurse asked about any enjoyable activities she thought she might be able to do.
>
> Pam had been good at crochet and thought she might try this again if the pain was not so severe. Rob agreed to buy some thread for her to try. The nurse then mentioned the possibility of getting a dog trained to help people with physical disabilities.

In addition to the practical help such a dog might afford, it would provide company, occupation and unconditional love (see humanistic psychology, Chapter 1). It might also provide an incentive for Pam to walk outside and meet people. Conversations with strangers are easier when conducted through an animal.

The interview had covered a lot of ground and much of it might be forgotten by the time Pam and Rob arrived home, therefore a written summary was given (Chapter 4). This also gave the opportunity to check agreement.

> The nurse wrote out a list of key points for Pam and Rob to take home, their action plan, and contact details including web addresses for further support. This might encourage Pam to learn computer skills.

Continued support is important. The nurse would have considered referral to a clinical psychologist specializing in chronic pain and depression if Pam had shown a complete lack of motivation (Chapter 6). If at further appointments she was unable to demonstrate progress, this would be considered.

During the one-hour interview, the nurse had begun to establish a therapeutic relationship; identified reasons for Pam's current state of hopelessness and low self-esteem; assessed her goals, coping strategies, coping resources and barriers; negotiated an action plan and provided information for continuing support.

> Rob and Pam thanked the nurse for her time and interest and left smiling. They made an appointment to share their progress and review the likelihood of having minor surgery to help control the pain.

This case study illustrates how a seemingly bleak situation can turn out to have many positive aspects and generate optimism. As often happens in health care, the nurse did not meet Pam or her husband again and this highlighted the problem of lack of continuity. As a result, the nurse now writes a letter detailing the key issues agreed, along with the agreed goals and action plan, including the support and resources needed to achieve it. The letter is sent to the referring pain consultant, with a copy to the patient and one to the family doctor. Evaluation indicates a reduction in medical consultations, and colleagues report that patient motivation to engage in self-management is considerably increased as a result of this motivational approach.

Summary of key points

- Pain and suffering are not the same thing.
- The gate control theory of pain explains how pain is influenced by stress and distress.
- The placebo response can be enhanced by establishing a therapeutic relationship.
- Pain assessment needs to focus on the concerns of the patient and the beliefs and contexts that influence pain, and not just on pain intensity.
- It is important to agree the patient's goals and priorities, and focus on these when preparing an action plan for pain management.

Exercise

See next section.

Further reading

Anand, K.J.S. and the International Evidence-Based Group for Neonatal Pain (2001) Consensus statement for the prevention and management of pain in the newborn, *Archives of Pediatric and Adolescent Medicine*, 155: 173–80.

Benedetti, F. (2006) Placebo analgesia, *Neurological Science*, 27: S100–2

Carr, D.B. and Goudas, L.C. (1999) Acute pain, *The Lancet*, 353: 2051–8.

Carter, B. (ed.) (1998) *Perspectives on Pain: Mapping the Territory*. London: Arnold.

Cheng, S.F., Foster, R.L. and Hester, N.O. (2003) A review of factors predicting children's pain experiences, *Issues in Comprehensive Pediatric Nursing*, 26: 203–16.

Eccleston, C. (2001) Role of psychology in pain management, *British Journal of Anaesthesia*, 87(1): 144–52.

Halimaa, S-L. (2003) Pain management in nursing procedures on premature babies, *Journal of Advanced Nursing*, 42(6): 587–97.

Hodgins, M.J. (2002) Interpreting the meaning of pain severity scores, *Pain Research and Management*, 7(4): 192–8.

Keefe, F.J., Abernethy, A.P. and Campbell, L.C. (2005) Psychological approaches to understanding and treating disease-related pain, *Annual Review of Psychology*, 56: 601–30.

Main, C.J. and Williams, A.C. de C. (2002) ABC of psychological medicine: musculoskeletal pain, *British Medical Journal*, 325: 534–7.

Rollnick, S. and Miller, W.R. (1995) What is motivational interviewing?, *Behavioural and Cognitive Psychotherapy*, 23(4): 325–34.

Strong, J., Unruh, A.M., Wright, A., Baxter, G.D. and Wall, P.D. (2001) *Pain: Textbook for Therapists*. Amsterdam: Elsevier.

Wall, P. (1999) *Pain: The Science of Suffering*. London: Weidenfeld & Nicholson.

Zaza, C. and Baine, N. (2002) Cancer pain and psychosocial factors: a critical review of the literature, *Journal of Pain and Symptom Management*, 24(5): 526–42.

Useful web addresses

www.dipex.org/DesktopDefault.aspx
Patients share information about illness experiences.

www.action-on-pain.co.uk/
Information about self-help groups for people with chronic pain, with links to other information sources.

www.cancerbackup.org.uk/Resourcessupport/Symptomssideeffects/Pain
Information for patients about all aspects of the management of cancer pain.

www.jr2.ox.ac.uk/bandolier/painres/acpnconc/acpnconc.html
Evidence-based information on all aspects of acute pain management.

www.rcn.org.uk/publications/pdf/guidelines/cpg_contents.pdf
RCN guidelines on the assessment and management of pain in children.

www.canceradvice.co.uk/support.cfm
Provides information on UK support groups for many types of cancer.

EXERCISES

Some exercises involve talking with patients or clients, or observing episodes of care. Before you do any of these, be sure to discuss it with your clinical supervisor and/or tutor and agree ground rules before starting. These should address the following considerations:

- How best to present yourself (this is not part of routine care).
- How to respect the person's privacy.
- How to respect the right of all concerned (patients/clients and staff) to choose whether or not to participate.
- What to do if the person becomes distressed at any point.
- How to communicate with those who have communication difficulties.
- What to do if a patient or client divulges information not generally known to staff or recorded in their notes.
- What to do if they divulge information that might harm their own health or the well-being of someone else.

Social care professionals may prefer to substitute well-being and social problems for health and illness.

Chapter 1. Think about what 'being healthy' means to you. Compare your ideas with those of your friends and colleagues and even some of your patients or clients. What have you learned about differences in health-related goals and priorities?

Chapter 2. Identify a patient or client who is willing to talk to you about the changes that their illness has brought about. Find out how their illness has affected their body image, their self-image and their self-esteem. What have you learned about what is important to them?

Chapter 3. Repeat the previous exercise with a patient who has a similar illness but is in a different age group. What are the similarities and what are the differences? Why do you think these differences might have arisen?

Chapter 4. Select a patient or client as above. Ask them to tell you about their illness, what caused it, what has happened to them, and what they understand about it. How does this compare with your own understanding of their illness and what is written in their notes?

Chapter 5. Observe the ways members of staff from different professional groups behave towards each other. Do you always act in accordance with the way you were taught? If not, what factors do you think have influenced your behaviour?

Chapter 6. Agree a time to sit with a patient and encourage them to tell you the story of their illness or problem, starting where they feel their story begins. What worries and/or losses, if any, have they experienced? Is their story coherent or chaotic? What have you learned about the things that have affected their current emotional state?

Chapter 7. Shadow one of your colleagues as they interact with patients, parents or clients, as they undertake their daily work. Observe their verbal and non-verbal behaviour. What impact did this have on each person and how could you tell if this had a positive or negative effect? Can you suggest any ways in which this might have been improved?

Chapter 8. Ask patients, parents or clients about the things that cause them most stress in their present situation and why. What small changes that involve little extra time or cost might make the biggest improvement in their lives?

Chapter 9. Identify a patient, parent or client who engages in a behaviour that is associated with a known health risk and is contemplating change. Ask them to imagine making the change and identify all the actual and potential barriers. How might this help to develop an action plan?

Chapter 10. Find a patient or client who has pain, but is not in too much pain to talk to you. Use the Brief Pain Inventory (short form) to assess their pain. Does this tell you anything that you did not previously know (look in their notes)? If they are able, ask them to tell you the story of their pain. What does this tell you about the effect of pain on their present life, or the possible effects of distressing life experiences on their pain?

GLOSSARY

A priori: refers to an assumption, hypothesis or prediction produced before an experiment or intervention takes place.

Active versus passive coping: doing something versus doing nothing when faced with a problem.

Adaptation: a process of change that achieves a desired outcome or has survival value.

Adherence: following an agreed plan of action developed with a doctor or health care professional.

Amnesia: memory loss.

Anxiety: a state of emotional and physiological arousal associated with perceptions of threat or lack of control.

Appraisal: thought processes used to evaluate a potential stressor (from Lazarus 1966).

Approach/avoidance: ways of coping with problems, either by confronting them (approach) or avoiding them.

Attachment: a strong emotional bond between two people that elicits caring behaviours.

Attribution theory: from social psychology, a theory of how people make inferences about the causes of behaviour.

Avoidance: behaviours associated with ignoring the existence of problems and any negative consequences.

Behaviourism: an approach to psychology that proposes that all behaviour is determined by its antecedents (cues) and its consequences.

Behaviourist, behavioural: based on the principles of behaviourism.

Bereavement: a perception of loss caused by death.

Biopsychosocial: an approach that views biological, psychological and social systems in combination, rather than separately.

Bipolar: refers to a scale of measure that has a positive and negative pole (e.g. a Likert scale).

Bonding: the formation of a strong attachment relationship.

Burnout: a response to stress in the caring professions that leads to feelings of emotional exhaustion and depersonalizing behaviours towards patients.

Catharsis: a term from psychoanalysis used to describe the therapeutic release of negative emotions.

CBT: Cognitive behaviour therapy.

Classical conditioning: from behaviourism, a simple form of associative learning in which reflex behaviours come under the unconscious control of an external stimulus.

Cognition: thought processes, including perception, memory and information processing.

Cognitive behaviour therapy: a structured therapy based on principles from behavioural and cognitive psychology.

Cognitive dissonance: a state of emotional tension created by two inconsistent beliefs, or between an incompatibility between the individual's beliefs and their behaviour (from Festinger 1957).

Compliance: actions undertaken in accordance with the instructions of others.

Conditioning: a process by which simple associative learning takes place.

Conformity: the tendency for perceptions, attitudes and behaviours to conform to those of powerful others, or the majority, in social situations.

Coping strategies: conscious methods of dealing with problems.

Coping: ways of dealing with problems.

Daily hassles: minor events that disrupt or interrupt daily routines.

Decentre: the ability to see or feel things from the point of view of another person.

Defence mechanisms: from psychoanalysis, the term used to describe unconscious processes that are assumed to defend the ego from unmanageable threats and anxiety.

Denial: from psychoanalysis, a defence mechanism by which the individual fails to accept the reality of a situation.

Depersonalization: the treatment of an individual as an object, rather than a person.

Depression: a state of hopelessness and helplessness.

Determinism: a doctrine that assumes that every event has a cause. Therefore all human behaviour is a response to some external stimulus or occurrence.

Dualism: philosophical position that separates mind from body.

Eclectic: in psychotherapy, a mix of psychological approaches drawn from different schools of thought.

Ego: in psychoanalysis, the part of the mind concerned with conscious self-regulation.

Egocentrism: the inability to see or feel things from the point of view of another individual.

Emotional support: helping people to feel loved, cared for and valued.

Emotion-focused coping: a form of coping that is intended to relieve unpleasant emotions such as anxiety or fear.

Empiricism: a philosophical belief that all knowledge is gained from experience (the opposite of nativism).

Fight or flight response: state of immediate readiness for action, stimulated by a perception of threat (from Cannon 1932).

Focus groups: a group of people who share an experience, brought together to identify common problems and solutions.

Functional analysis: from behaviourism, a systematic analysis of immediate cues and consequences that influence behaviour.

Fundamental attribution error: tendency to blame people for their own problems or mistakes, rather than looking for situational causes.

Generalized/generalizable: implies that findings from a sample, or situation, are applicable to the whole population, or to all situations.

Grief: the emotional response to feelings of loss.

Groupthink: group interaction that can lead to erroneous beliefs in the correctness of group decisions (from Janis 1982).

Habit, habitual: a routine pattern of behaviour, not subject to deliberation or conscious awareness.

HBM: Health belief model.

Health behaviour: a behaviour directed towards achieving a health goal.

Health-related behaviour: a behaviour that has an impact on health, but is not necessarily directed towards achieving a health goal.

Homeostasis: process by which physiological systems are maintained in a state of balance.

Hypothesis: a prediction that a particular action will lead to a particular outcome.

Iatrogenesis: medically induced illness.

Illness behaviour: behavioural responses to illness that include signalling the need for help.

Inductive: a process of generating theory from observational data.

Informational support: giving advice or information to enhance well-being.

Instrumental support: practical or tangible help.

Intervention: used in research to refer to any action or change likely to have an effect on an individual or group.

Introspection: examination of one's own mental experiences.

Learned helplessness: a state of depression caused by perceived uncontrollability and associated with cognitive, motivational and behavioural deficits (from Seligman 1975).

Life events: events involving loss or change that require major adjustment or adaptation.

Likert scale: a measure of agreement versus disagreement that is scaled for the purpose of statistical analysis, e.g. Strongly agree Agree Neutral Disagree Strongly disagree

LOC: Locus of control.

Locus of control: a set of beliefs about internal (personal) or external (other or chance) responsibility for achieving a desired outcome (from Rotter 1966).

Loss: an unpleasant experience caused by separation from a loved person or object.

Maladaptation: responses to change that lead to adverse outcomes or unintended consequences.

Meta-analysis: analysis of combined data from all good quality randomized controlled trials of a specific intervention.

Mnemonic: a technique of visual or verbal association used to improve memory for facts.

Modelling: the learning of new skills by observing and copying others (from Bandura 1977a).

Mourning: the behavioural expression of grief, shaped by cultural expectations.

Narrative psychology: psychology based on the belief that our biographical stories constitute our sense of self.

Narrative therapy: therapy that uses therapeutic writing or verbal storytelling, with or without the presence of a therapist.

Nativism: a philosophical belief that humans are born with unique abilities to organize knowledge and respond to their environment.

Non-verbal communication: communication by facial expression and body movement.

Normative: in social psychology, social influences to conform.

Operant conditioning: learning by which voluntary behaviours and activities are brought under the control of external stimuli.

PCA: Patient controlled anagesia.

Peer Teaching: refers to education delivered by lay people who have gained knowledge from similar types of experience.

Phenomenology: a philosophical doctrine that advocates the study of subjective or 'lived' experience.

Placebo response: physiological change brought about by expectation.

Placebo: an inert substance that elicits an expectation of an effect and leads to physiological change.

Positivism: philosophical stance which holds that legitimate knowledge can only be obtained using scientific methods of inquiry.

Post hoc: refers to an explanation given after the event (opposite of a priori).

Primacy effect: information given first is remembered best.

Primary appraisal: cognitive process by which the individual determines if there is a threat (from Lazarus 1966).

Primary prevention: preventive actions to maintain health in the absence of any signs or symptoms of disease.

Problem-focused coping: a response to stress that focuses on resolving the cause of the problem.

Pseudoscience: a body of theory that is not testable using scientific methods.

Psychoanalysis: a method of investigation, theory of mind, and form of treatment invented by Sigmund Freud.

Psychodynamic: refers to psychological systems that emphasize processes of development and change across the lifespan.

Psychogenic: a disease that has a psychological origin.

Psychoneuroimmunology: study of psychological factors that affect the immune system.

Psychosocial: an approach that views psychological and social systems in combination, rather than separately.

Psychosomatic: a disease that has a psychological component, as cause or effect.

Punishment: in behaviourism, an intervention that decreases the likelihood that the target behaviour will occur.

Qualitative research: focuses on subjective experience.

Quantitative research: based on objective and measurable data.

Random: occurs by chance.

Randomized controlled trial: a research method used to test a new intervention; attempts to control for effects not attributable to the intervention by random allocation of participants to receive either a new (test) intervention or a comparable alternative treatment.

Recency effect: information given last is remembered best.

Reductionism: the belief that complex phenomena can be understood by breaking them down into more simple fundamental elements.

Reference group: a group of people who share desired attributes and goals.

Reinforcement: in behaviourism, an intervention that increases the likelihood that the target behaviour will occur.

Reliablity: when applied to a psychological measurement tool, consistency in producing the same result on separate occasions in similar circumstances.

Repertory grid: a method used to measure the self concept (from Kelly 1955).

Repression: from psychoanalysis, a defence mechanism that suppresses memories that cause anxiety.

Rogerian counselling: based on the work of Carl Rogers, non-directive client-centred therapy provided in an atmosphere of 'unconditional positive regard'.

Schedule of reinforcement: from behaviourism, the frequency or regularity by which reinforcement is received.

Schema: mental representation that informs understanding.

Secondary appraisal: cognitive process by which the individual determines what to do about a perceived threat (from Lazarus 1966).

Secondary prevention: preventive actions designed to detect and treat illness or disease at an early stage, as in attending for screening tests.

Self: personal identity.

Self-actualization: from humanistic psychology, a process of personal growth, or the pinnacle of achievement.

Self-efficacy: belief on one's ability to achieve a desired outcome (from Bandura 1977b).

Self-esteem: feeling good about oneself.

Self-management: learning to deal with an illness and its consequences through one's own actions.

Self-regulation: conscious efforts to achieve a desired goal in a changing environment.

Semantic differential scale: bipolar measure using a five- or seven-point scale, e.g. Happy I__I__I__I__I__I Sad I__I__I__I__I__I.

Sense of coherence: the feeling that one's life is meaningful, from Antonovsky (1985).

Social cognition: study of thought processes in the context of the social environment in which they arise.

Social norm: expected standards of belief or behaviour determined by one's social or cultural reference group.

Social support: actions that impact on the well-being of others.

Socialization: process of learning about socially and culturally acceptable norms of behaviour.

Stigma: distinguishing features that have a negative impact on the attitudes of others (from Goffman 1963).

Stimulus control: from behavioural psychology, the automatic triggering of a response by an external event or situational cue.

Stimulus: from behavioural psychology, an internal or external event or change that alerts attention and precipitates arousal.

Stressor: an internal of external event that is perceived as a potential cause of threat or harm.

Systematic review: review of all research data on a particular topic, including unpublished data.

Tangible support: see instrumental support.

Tertiary prevention: actions to promote or preserve well-being and quality of life after the onset of illness or disease.

Threat: any event that potentially threatens physical or psychological well-being.

TPB: Theory of planned behaviour.

Unconditional positive regard: from humanistic psychology, esteem that is freely given, regardless of the behaviour or demeanour of the other.

Validity: when applied to a psychological measure, the extent to which it measures what it is intended to measure, and not something else.

Variable: in statistics, a measurable factor that is subject to variation or change.

Whitehall studies: a series of studies over several decades to identify causes of morbidity and mortality in UK civil servants.

REFERENCES

Abrams, D. and Hogg, M.A. (2004) Collective identity: group membership and self-conception, in M.B. Brewer and M. Hewstone (eds) *Self and Social Identity*, pp. 147–81. Oxford: Blackwell.

Ader, R., Cohen, N. and Felton, D. (1995) Psychoneuroimmunology: interactions between the nervous system and the immune system, *The Lancet*, 345: 99–103.

Ainsworth, M.D.S., Blehar, M.C., Waters, E. and Wall, S. (1978) *Patterns of Attachment*. Hillsdale, NJ: Lawrence Erlbaum Associates.

Ajzen, I. (1988) *Attitudes, Personality and Behaviour*. Milton Keynes: Open University Press.

Ajzen, I. (1991) The theory of planned behavior, *Organizational Behavior and Human Decision Processes*, 50: 179–211.

Ajzen, I. and Fishbein, M. (1980) *Understanding Attitudes and Predicting Social Behavior*. Englewood Cliffs, NJ: Prentice Hall.

Al-Ghazal, S.K., Fallowfeld, L. and Blamey, R.W. (2000) Comparison of psychological aspects and patient satisfaction following breast conserving surgery, simple mastectomy and breast reconstruction, *European Journal of Cancer*, 36: 1938–43.

American Academy of Pediatrics (2006) Prevention and management of pain in the neonate: an update, *Pediatrics*, 118(5): 2231–41.

Andersen, B.L., Farrar, W.B., Golden-Kreutz *et al.* (2004) Psychological, behavioral, and immune changes after a psychological intervention: a clinical trial, *Journal of Clinical Oncology*, 22(17): 3671–9.

Anderson, M.C. (2003) Rethinking interference theory: executive control and the mechanisms of forgetting, *Journal of Memory and Language*, 9(4): 415–45.

Anderson, R.M. and Funnell, M.M. (2000) Compliance and adherence are dysfunctional concepts in diabetes care, *Diabetes Educator*, 26(4): 597–604.

Antonovsky, A. (1985) *Health, Stress and Coping*. San Francisco: Jossey-Bass.

APA (American Psychiatric Association) (2000) *Diagnostic and Statistical Manual of Mental Disorders: DSM-IVfi-TR*, 4th edition. Washington, DC: APA.

Armitage, C.J. and Conner, M. (2001) Efficacy of the theory of planned behaviour: a meta-analytic review, *British Journal of Social Psychology*, 40(4): 471–99.

Aronson, E. (1988) *The Social Animal*, 5th edn. New York: W.H. Freeman.

Asarnow, J.R., Jaycox, L.H. and Tompson, M.C. (2001) Depression in youth: psychosocial interventions, *Journal of Clinical Child Psychology*, 30(1): 33–47.

Asbring, P. (2001) Chronic illness – a disruption in life: identity-transformation among women with chronic fatigue syndrome and fibromyalgia, *Journal of Advanced Nursing*, 34(3): 312–19.

Asch, S.E. (1956) Studies of independence and submission to group pressure: 1: a minority of one against unanimous majority, *Psychological Monographs*, 70: 416.

Baer, R. (2003) Mindfulness training as a clinical intervention: a conceptual and empirical review, *Clinical Psychology: Science and Practice*, 10(2): 125–43.

Bajor, J.K. and Baltes, B.B. (2003) The relationship between selection optimization with compensation, conscientiousness, motivation, and performance, *Journal of Vocational Behavior*, 63: 347–67.

Bandura, A. (1977a) *Social Learning Theory*. Englewood Cliffs, NJ: Prentice Hall.

Bandura, A. (1977b) Self-efficacy: towards a unifying theory of behavioural change, *Psychological Review*, 84(2): 191–215.

Bandura, A. (1997) *Self-efficacy: The Exercise of Control*. New York: W.H. Freeman.

Bandura, A. (2000) Health promotion from the perspective of social cognitive theory, in P. Norman, C. Abraham and M. Conner (eds) *Understanding and Changing Health Behaviour: From Health Beliefs to Self-regulation*, pp. 299–342. Amsterdam: Harwood.

Bandura, A. (2005) The primacy of self-regulation in health promotion, *Applied Psychology: An International Review*, 54(2): 245–54.

Bandura, A., Ross, D., and Ross, S.A. (1961) Transmission of aggression through imitation of aggressive models, *Journal of Abnormal and Social Psychology*, 63: 575–82.

Bartlett, G. (1932) *Remembering*. Cambridge: Cambridge University Press.

Baumrind, D. (1967) Child care practices anteceding three patterns of preschool behaviour, *Genetic Psychology Monographs*, 75: 43–8.

Baumrind, D. (1971) Current patterns of parental authority, *Developmental Psychology Monograph, Part 2*, 4(1), 1–103.

Baumrind, D. (1991) The influence of parenting style on adolescent competence and substance use, *Journal of Early Adolescence*, 11(1): 56–95.

Beaver, K., Luker, K.A., Owens, R.G., Leinster, S.J., Degner, L.F. and Sloan, J.A. (1996) Treatment decision making in women newly diagnosed with breast cancer, *Cancer Nursing*, 19(1): 8–19.

Beck, A.T. (1976) *Cognitive Therapy and Emotional Disorders*. Harmondsworth: Penguin.

Beck, A.T., Ward, C.H., Mendelson, M., Mock, J. and Erbaugh, J. (1961) An inventory for measuring depression, *Archives of General Psychiatry*, 4: 561–71.

Beck, J. (1995) *Cognitive Therapy: Basics and Beyond*. London: The Guilford Press.

Becker, M.H. and Maiman, L.A. (1975) Sociobehavioural determinants of compliance with health and medical care recommendations, *Medical Care*, 13: 10–24.

Beecher, H.K. (1959) *Measurement of Subjective Responses*. New York: Oxford University Press.

Bendelow, G.A. (2006) Pain, suffering and risk, *Health, Risk & Society*, 8(1): 59–70.

Benedetti, F. (2006) Placebo analgesia, *Neurological Science*, 27: S100–2.

Benedetti, F., Claudia Arduino, C. and Martina Amanzio, M. (1999) Somatotopic activation of opioid systems by target-directed expectations of analgesia, *The Journal of Neuroscience*, 19(9): 3639–48.

Benedetti, F., Mayberg, H.S., Wager, T.D., Stohler, C.S., and Jon-Kar Zubieta, J-K. (2005) Neurobiological mechanisms of the placebo effect, *The Journal of Neuroscience*, 25(45): 10390–402.

Benedetti, F., Arduino, C., Costa, S., Vighetti, S., Tarenzi, L, Rainero, I. and Asteggiano, G. (2006) Loss of expectation-related mechanisms in Alzheimer's disease makes analgesic therapies less effective, *Pain*, 121(1–2): 133–44.

Benner, P. and Wrubel, J. (1989) *The Primacy of Caring: Stress and Coping in Health and Illness*. Menlo Park, CA: Addison-Wesley.

Berde, C.B., Lehn, B.M., Yee, J.D., Sethna, N.F. and Russo, D. (1991) Patient-controlled analgesia in children and adolescents: a randomized prospective comparison with intramuscular administration of morphine for postoperative analgesia, *Journal of Pediatrics*, 118(3): 460–6.

Beutler, L.E. and Malik, M.I. (2002) *Rethinking the DSM: A Psychological Perspective*. Washington, DC: APA Books.

Bhawuk, D.P.S. and Brislin, R.W. (2000) Cross-cultural training: a review, *Applied Psychology: An International Review*, 49(1): 162–91.

Birtwistle, J., Payne, S., Smith, P. and Kendrick, T. (2002) The role of the district nurse in bereavement support, *Journal of Advanced Nursing*, 38(5): 467–78.

Bishop, G.D., Kaur, D., Tan, V.L., Chua, Y.L., Liew, S.M. and Mak, K.H. (2005) Effects of a psychosocial skills training workshop on psychophysiological and psychosocial risk in patients undergoing coronary artery bypass grafting, *American Heart Journal*, 150(3): 602–9.

Bisson, J. and Andrew, M. (2006) Psychological treatment of post-traumatic stress disorder (PTSD), *Cochrane Database of Systematic Reviews*, 2, art. no.: CD003388.

Blaxter, M. (1990) *Health and Lifestyles*. London: Tavistock/Routledge.

Boersma, K., Linton, S., Overmeer, T., Jansson, M., Vlaeyen, J. and de Jong, J. (2004) Lowering fear-avoidance and enhancing function through exposure in vivo: a multiple baseline study across six patients with back pain, *Pain*, 108: 8–16.

Bohlmeijer, E., Smit, F. and Cuijpers, P. (2003) Effects of reminiscence and life review on late-life depression: a meta-analysis, *International Journal of Geriatric Psychiatry*, 18(12): 1088–94.

Bonanno, G.A. (2004) Loss, trauma, and human resilience: have we underestimated the human capacity to thrive after extremely aversive events? *American Psychologist*, January: 1–28.

Borkenau, P., Riemann, R., Angleitner, A. and Spinath, F.M. (2001) Genetic and environmental influences on observed personality: evidence from the German observational study of adult twins, *Journal of Personality and Social Psychology*, 80(4): 655–68.

Boulos, M.N. (2005) British internet-derived patient information on diabetes mellitus: is it readable? *Diabetes Technology and Therapy*, 7(3): 528–35.

Bowlby, J. (1969) *Attachment and Loss: Vol. 1. Attachment*. London: Hogarth Press.

Bowling, A. (2004) *Measuring Health*, 2nd edn. Buckingham: Open University Press.

Boyd, D. and Bee, H. (2006) *Lifespan Development*, 4th edn. Boston, MA: Allyn & Bacon.

Brehm, S.S., Kassin, S.M. and Fein, S. (2002) *Social Psychology*, 5th edn. Boston, MA: Houghton Mifflin.

Brewin, C.R., Dagleish, T. and Joseph, S. (1996) A dual representation theory of posttraumatic stress disorder, *Psychological Review*, 103(4): 670–86.

Briner, R. (1994) Stress: the creation of a modern myth, paper presented at the Annual Conference of the British Psychological Society, Brighton, March.

Brissette, I., Scheier, M.F. and Carver, C.S. (2002) The role of optimism in social network development, coping, and psychological adjustment during a life transition, *Journal of Personality and Social Psychology*, 82(1): 102–11.

Britt, E., Hudson, S.M. and Blampied, N.M. (2004) Motivational interviewing in health settings: a review, *Patient Education and Counseling*, 53: 147–55.

Bury, M. (1982) Chronic illness as biographical disruption, *Sociology of Health and Illness*, 4: 167–82.

Bushnell, I.W.R. (2001) Mother's face recognition in newborn infants: learning and memory, *Infant and Child Development*, 10: 67–74.

Butler, R.N. (1974) Successful aging and the role of the life review, *Journal of the American Geriatrics Society*, 22(12): 529–35.

Cameron, L.D., Petrie, K.J., Ellis, C.J., Buick, D. and Weinman, J.A. (2005) Trait negative affectivity and responses to a health education intervention for myocardial infarction patients, *Psychology and Health*, 20(1): 1–18.

Campbell, C. and MacPhail, C. (2002) Peer education, gender and the development of critical consciousness: participatory HIV prevention by South African youth, *Social Science and Medicine*, 55(2): 331–45.

Caris-Verhallen, W.M., de Gruijter, I.M., Kerkstra, A. and Bensing, J.M. (1999) Factors related to nurse communication with elderly people, *Journal of Advanced Nursing*, 30(5): 11(6): 1117.

Carman, M.B. (1997) The psychology of normal aging, *Psychiatric Clinics of North America*, 20(1): 15–24.

Carr, D.B. and Goudas, L.C. (1999) Acute pain, *The Lancet*, 353: 2051–8.

Carroll, D., Moore, R.A., McQuay, H.J., Fairman, F., Gramer, M. and Leijon, G. (2006) Transcutaneous electrical nerve stimulation (TENS) for chronic pain, *The Cochrane Database of Systematic Reviews*, issue 4. Chichester: Wiley.

Cassidy, J. and Shaver, P.R. (1999) *Handbook of Attachment: Theory, Research and Applications*. New York: Guilford Press.

Champion, V.L. (1984) Instrument development for health belief model constructs, *Advances in Nursing Science*, 6: 73–85.

Chapman, C.R., Nakamura, Y. and Flores, L.Y. (1999) Chronic pain and consciousness: a constructivist perspective, in R.J. Gatchel and D.C. Turk (eds) *Psychosocial Factors in Pain*. New York: The Guilford Press.

Chesney, M.A., Neilands, T.B., Chambers, D.B., Taylor, J.M. and Folkman, S. (2006) A validity and reliability study of the coping self-efficacy scale, *British Journal of Health Psychology*, 11: 421–37.

Christiana, J.M., Gilman, S.E., Guardino, M., Mickelson, K., Morselli, P.L., Olfson, M. and Kessler, R.C. (2000) Duration between onset and time of obtaining initial treatment among people with anxiety and mood disorders: an international survey of members of mental health patient advocate groups, *Psychological Medicine*, 30(3): 693–703.

Christie, D. and Wilson, C. (2005) CBT in paediatric and adolescent health settings: a review of practice-based evidence, *Pediatric Rehabilitation*, 8(4): 241–7.

Cignacco, E., Mueller, R., Hamers, J.P. and Gessler, P. (2004) Pain assessment in the neonate using the Bernese Pain Scale for Neonates, *Early Human Development*, 78(2): 125–31.

Clark, P. (2001) Narrative gerontology in clinical practice: current applications and future prospects, in G. Kenyon, P. Clark and B. de Vries (eds) *Narrative Gerontology: Theory, Research, and Practice*. New York: Springer.

Cleeland, C.S. (1991) The Brief Pain Inventory, www.mdanderson.org/pdf/bpi-long.pdf, accessed 10 January 2007.

Closs, S.J., Barr, B., Briggs, M., Cash, K. and Seers, K. (2004) A comparison of five pain assessment scales for nursing home residents with varying degrees of cognitive impairment, *Journal of Pain and Symptom Management*, 27(3): 196–205.

Cobb, S. (1976) Social support as a moderator of life stress, *Psychosomatic Medicine*, 38(5): 300–14.

Cohen, D.A., Richardson, J. and Labree, L. (1994) Parenting behaviors and the onset of smoking and alcohol use: a longitudinal study, *Paediatrics*, 94(3): 368–75.

Cohen, F., Kearney, K.A., Zegans, L.S., Kemeny, M.E., Neuhaus, J.M. and Stites, D.P. (1999) Differential immune system changes with acute and persistent stress for optimists vs pessimists, *Brain, Behaviour and Immunity*, 13: 155–74.

Coleman, L.M. and Ingham, R. (1999) Contraception: how can we encourage more discussion between partners? *Health Education Research*, 14(6): 741–50.

Coleman, P.G. (1999) Creating a life story: the task of reconciliation, *The Gerontologist*, 39(2): 133–9.

Coleman, P.G. and O'Hanlon, A. (2004) *Ageing and Development*. London: Arnold.

Conner, M. and Norman, P. (1995) The role of social cognition in health behaviours, in M. Conner and P. Norman (eds) *Predicting Health Behaviour: Research and Practice with Social Cognition Models*. Buckingham: Open University Press.

Connolly, D. (2004) Posttraumatic stress disorder in children after cardiac surgery, *Journal of Pediatrics*, 144(4): 480–4.

Cooper, C.L. and Cartright, S. (1997) An intervention strategy for workplace stress, *Journal of Psychosomatic Research*, 43(1): 7–16.

Costa, P.T. and McCrae, R.R. (1992) The five-factor model of personality and its relevance to personality disorders, *Journal of Personality Disorders*, 6(4): 343–59.

Coull, F. (2003) Personal story offers insight into living with facial disfigurement, *Journal of Wound Care*, 12(7): 254–8.

Courneya, K.S., Nigg, C.R. and Estabrooks, P.I.A. (2000) Relationships among the theory of planned behaviour, stages of change and exercise behaviour in older persons over a three year period, in P. Norman, C. Abraham and M. Conner (eds) *Understanding and Changing Health Behaviour*, pp. 189–206. Amsterdam: Harwood.

Coward, D.D. and Wilkie, D.J. (2000) Metastatic bone pain: meanings associated witih self-report and self-management decision making, *Cancer Nursing*, 23(2): 101–8.

Cowen, E.L. (1994) The enhancement of psychological wellness: challenges and opportunities, *American Journal of Community Psychology*, 22(2): 149–79.

Cowin, L., Davies, R., Estall, G., Fitzerald, M. and Hoot, S. (2003) De-escallating aggression and violence in the mental health setting, *International Journal of Mental Health Nursing*, 12(1): 64.

Craig, K.D. (2004) Social communication of pain enhances protective functions: a comment on Deyo, Prkachin and Mercer (2004), *Pain*, 107: 5–6.

Crane, C. and Martin, M. (2002) Adult illness behaviour: the impact of childhood experience, *Personality and Individual Differences*, 32: 785–98.

Creer, T.L., Stein, R.E., Rappaport, L. and Lewis, C. (1992) Behavioural consequences of illness: childhood asthma as a model, *Pediatrics*, 90(5): 808–15.

Cross, M.J., March, L.M., Lapsley, H.M., Byrne, E. and Brooks, P.M. (2006) Patient self-efficacy and health locus of control: relationships with health status and arthritis-related expenditure, *Rheumatology*, 45: 92–6.

Crossley, M. (2003) 'Let me explain': narrative emplotment and one patient's experience of oral cancer, *Social Science and Medicine*, 56: 439–48.

Crowne, D.P. and Marlowe, D. (1960) A new scale of social desirability independent of psychopathology, *Journal of Consulting Psychology*, 24: 349–54.

Cumming, E. and Henry, W.E. (1961) *Growing Old: The Process of Disengagement*. New York: Basic Books.

Dalgleish, T. (2004) Cognitive approaches to posttraumatic stress disorder: the evolution of multirepresentational theorizing, *Psychological Bulletin*, 130(2): 228–60.

De Beni, R. and Palladino, P. (2004) Decline in working memory updating through ageing: intrusion error analysis, *Memory*, 12(1): 75–89.

de Melker, R.A., Touw-Otten, F.W. and Kuyvenhoven, M.M. (1997) Transcultural differences in illness behaviour and clinical outcome: an underestimated aspect of general practice? *Family Practice*, 14(6): 472–7.

DeCharms, R. (1968) *Personal Causation: The Internal Affective Determinants of Behaviour*. New York: Academic Press.

DiClemente, C.C. (1993) Changing addictive behaviours: a process perspective, *Current Directions in Psychological Science*, 2: 101–6.

Dixon, M., Benedict, H. and Larson, T. (2001) Functional analysis and treatment of inappropriate verbal behaviour, *Journal Of Applied Behavior Analysis*, 34: 361–3.

DoH (Department of Health) (1999) *Saving Lives: Our Healthier Nation*. London: DoH.

DoH (Department of Health) (2000) *Adding Life to Years: Report of the Expert Group on Healthcare of Older People*. London: DoH.

DoH (Department of Health) (2001a) *Seeking Consent: Working with Children*. London: The Stationery Office.

DoH (Department of Health) (2001b) *The Expert Patient: A New Approach to Chronic Disease Management for the 21st Century*. London: DoH.

DoH (Department of Health) (2002) *Self-management of Long-term Health Conditions: A Handbook for People with Chronic Disease*. Boulder, CO: Bull Publishing.

DoH (Department of Health) (2006) *The Expert Patients Programme*. London: DoH.

Dolbier, C.L., Cocke, R.R., Leiferman et al. (2001) Differences in functional immune responses of high versus low hardy healthy individuals, *Journal of Behavioral Medicine*, 24(3): 219–29.

Donaldson, M. (1978) *Children's Minds*. London: Fontana.

Donaldson, M. (1990) *Children's Minds*, 2nd edn. Glasgow: Fontana.

Donovan, J.L. and Blake, D.R. (1992) Patient non-compliance: deviance or reasoned decision-making? *Social Science and Medicine*, 34(5): 507–13.

Eccleston, C. (2001) Role of psychology in pain management, *British Journal of Anaesthesia*, 87(1): 144–52.

Ehlers, A. and Clark, D.M. (2000) A cognitive model of post-traumatic stress disorder, *Behaviour Research and Therapy*, 38(4): 319–45.

Eisenberg, L. (1977) Disease and illness: distinctions between professional and popular ideas of sickness, *Cultural Medical Psychiatry*, 1(1): 9–23.

Ekman, P. and Davidson, R.J. (1994) *The Nature of Emotion: Fundamental Questions*. Oxford: Oxford University Press.

Elkin, A.J. and Rosch, P.J. (1990) Promoting mental health at the workplace: the prevention side of stress management, *Occupational Medicine*, 5(4): 739–54.

Erikson, E.H. (1980) *Identity and the Life Cycle*. New York: Norton.

Evans, A. (1994) Anticipatory grief: a theoretical challenge, *Palliative Medicine*, 8: 159–65.

Ezzo, J., Berman, B., Hadhazy, V.A. Jadad, A.R., Lao, L. and Singh, B.B. (2000) Is acupuncture effective for the treatment of chronic pain? A systematic review, *Pain*, 86: 217–25.

Fallowfield, L. and Jenkins, V. (1999) Effective communication skills are the key to good cancer care, *European Journal of Cancer*, 35(11): 1592–7.

Fallowfield, L.J., Jenkins, V.A. and Beveridge, H.A. (2002) Truth may hurt but deceit hurts more: communication in palliative care, *Palliative Medicine*, 16(4): 297–303.

Faulkner, T.M. and de Luce, J. (1992) A view from antiquity: Greece, Rome and elders, in T.R. Cole, D. van Tussel and R. Kastenbaum (eds) *Handbook of the Humanities and Aging*, pp. 3–39. New York: Springer.

Ferner, R.E. (2003) Is concordance the primrose path to health? *British Medical Journal*, 327(7419): 821–2.

Ferrell, B.A., Ferrell, B.R. and Rivera, L. (1995) Pain in cognitively impared nursing home patients, *Journal of Pain and Symptom Management*, 10(8): 591–8.

Ferri, C.P., Prince, M., Bravne, C. *et al.* for Alzheimer's Disease International (2005) Global prevalence of dementia: a Delphi consensus study, *The Lancet*, 366: 2112–17.

Festinger, L. (1954) A theory of social comparison, *Human Relations*, 7: 117–40.

Festinger, L. (1957) *A Theory of Cognitive Dissonance*. Stanford, CA: Stanford University Press.

Fogarty, J.S. (1997) Reactance theory and patient noncompliance, *Social Science and Medicine*, 45(8): 1277–88.

Folkman, S. and Lazarus, R.S. (1985) If it changes it must be a process: study of emotion and coping during three stages of a college examination, *Journal of Personal and Social Psychology*, 48(1): 150–70.

Folkman, S. and Lazarus, R.S. (2003) Ways of Coping Questionnaire (WAYS), www.mindgarden.com/Assessments/Info/waysinfo.htm.

Folstein, M.F., Folstein, S.E. and McHugh, P.R. (1975) Mini Mental State, *Journal of Psychosomatic Research*, 12: 196–8.

Fordyce, W.E. (1982) A behavioural perspective on chronic pain, *British Journal of Clinical Psychology*, 21: 313–20.

Fox, N.A. and Card, J.A. (1999) Psychophysiological measures in the study of attachment, in J. Cassidy and P.R. Shaver (eds) *Handbook of Attachment: Theory, Research and Clinical Applications*. New York: Guilford Press.

Frank, A.W. (1995) *The Wounded Storyteller: Body, Illness and Ethics*. Chicago: University of Chicago Press.

Friedman, H.S. (2000) Long-term relations of personality and health: dynamisms, mechanisms, tropisms, *Journal of Personality*, 68(6): 1089–107.

Friedman, J. and Combs, G. (1996) *Narrative Therapy: The Social Construction of Preferred Realities*. London: W.W. Norton.

Friedman, M. and Rosenman, R.H. (1974) *Type A Behaviour and Your Heart*. New York: Knopf.

Galvin, K.T. (1992) A critical review of the health belief model in relation to cigarette smoking behaviour, *Journal of Clinical Nursing*, 1(1): 13–18.

Garand, L., Buckwalter, K.C., Lubaroff, D., Tripp-Reimer, T., Frantz, R.A. and Ansley, T.N. (2002) A pilot study of immune and mood outcomes of a community-based intervention for dementia caregivers: the PLST intervention, *Archives of Psychiatric Nursing*, XVI (4): 156–67.

Garcia, J., Ervin, F.R. and Koelling, R.A. (1966) Learning with prolonged delay to reinforcement, *Psychonomic Science*, 5(3): 121–2.

Garley, D., Gallop, R. and Johnston, N. (1997) Children of the mentally ill: a qualitative focus group approach, *Journal of Psychiatric and Mental Health Nursing*, 4: 97–103.

Gaston, C.M. and Mitchell, G. (2005) Information giving and decision-making in patients with advanced cancer: a systematic review, *Social Science & Medicine*, 61: 2252–64.

Gilbert, P. (1992) *Depression: The Evolution of Powerlessness*. Hove: Lawrence Erlbaum Associates.

Gilbert, P. (2005) Evolution and depression: issues and implications, *Psychological Medicine*, 35: 1–11.

Goffman, E. (1959) *The Presentation of Self in Everyday Life*. London: Penguin.

Goffman, E. (1963) *Stigma: Notes on the Management of Spoiled Identity*. Harmondsworth: Penguin.

Gollwitzer, P.M. and Oettingen, G. (2000) The emergence and implementation of health goals, in P. Norman, C. Abraham and M. Conner (eds) *Understanding and Changing Health Behaviour*, pp. 229–60. Amsterdam: Harwood.

Goodwin, R.D., Hoven, C.W., Lyons, J.S. and Stein, M.B. (2002) Mental health service utilization in the United States: the role of personality factors, *Social Psychiatry and Psychiatric Epidemiology*, 37(12): 561–6.

Gracely, R.H. (2000) Charisma and the art of healing, in M. Devor, M.C. Rowbotham and Z. Wiesenfed-Hallin (eds) *Proceedings of the 9th World Congress on Pain*. Seattle, WA: IASP Press.

Graham, H. (1993) *Hardship and Health in Women's Lives*. New York: Harvester Wheatsheaf.

Greenberg, M.T., O'Brien, M.U., Zins, J.F., Fredericks, L., Rosnik, J. and Elias, M.J. (2003) Enhancing school-based prevention and youth development through coordinated social, emotional, and academic learning, *American Psychologist*, 58(6–7): 466–74.

Griffin, J.M., Fuhrer, R., Stansfeld, S.A. and Marmot, M. (2002) The importance of low control at work and home on depression and anxiety: do these effects vary by gender and social class? *Social Science and Medicine*, 54(5): 783–98.

Grimby, A. and Wiklund, I. (1994) Health-related quality of life in old age: a study among 76-year-old Swedish urban citizens, *Scandivanian Journal of Social Medicine*, 22(1): 7–14.

Grossman, P., Niemann, L., Schmidtc, S. and Walach, H. (2004) Mindfulness-based stress reduction and health benefits: a meta-analysis, *Journal of Psychosomatic Research*, 57: 35–43.

Grunau, R.E., Holsti, L and Peters, J.W.B. (2006) Long-term consequences of pain in human neonates, *Seminars in Fetal and Neonatal Medicine*, 11: 268–275.

Grunfeld, E.A., Hunter, M.S., Ramirez, A.J. and Richards, M.A. (2003) Perceptions of breast cancer across the lifespan, *Journal of Psychosomatic Research*, 54(2): 141–6.

Haight, B.K. and Olson, M. (1989) Teaching home health aides the use of life review, *Journal of Nursing Staff Development*, 5(1): 11–16.

Halimaa, S-L. (2003) Pain management in nursing procedures on premature babies, *Journal of Advanced Nursing*, 42(6), 587–97.

Hall, S., Abramsky, L. and Marteau, T.M. (2003) Health professionals' reports of information given to parents following the prenatal diagnosis of sex chromosome anomalies and outcomes of pregnancies: a pilot study, *Prenatal Diagnosis*, 23(7): 535–8.

Harlow, H.F. (1959) Love in infant monkeys, *Scientific American*, 200: 68–74.

Hay, P.J., Bacaltchuk, J. and Stefano, S. (2006) Psychotherapy for bulimia nervosa and bingeing (Cochrane Review). *The Cochrane Library*, issue 3. Chichester: Wiley.

Hayward, J. (1994) *Information – A Prescription Against Pain*. London: Scutari.

Hazan, C. and Zeifman, D. (1999) Pair bonds as attachments: evaluating the evidence, in J. Cassidy and P.R. Shaver (eds) *Handbook of Attachment: Theory, Research and Clinical Applications*, pp. 336–54. New York: Guilford Press.

Helson, R., Jones, C. and Kwan, V.S.Y. (2002) Personality change over 40 years of adulthood: hierarchical linear modeling analyses of two longitudinal samples, *Journal of Personality and Social Psychology*, 83(3): 752–66.

Hewison, D. (1997) Coping with loss of ability: 'good grief' or episodic stress responses? *Social Science and Medicine*, 44(8): 1129–39.

Hewstone, M. (1989) *Causal Attribution: From Cognitive Processes to Collective Beliefs*. Oxford: Blackwell.

Higgins, I. (2005) The experience of chronic pain in elderly nursing home residents, *Journal of Research in Nursing*, 10(4): 369–82.

Hobfoll, S.E. (1988) *The Ecology of Stress*. New York: Hemisphere.

Hodgins, M.J. (2002) Interpreting the meaning of pain severity scores, *Pain Research and Management*, 7(4): 192–8.

Hodgins, D. (2005) Weighing the pros and cons of changing change models: a comment on West (2005), *Addiction*, 100: 1042–3.

Hoffman, G.A., Harrington, A. and Fields, H.L. (2005) Pain and the placebo: what we have learned, *Perspectives in Biology and Medicine*, 48(2): 248–65.

Hofling, C.K., Brotzman, E., Dalrymple, S., Graves, N. and Pierce, C.M. (1966) An experimental study in nurse–physician relationships, *Journal of Nervous and Mental Disease*, 143(2): 171–80.

Hogbin, B. and Fallowfield, L. (1989) Getting it taped: the 'bad news' consultation with cancer patients, *British Journal of Hospital Medicine*, 41(4): 330–3.

Holloway, I., Sofaer, B. and Walker, J. (in press) The stigmatisation of people with chronic back pain, *Disability and Rehabilitation*.

Holmes, T.H. and Rahe, R.H. (1967) The Social Readjustment Rating Scale, *Journal of Psychsomatic Research*, 11: 213–18.

Holt, C.L., Clark, E.M., Krueter, M.W. and Scharff, D.P. (2000) Does locus of control moderate the effects of tailored health education materials? *Health Education Research*, 15(4): 393–403.

Houston, V. and Bull, R. (1994) Do people avoid sitting next to someone who is facially disfigured? *European Journal of Social Psychology*, 24(2): 279–84.

Hudcova, J. *et al.* (2005) Patient controlled opioid analgesia versus conventional opioid analgesia for postoperative pain, *Cochrane Database of Systematic Reviews*, 18(4): CD003348.

Hunt, S.M. and Martin, C.J. (1988) Health-related behavioural change – a test of a new model, *Psychology and Health*, 2: 209–30.

Igoe, J.B. (1988) Healthy long-term attitudes on personal health can be developed in school-age children, *Pediatrician*, 15(3): 127–36.

Igoe, J.B. (1991) Empowerment of children and youth for consumer self-care, *American Journal of Health Promotion*, 6(1): 55–64.

Ingham, R. (1993) Old bodies in older clothes, *Health Psychology Update*, 14: 31–6.

James, A., Soler, A. and Weatherall, R. (2006) Cognitive behavioural therapy for anxiety disorders in children and adolescents (Cochrane Review), *The Cochrane Library*, issue 3. Chichester: Wiley.

Janis, I.L. (1982) *Groupthink: Psychological Studies of Policy Decisions and Fiascos*, 2nd edn. Boston, MA: Houghton Mifflin.

Janssen, C.G., Schuengel, C. and Stolk, J. (2002) Understanding challenging behaviour in people with severe and profound intellectual disability: a stress-attachment model, *Journal of Intellectual Disability Research*, 46(6): 445–53.

Janz, N. and Becker, M.H. (1984) The health belief model: a decade later, *Health Education Quarterly*, 11: 1–47.

Johnson, M.H. and Morton, J. (1991) *Biology and Cognitive Development*. Oxford: Blackwell.

Johnson, M. and Webb, C. (1995) Rediscovering the unpopular patients: the concept of social judgement, *Journal of Advanced Nursing*, 21(3): 466–74.

Johnson, N. (2004) *Cancer – My Partner*. Southampton: Paul Cave Publications.

Jones, D. (2003) Pain management and people with learning disabilities: a complex challenge, *Journal of Learning Disabilities*, 7(4): 294–5.

Jordan, J.R. and Neimeyer, R.A. (2003) Does grief counseling work? *Death Studies*, 27(9): 765–86.

Kabat-Zinn, J., Lipworth, L. and Burney, R. (1985) The clinical use of mindfulness meditation for the self-regulation of chronic pain, *Journal of Behavioural Medicine*, 8(2): 163–90.

Kain, Z.N., Mayes, L.C. and Caramico, L.A. (1996) Preoperative preparation in children: a cross-sectional study, *Journal of Clinical Anesthesia*, 8: 508–14.

Keijsers, G.P., Schaap, C.P. and Hoogduin, C.A. (2000) The impact of interpersonal patient and therapist behavior on outcome in cognitive-behavior therapy: a review of empirical studies, *Behavior Modification*, 24(2): 264–97.

Kelly, G.A. (1955) *A Theory of Personality: The Psychology of Personal Constructs*. New York: W.W. Norton.

Kelly, P. (1998) Loss experienced in chronic pain and illness, in J.H. Harvey (ed.) *Perspectives on Loss: A Sourcebook*. Philadelphia, PA: Brunner Mazel.

Kentsch, M., Rodemerk, U., Müller-Esch, G., Schnoor, U., Münzel, T., Ittel, T.-H. and Mitusch, R. (2002) Emotional attitudes toward symptoms and inadequate coping strategies are major determinants of patient delay in acute myocardial infarction, *Zeitschrift für Kardiologie*, 91(2): 147–55.

Kiecolt-Glaser, J.K., McGuire, L., Robles, T.F. and Glaser, R. (2002) Psychoneuroimmunology: psychological influences on immune function and health, *Journal of Consulting and Clinical Psychology*, 70(3): 537–47.

Kiecolt-Glaser, J. Preacher, K.J., MacCallum, R.C., Atkinson, C., Malarkey, W.B. and Glaser, R. (2003) Chronic stress and age-related increases in the proinflammatory cytokine IL-6, *Proceedings of the National Academy of Science*, USA, 100(15): 9090–5.

Kitwood, T. (1997) *Dementia Reconsidered*. Buckingham: Open University Press.

Kivimäki, M., Elovainio, M., Kokko, K., Pulkkinen, L., Kortteinen, M. and Tuomikoski, H. (2003) Hostility, unemployment and health status: testing three theoretical models, *Social Science and Medicine*, 56(10): 2139–52.

Klaus, H.M. and Kennell, J.H. (1976) *Maternal-Infant Bonding*. St Louis, MO: Mosby.

Kleinhesselink, R.R. and Edwards, R.E. (1975) Seeking and avoiding belief-discrepant information as a function of its perceived refutability, *Journal of Personality and Social Psychology*, 31: 787–90.

Kleinman, A. (1988) *The Illness Narratives: Suffering, Healing and the Human Condition*. New York: Basic Books.

Kobasa, S.C. (1979) Stressful life events, personality and health: an inquiry into hardiness, *Journal of Personality and Social Psychology*, 37: 1–11.

Koenig, H.G. and Cohen, H.J. (eds) (2002) *The Link Between Religion and Health: Psychoneuroimmunology*. Oxford: Oxford University Press.

Kohlberg, L. (1969) Stage and sequence: the cognitive-developmental approach to socialization, in D.A. Goslin (ed.) *Handbook of Socialization Theory and Research*. Skokie, IL: Rand McNally.

Kotses, H. and Harver, A. (eds) (1998) *Self-management of Asthma*. New York: Marcel Dekker.

Kübler-Ross, E. (1969) *On Death and Dying*. London: Tavistock/Routledge.

Kwekkeboom, K.L. and Gretarsdottir, E. (2006) Systematic review of relaxation interventions for pain, *Journal of Nursing Scholarship*, 38(3): 269–77.

Lam, D. and Gale, J. (2000) Cognitive behaviour therapy: teaching a client the ABC model – the first step towards the process of change, *Journal of Advanced Nursing*, 31(2): 444–51.

Langer, E.J., Janis, I.L. and Wolfer, J.A. (1975) Reduction of psychological stress in surgical patients, *Journal of Experimental Social Psychology*, 11: 155–65.

Lasch, K.E. (2000) Culture, pain, and culturally sensitive pain care, *Pain Management Nursing*, 1(3), Suppl. 1: 16–22.

Latané, B. and Darley, J.M. (1968) Group inhibition of bystander intervention in emergencies, *Journal of Personality and Social Psychology*, 10: 215–21.

Lau, R.R. and Hartman, K.A. (1983) Common sense representations of common illness, *Health Psychology*, 2: 319–32.

Lazarus, R.S. (1966) *Psychological Stress and the Coping Process*. New York: McGraw-Hill

Lazarus, R.S. and Averill, J.R. (1972) Emotion and cognition: with special reference to anxiety, in C.D. Spielberger (ed.) *Anxiety: Current Trends in Therapy and Research Volume II*. New York: Academic Press.

Lazarus, R.S. and Folkman, S. (1984) *Stress, Appraisal and Coping*. New York: Springer-Verlag.

LeBlanc, M. and Ritchie, M. (2001) A meta-analysis of play therapy outcomes, *Psychology Quarterly*, 14(2): 149–63.

LeFort, S.M., Gray-Donald, K., Rowat, K.M. and Jeans, M.E. (1998) Randomized controlled trial of a community-based psychoeducation program for the self-management of chronic pain, *Pain*, 74(2–3): 297–306.

Levenson, H. (1974) Activism and powerful others: distinctions within the concept of internal-external control, *Journal of Personality Assessment*, 38: 377–83.

Leventhal, H. and Nerenz, D. (1982) Representations of threat and the control of stress, in D. Meichenbaum and J. Jaremki (eds) *Stress Management and Presention: A Cognitive-Behavioural Approach*. New York: Plenum Press.

Levin, J. (2003) Spiritual determinants of health and healing: an epidemiologic perspective on salutogenic mechanisms, *Alternative Therapies in Health and Medicine*, 9(6): 48–57.

Levinson, D.J., Darrow, D.N., Klein, E.B., Levinson, M.H. and McKee, B. (1978) *The Seasons of a Man's Life*. New York: A.A. Knopf.

Lewinsohn, P.M. (1974) A behavioural approach to depression, in R.J. Freidman and M.M. Katz (eds) *The Psychology of Depression: Contemporary Theory and Reseach*, pp. 157–86. Washington, DC: V.H. Winston.

Ley, P. (1997) *Communicating with Patients: Improving Satisfaction and Compliance*. Cheltenham: Stanley Thornes.

Link, B.G. and Phedan, J.C. (2006) Stigma and its public health implications, *The Lancet*, 367: 528–9.

Linville, P.W. (1987) Self-complexity as a cognitive buffer against stress-related illness and depression, *Journal of Personality and Social Psychology*, 52(4): 663–76.

Litz, B.T., Gray, M.J., Bryant, R.A. and Adler, A.B. (2002) Early intervention for trauma: current status and future directions, *Clinical Psychology: Science and Practice*, 9(2): 112.

Loftus, E. (2002) Memory faults and fixes, *Issues In Science And Technology*, 18(4): 41–50.

Loftus, E. (2005) Planting misinformation in the human mind: a 30-year investigation of the malleability of memory, *Learning and Memory*, 12.

Lorig, K. and Holman, H. (1989) Arthritis self-management studies: a twelve year review, *Health Education Quarterly*, 20: 17–28.

Lorig, K., Mazanson, P.D. and Holman, H.R. (1993) Evidence suggesting that health education for self-management in patients with chronic arthritis has sustained health benefits while reducing health costs, *Arthritis and Rheumatism*, 36(4): 439–46.

Lund, M.L. and Tamm, M. (2001) How a group of disabled persons experience rehabilitation over a period of time, *Scandinavian Journal of Occupational Therapy*, 8(2): 96–104.

Maccoby, E.E. (1980) *Social Development: Psychological Growth and the Parent-Child Relationship*. New York: Harcourt Brace Jovanovich.

Maddux, J.E. (1993) Social cognitive models of health and exercise behavior: an introduction and review of conceptual issues, *Journal of Applied Sport Psychology*, 5(2): 116–40.

Main, C.J. and Williams, A.C de C. (2002) ABC of psychological medicine: musculo-skeletal pain. *British Medical Journal*, 325: 534–7.

Marks, D.F., Murray, M., Evans, B. and Willig, C. (2005) *Health Psychology: Theory, Research and Practice*, 2nd edn. London: Sage.

Marmot, M., Siegrist, J., Theorell, T. and Feeney, A. (1999) Health and the psycho-social environment at work, in M. Marmot and R.G. Wilkinson (eds) *Social Determinants of Health*, pp. 105–31. Oxford: Oxford University Press.

Marsland, A.L., Bachen, E.A., Cohen, S., Rabin, B. and Manuck, S.B. (2002) Stress, immune reactivity and susceptibility to infectious disease, *Physiology and Behaviour*, 77: 711–16.

Maslach, C., Schaufeli, W.B. and Leiter, M.P. (2001) Job burnout, *Annual Review of Psychology*, 52: 397–422.

Maslow, A.H. (1970) *Motivation and Personality*, 2nd edn. New York: Harper & Row.

Matthews, S., Stansfeld, S. and Power, C. (1999) Social support at age 33: the influence of gender, employment status and social class, *Social Science and Medicine*, 49(1): 133–42.

McCambridge, J. and Strang, J. (2004) The efficacy of single-session motivational interviewing in reducing drug consumption and perceptions of drug-related risk and harm among young people: results from a multi-site cluster randomized trial, *Addiction*, 99(1): 39–52.

McCann, M.E. and Kain, Z.N. (2001) The management of preoperative anxiety in children: an update, *Anesthesia-Analgesia*, 93: 98–105.

McDermut, W., Miller, I.W. and Brown, R.A. (2001) The efficacy of group psycho-therapy for depression: a meta-analysis and review of the empirical research, *Clinical Psychology: Science and Practice*, 8(1): 98–116.

McGaugh, J.L. (2003) *Memory and Emotion: The Making of Lasting Memories*. London: Weidenfeld & Nicolson.

McGrath, J.E. (1970) A conceptual formulation for research on stress, in J.E. McGrath (ed.) *Social and Psychological Factors in Stress*. New York: Holt, Rinehart & Winston.

Meadows, S. (1993) *The Child as Thinker*. London: Routledge.

Melzack, R. (2005) The McGill Pain Questionnaire from description to measurement, *Anesthesiology*, 103: 199–202.

Melzack, R. and Wall, P.D. (1965): Pain mechanisms: a new theory, *Science*, 150: 971–9.

Merritt, M.M., Bennett, G.G., Williams, R.B., Sollers, J.J. and Thayer, J.F. (2004) Low educational attainment, John Henryism, and cardiovascular reactivity to and recovery from personally relevant stress, *Psychosomatic Medicine*, 66: 49–55.

Miller, G.A. (1956) The magical number seven, plus or minus two: some limits to our capacity for processing information, *Psychological Review*, 63: 81–97.

Miller, J.F. (1992) Analysis of coping with illness, in J.F. Miller (ed.) *Coping with Chronic Illness: Overcoming Powerlessness*, 2nd edn. Philadelphia, PA: F.A. Davis.

Miller, W.R. and Rollnick, S. (2002) *Motivational Interviewing: Preparing People to Change Addictive Behaviour*, 2nd edn. New York: The Guilford Press.

Mills, M. and Walker, J.M. (1994) Memory, mood and dementia, *Journal of Aging Studies*, 8(1): 17–27.

Mirowsky, J. and Ross, C.E. (2003) *Social Causes of Psychological Distress* 2nd edn. New York: Aldine de Gruyter.

Monat, A. and Lazarus, R.S. (1991) *Stress and Coping: An Anthology*, 3rd edn. New York: Columbia University Press.

Morley, S., Eccleston, C. and Williams, A. (1999) Systematic review and meta-analysis of randomized controlled trials of cognitive behaviour therapy and behaviour therapy for chronic pain in adults, excluding headache, *Pain*, 80: 1–13.

Morris, J. and Ingham, R. (1988) Choice of surgery for early breast cancer: psychosocial considerations, *Social Science and Medicine*, 27(11): 1257–62.

Muntner, P. Sudre, P., Uldry, C., Rochat, T., Courteheuse, C., Naef, A.F. and Perneger, T.V. (2001) Predictors of participation and attendance in a new asthma patient self-management education program, *Chest*, 120(3) 778–84.

Murray, M. (2003) Narrative psychology, in J.A. Smith (ed.) *Qualitative Psychology: A Practical Guide to Research Methods*, pp. 111–31. Thousand Oaks, CA: Sage.

Newell, R. (2002a) Living with disfigurement, *Nursing Times*, 98(15): 34–5.

Newell, R. (2002b) The fear-avoidance model: helping patients to cope with disfigurement, *Nursing Times*, 98(16): 39–9.

NICE (National Institute for Health and Clinical Excellence) (2004a) *Anxiety: Management of Anxiety (Panic Disorder, with or without Agoraphobia, and Generalised Anxiety Disorder) in Adults in Primary, Secondary and Community Care*. London: NICE.

NICE (National Institute for Health and Clinical Excellence) (2004b) *Depression: Management of Depression in Primary and Secondary Care – NICE Guidance*. London: NICE.

NICE (National Institute for Health and Clinical Excellence) (2005a) Depression in Children and Young People: Identification and *Management in Primary, Community and Secondary Care*. London: NICE.

NICE (National Institute for Health and Clinical Excellence) (2005b) *Post-traumatic Stress Disorder (PTSD): The Management of PTSD in Adults and Children in Primary and Secondary Care, Clinical Guideline* no. 26. London: National Institute for Clinical Excellence.

Nicholas, P.K. (1993) Hardiness, self-care practices and perceived health status in older adults, *Journal of Advanced Nursing*, 18(7): 1085–94.

Nunes, E. and Cutler, J. (2000) *The Psychiatric Interview: A Guide to History Taking and the Mental State Examination*. Amsterdam: Harwood.

O'Connell, K., Skevington, S. and Saxena, S. (2003) Preliminary development of the World Health Organsiation's Quality of Life HIV instrument (WHOQOL-HIV): analysis of the pilot version, *Social Science and Medicine*, 57(7): 1259–75.

Omoto, A.M. and Snyder, M. (1995) Sustained helping without obligation: motivation, longevity of service, and perceived attitude change among AIDS volunteers, *Journal of Personality and Social Psychology*, 68(4): 671–86.

Osiri, M., Welch, V., Brosseau, L., Shea, B., McGowan, J., Tugwell, P. and Wells, G. (2000) Transcutaneous electrical nerve stimulation for knee osteoarthritis, *The Cochrane Database of Systematic Reviews*, issue 4. Chichester: Wiley.

Oterhals, K., Hanestad, B.R., Eide, G.E., and Hanssen, T.A. (2006) The relationship between in-hospital information and patient satisfaction after acute myocardial infarction, *European Journal of Cardiovascular Nursing*, 5: 303–10.

Overmier, J.B. and Murison, R. (2000) Anxiety and helplessness in the face of stress predisposes, precipitates and sustains gastric ulceration, *Behavioural Brain Research*, 110: 161–74.

Palmer, S., Cooper, C.L. and Thomas, K. (2003) *Creating a Balance: Managing Stress*. London: British Library Publishing.

Park, C.L., Folkman, S. and Bostrom, A. (2001) Appraisals of controllability and coping in caregivers and HIV+ men: testing the goodness-of-fit hypothesis, *Journal of Consulting and Clinical Psychology*, 69(3): 481–8.

Park, D.C., Hertzog, C., Leventhal, H., Morrell, R.W., Leventhal, E., Birchmore, D., Martin, M. and Bennett, J. (1999) Medication adherence in rheumatoid arthritis patients: older is wiser (comments), *Journal of the American Geriatrics Society*, 48(4): 457–9.

Parkes, C.M. (1972) *Bereavement: Studies of Grief in Adult Life*. Harmondsworth: Penguin.

Parsons, S., Neale, H.R., Reynard, G. *et al*. (2000) Development of social skills amongst adults with Asperger's Syndrome using virtual environments: the 'AS Interactive' project, *Proceedings of the 3rd International Conference in Disability, Virtual Reality and Associated Technologies*, pp. 163–70. Alghero, Italy.

Pascalis, O., de Schonen, S., Morton, J., Derulle, C. and Fabre-Grenet, M. (1995) Mother's face recognition by neonates: a replication and extension, *Infant Behavior and Development*, 18: 79–85.

Paterson, C. (1996) Measuring outcomes in primary care: a patient generated measure, MYMOP, compared with the SF–36 health survey, *British Medical Journal*, 312: 1016–20.

Paterson, C. (2003) MYMOP2, http://www.hsrc.ac.uk/mymop/entrymymop.htm.

Payne, S.A., Dean, S.J. and Kalus, C. (1998) A comparative study of death anxiety in hospice and emergency nurses, *Journal of Advanced Nursing*, 28(4): 700–6.

Peters, M.L., Godaert, G.L.R., Balliieux, R.E. *et al*. (1999) Immune response to experimental stress: effects of mental effort and uncontrollability, *Psychosomatic Medicine*, 61: 513–24.

Petty, R.E. and Cacioppo, J.T. (1986) *Communication and Persuasion: Central and Peripheral Routes to Attitude Change*. New York: Springer-Verlag.

Piaget, J. (1952) *The Origins of Intelligence in Children*. New York: Norton.

Piaget, J. and Inhelder, B. (1956) *The Child's Conception of Space*. London: Routledge & Kegan Paul.

Powell, H. and Gibson, P.G. (2003) Options for self-management education for adults with asthma, *Cochrane Database Systematic Review*, 3(1): CD004107.

Price, J.R. and Couper, J. (2003) Cognitive behaviour therapy for chronic fatigue syndrome in adults (Cochrane Review), *The Cochrane Library*, issue 4. Chichester: Wiley.

Prochaska, J.O. (2006) Moving beyond the transtheoretical model: further commentaries on West, *Addiction*, 101(6): 6.

Prochaska, J.O. and DiClemente, C.C. (1983) Stages and processes of self change in smoking: towards an integrative model of change, *Journal of Consulting and Clinical Psychology*, 51: 390–5.

Prochaska, J.O. and Norcross, J.C. (2001) Stages of change, *Psychotherapy*, 38(4): 443–8.

Purdie, N. and McCrindle, A. (2002) Self-regulation, self-efficacy and health behavior change in older adults, *Educational Gerontology*, 28(5): 379–400.

Radley, A. (1994) *Making Sense of Illness: The Social Psychology of Health and Disease*. London: Sage.

Radloff, L.S. (1977) The CES-D scale : a self-report depression scale for research in the general population, *Applied Psychological Measurement*, 1: 385–401.

Reason, J. (1990) *Human Error*. Cambridge: Cambridge University Press.

Rief, W., Ihle, D. and Pilger, F. (2003) A new approach to assess illness behaviour, *Journal of Psychosomatic Research*, 54(5): 415–16.

Riemsma, R.P., Pattenden, J., Bridle, C., Sowden, A.J., Mather, L., Watt, I.S. and Walker, A. (2003) Systematic review of the effectiveness of stage based interventions to promote smoking cessation, *British Medical Journal*, 326(7400): 1175–7.

Robertson, J. and Robertson, J. (1967–73) Young children in brief separation (videos), http://www.childdevmedia.com/.

Rose, S., Bisson, J. and Wessely, S. (2004) Psychological debriefing for preventing post traumatic stress disorder (PTSD) (Cochrane Review), *The Cochrane Library*, issue 1. Chichester: Wiley.

Rosenhan, D.L. (1973) On being sane in insane places. *Science*, 179: 365–9.

Rosenstiel, A.K. and Keefe, F.J. (1983) The use of coping strategies in chronic low back pain patients: relationship to patient characteristics and current adjustment, *Pain*, 17: 33–44.

Rosenstock, I.M. (1974a) Historical origins of the health belief model, *Health Education Monographs*, 2: 328–35.

Rosenstock, I.M. (1974b) The health belief model and preventive health behaviour, *Health Education Monographs*, 2: 354–86.

Rosenstock, I.M., Strecher, V.J. and Becker, M.H. (1988) Social learning theory and the health belief model, *Health Education Quarterly*, 15: 175–83.

Rosenthal, R. and Jacobson, L. (1968) *Pygmalion in the Classroom: Teacher Expectations and Pupils' Intellectual Development*. New York: Holt, Rinehart & Winston.

Ross, C.E. and Mirowsky, J. (1989) Explaining the social patterns of depression: control and problem solving – or support and talking? *Journal of Health and Social Behavior*, 30(2): 206–19.

Ross, L. (1977) The intuitive psychologist and his shortcomings: distortions in attribution process, in L. Berkowitz (ed.) *Advances in experimental social psychology*. Vol 10. New York: Academic Press

Roth, A. and Fonagy, P. (1996) *What Works for Whom: A Critical Review of Psychotherapy Research*. London: The Guilford Press.

Roth, S. and Cohen, L.J. (1986) Approach, avoidance and coping with stress, *American Psychologist*, 41(7): 813–9.

Rotter, J.B. (1966) Generalized expectancies for internal versus external control of reinforcement, *Psychological Monographs: General and Applied*, 80(1): 1–28.

Rubak, S., Sandbaek, A., Lauritzen, T. and Christensen, B. (2005) Motivational interviewing: a systematic review and meta-analysis, *British Journal of General Practice*, 55(513): 305–12.

Rubin, M. and Hewstone, M. (1998) Social identity theory's self-esteem hypothesis: a review and some suggestions for clarification, *Personality and Social Psychology Review*, 2(1): 40–62.

Rumsey, N. (2004) Psychological aspects of face transplantation: read the small print carefully, *The American Journal of Bioethics*, 4(3): 22–5.

Rumsey, N. and Harcourt, D. (2004) Body image and disfigurement: issues and interventions, *Body Image*, 1: 83–97.

Rushforth, H. (1999) Practitioner review: communicating with hospitalized children: review and application of research pertaining to children's understanding of health and illness, *Journal of Child Psychology and Psychiatry*, 40(5): 683–91.

Rutter, M. (1979) Maternal deprivation, 1972–1978: new findings, new concepts, new approaches, *Child Development*, 50: 282–305.

Sahler, O.J., Fairclough, D.L., Phipps, S. *et al.* (2005) Using problem-solving skills training to reduce negative affectivity in mothers of children with newly diagnosed cancer: report of a multisite randomized trial, *Journal of Consulting and Clinical Psychology*, 73(2): 272–83.

Sanders-Dewey, N.E.J., Mullins, L.L. and Chaney, J.M. (2001) Coping style, perceived uncertainty in illness, and distress in individuals with Parkinson's disease and their caregivers, *Rehabilitation Psychology*, 46(4): 363–81.

Sanz, E.J. (2003) Concordance and children's use of medicines, *British Medical Journal*, 327(7419): 858–60.

Schachter, S. and Singer, J.E. (1962) Cognitive, social and physiological determinants of emotional state, *Psychological Review*, 69: 379–99.

Schumacher, K. (2002) Putting cancer pain management regimens into practice at home, *Journal of Pain and Symptom Management*, 2(5): 369–82.

Seligman, M.E. (1972) *Biological Boundaries of Learning*. New York: Academic Press.

Seligman, M.E. and Csikszentmihalyi, M. (2000) Positive psychology: an introduction, *American Psycholologist*, 55(1): 5–14.

Seligman, M.E.P. (1975) *Helplessness: On Development, Depression and Death*. New York: Freeman.

Seligman, M.E.P. and Maier, S.F. (1967) Failure to escape traumatic shock, *Journal of Experimental Psychology*, 74: 1–9.

Selye, H. (1956) *The Stress of Life*. New York: McGraw-Hill.

Sephton, S.E., Koopman, C., Schaal, M., Thorsens, C. and Spiegel, D. (2001) Spiritual expression and immune status in women with metastic breast cancer: an exploratory study, *The Breast Journal*, 7(5): 345–53.

Sepúlveda, C., Marlin, A., Yoshida, T. and Ullrich, A. (2002) Palliative care: the World Health Organization's global perspective, *Journal of Pain and Symptom Management*, 24(2): 91–6.

Shapiro, F. (1996), Eye movement desensitization and reprocessing (EMDR): evaluation of controlled PTSD research, *Journal of Behavioural Theory and Experimental Psychiatry*, 27(3): 209–18.

Shaw, J. and Baker, M. (2004) 'Expert patient' – dream or nightmare? The concept of a well informed patient is welcome, but a new name is needed, *British Medical Journal*, 328(7442): 723–4.

Sheeran, P. and Abraham, C. (1996) The health belief model, in M. Conner and P. Norman (eds) *Predicting Health Behaviour: Research and Practice with Social Cognition Models*. Buckingham: Open University Press.

Sitzer, D.L., Twamley, E.W. and Jeste, D.V. (2006) Cognitive training in Alzheimer's disease: a meta-analysis of the literature, *Acta Psychiatrica Scandinavica*, 114: 75–90.

Skevington, S.M., Bradshaw, J. and Saxena, S. (1999) Selecting national items for the WHOQOL: conceptual and psychometric considerations, *Social Science and Medicine*, 48(4): 473–87.

Sliwinski, M.J., Hofer, S.M., Hall, C., Buschke, H. and Lipton, R.B. (2003) Modeling memory decline in older adults: the importance of preclinical dementia, attrition, and chronological age, *Psychology and Aging*, 18(4): 658–71.

Snyder, C.R. (1998) A case for hope in pain, loss and suffering, in J.H. Harvey (ed.) *Perspectives on Loss: A Sourcebook*. Philadelphia, PA: Brunner Mazel.

Spector, P.E., Zapf, D., Chen, P.Y. and Frese, M. (2000) Why negative affectivity should not be controlled in job stress research: don't throw out the baby with the bath water, *Journal of Organizational Behavior*, 21: 79–95.

Spieker, S.J. and Bensley, L. (1994) Roles of living arrangements and grandmother social support in adolescent mothering and infant attachment, *Developmental Psychology*, 30(1) : 102–11.

Srivastava, S., John, O.P., Gosling, S.D. and Potter, J. (2003) Development of personality in early and middle adulthood: set like plaster or persistent change? *Journal of Personality and Social Psychology*, 84(5): 1041–53.

Stansfield, S.A. (1999) Social support and social cohesion, in M. Marmot and R.G. Wilkinson (eds) *Social Determinants of Health*, pp. 155–78. Oxford: Oxford University Press.

Steinberg, L. (2004) Risk-taking in adolescence: what changes, and why? *Annual New York Academy of Science*, 1021: 51–8.

Stephenson, N.L. and Herman, J. (2000) Pain measurement: a comparison using horizontal and vertical visual analogue scales, *Applied Nursing Research*, 13(3): 157–8.

Stewart, K. (2002) *Helping a Child with Nonverbal Learning Disorder or Asperger's Syndrome: A Parent's Guide*. Oakland, CA: New Harbinger Publications.

Stockwell, F. (1984) *The Unpopular Patient*. London: Croom Helm.

Stroebe, M.S. and Schut, H. (1998) Culture and grief, *Bereavement Care*, 17(1): 7–10.

Stroebe, W. and Stroebe, M.S. (1987) *Bereavement and Health: The Psychological and Physical Consequences of Partner Loss*. New York: Cambridge University Press.

Sullivan, M.J. *et al.* (2001) Theoretical perspectives on the relation between catastrophizing and pain, *Clinical Journal of Pain*, 17(1): 52–64.

Szasz, T. (1996) *The Meaning of Mind: Language, Morality, and Neuroscience*. London: Praeger.

Tajfel, H. (1982) *Social Identity and Intergroup Relations*. Cambridge: Cambridge University Press.

Taris, T.W. and Bok, I.A. (1996) Effects of parenting style upon psychological well-being of young adults: exploring the relations among parental care, locus of control and depression, *Early Child Development and Care*, 132: 93–104.

Taylor, S.E. (1979) Patient hospital behaviour: reactance, helplessness, or control? *Journal of Social Issues*, 35: 156–84.

Taylor, S.E. and Brown, J.D. (1988) Illusion and well-being: a social psychological perspective on mental health, *Psychological Bulletin*, 103(2): 193–210.

Taylor, S.E. and Gollwitzer, P.M. (1995) Effects of mindset on positive illusions, *Journal of Personality and Social Psychology*, 69: 213–26.

Temoshok, L. (1987) Personality, coping style, emotion and cancer: towards an integrative model, *Cancer Surveys*, 6(iii): 545–67.

Teresi, J.A., Holmes, D., Ramirez, M., Gurland, B.J. and Lantigua, R. (2001) Performance of cognitive tests among different racial/ethnic and education groups: findings of differential item functioning and possible item bias, *Journal of Mental Health and Aging*, 7(1): 79–89.

Thieme, K., Spies, C., Sinha, P., Turk, D.C. and Flor, H. (2005) Predictors of pain behaviours in fibromyalgia syndrome, *Arthritis & Rheumatism*, 53(3): 343–50.

Thomsen, A.B., Sorensen, J., Sjogren, P. and Eriksen, J. (2001) Economic evaluation of multidisciplinary pain nanagement in chronic pain patients: a qualitative systematic review, *Journal of Pain and Symptom Management*, 22(2): 688–98.

Todd, S. and Shearn, J. (1997) Family dilemmas and secrets: parents' disclosure of information to their adult offspring with learning disabilities, *Disability and Society*, 12(3): 341–66.

Toth, E.L., Majumdar, S.R., Guirguis, L.M., Lewanczuk, R.Z., Lee, T.K. and Johnson, J.A. (2003) Compliance with clinical practice guidelines for type 2 diabetes in rural patients: treatment gaps and opportunities for improvement, *Pharmacotherapy*, 23(5): 659–65.

Twycross, R., Harcourt, J. and Bergl, S. (1996) A survey of pain in patients with advanced cancer, *Journal of Pain and Symptom Management*, 12(5): 273–82.

Uchino, B.N., Cacioppo, J.T. and Kiecolt-Glaser, J.K. (1996) The relationship between social support and physiological processes: a review with emphasis on underlying mechanisms and implications for health, *Psychological Bulletin*, 119(3): 488–531.

Vachon, M.L., Sheldon, A.R., Lancee, W.J., Lyall, W.A., Rogers, J. and Freeman, S.J. (1982) Correlates of enduring distress patterns following bereavement: social network, life situation and personality, *Psychological Medicine*, 12(4): 783–8.

Van der Spank, J.T., Cambier, D.C., De Paepe, H.M.C., Danneels, I.A.G., Witvrouw, E.E. and Beerens, L. (2000) Pain relief in labour by transcutaneous electrical nerve stimulation (TENS), *Archives of Gynecology and Obstetrics*, 264(3): 131–6.

Van Doorn, C., Kasl, S.V., Beery, L.C., Jacobe, H.G. and Prigerson, H.G. (1998) The influence of marital quality and attachment styles on traumatic grief and depressive symptoms, *Journal of Nervous and Mental Diseases*, 186(9): 566–73.

Vanltallie, T.B. (2002) Stress: a risk factor for serious illness, *Metabolism*, 51(6 suppl. 1): 40–5.

Vedhara, K., McDermott, M.P., Evans *et al.* (2002) Chronic stress in nonelderly caregivers: psychological, endocrine and immune implications, *Journal of Psychosomatic Research*, 53: 1153–61.

Veldtman, G.R., Matley, S.L., Kendall, L., Quirk, J., Gibbs, J.L., Parsons, J.M. and Hewison, J. (2000) Illness understanding in children and adolescents with heart disease, *Heart*, 84(4): 395–7.

Vlaeyen, J.W.S. and Linton, S.J. (2000) Fear-avoidance and its consequences in chronic musculoskeletal pain: a state of the art, *Pain*, 85: 317–32.

Vollrath, M. and Torgersen, S. (2000) Personality types and coping, *Personality and Individual Differences*, 29(2): 367–78.

Von Korff, M., Moore, J.E., Lorig, K., Cherkin, D.C., Saunders, K., Gonzalez, V.M., Laurent, D., Rutter, C. and Comite, F. (1998) A randomized trial of a lay person-led self-management group intervention for back pain patients in primary care, *Spine*, 23(23): 2608–15.

Vygotsky, L.S. (1978) *Mind in Society: The Development of Higher Mental Processes*. Cambridge, MA: Harvard University Press.

Waatkaar, T., Borge, A.I.H., Fundingsrudc, H.P., Christiea, H.J. and Torgersen, S. (2004) The role of stressful life events in the development of depressive symptoms in adolescence – a longitudinal community study, *Journal of Adolescence*, 27: 153–63.

Waddell, G. (1992) Biopsychosocial analysis of low back pain, *Bailliere's Clinical Rheumatology*, 6: 523–51.

Walker, J. (1989) The nursing management of pain in the elderly, unpublished Ph.D. thesis, Dorset Institute (Bournemouth University).

Walker, J. (1994) Caring for elderly people with persistent pain in the community: a qualitative perspective on the attitudes of patients and nurses, *Health and Social Care in the Community*, 2: 221–8.

Walker, J. (2000) Women's experiences of transfer from a midwife-led to a consultant-led maternity unit, *Journal of Midwifery and Women's Health*, 45(2): 161–8.

Walker, J. (2001) *Control and the Psychology of Health*. Buckingham: Open University Press.

Walker, J. and Sofaer, B. (1998) Predictors of psychological distress in chronic pain patients, *Journal of Advanced Nursing*, 27: 320–6.

Walker, J., Brooksby, A., McInerney, J. and Taylor, A. (1998) Patient perceptions of hospital care: building confidence, faith and trust, *Journal of Nursing Management*, 6: 193–200.

Walker, J., Holloway, I. and Sofaer, B. (1999) 'In the system': patients' experiences of chronic back pain, *Pain*, 80: 621–8

Walker, J., Sofaer, B. and Holloway, I. (2006) The experience of chronic back pain: accounts of loss in those seeking help from pain clinics, *European Journal of Pain*, 10: 199–207.

Wall, P. (1999) *Pain: The Science of Suffering*. London: Weidenfeld & Nicholson.

Wallhagen, M.I., Strawbridge, W.J., Kaplan, G.A. and Cohen, R.D. (1994) Impact of internal health locus of control on health outcomes for older men and women: a longitudinal perspective, *Gerontologist*, 34(3): 299–306.

Wallston, K.A., Wallston, B.S. and DeVellis, R. (1978) Development of the Multi-dimensional Health Locus of Control (MHLOC) scale, *Health Education Monographs*, 6: 161–70.

Walter, T. (1996) A new model of grief: bereavement and biography, *Mortality*, 1(1): 7–25.

Walter, T. (1999) *On Bereavement: The Culture of Grief*. Buckingham: Open University Press.

Wasserman, D. (2006) *Depression, the Facts: Expert Advice for Patients, Carers and Professionals*. Oxford: Oxford University Press.

Watson, A. and Visram, A. (2000) The developing role of play preparation in paediatric anaesthesia, *Paediatric Anaesthesia*, 10: 681–6.

Watson, D. and Pennebaker, J.W. (1989) Health complaints, stress, and distress: exploring the central role of negative affectivity, *Psychological Review*, 96(2): 234–54

Weinman, J., Petrie, K.J., Moss-Morris, R. and Horne, R. (1996) The illness perception questionnaire: a new method for assessing the cognitive representation of illness, *Psychology and Health*, 11: 431–5.

West, R. (2005) Time for a change: putting the Transtheoretical (Stages of Change) Model to rest, *Addiction*, 100: 1036–9.

WHO (World Health Organization) (1946) *Preamble to the Constitution of the World Health Organization as Adopted by the International Health Conference*, New York, 19–22 June 1946, and entered into force on 7 April 1948. Geneva: WHO, www.who.int/en/.

WHO (World Health Organization) (2001) *The World Health Report 2001. Mental*

Health: New Understanding, New Hope, www.who.int/whr2001/2001/main/en/chapter3/003d.htm.

WHO (World Health Organization) (2006) *International Statistical Classification of Diseases and Related Health Problems*, 10th revision, www.who.int/classifications/apps/icd/icd10online/, accessed 10 January 2007.

WHO (2007) Analgesic ladder, www.who.int/cancer/palliative/painladder, accessed 15 January 2007.

Wiebe, D.J. and Korbel, C. (2003) Defensive denial, self-regulation and health, in L.D. Cameron and H. Leventhal (eds) *The Self-regulation of Health and Illness Behaviour*. London: Routledge.

Wiese, B.S., Freund, A.M. and Baltes, P.B. (2002) Subjective career success and emotional well-being: longitudinal predictive power of selection, optimization, and compensation, *Journal of Vocational Behavior*, 60: 321–35.

Williams, L.M. and Payne, S. (2003) A qualitative study of clinical nurse specialists' views on depression in palliative care patients, *Palliative Medicine*, 17(4): 334–8.

Williams-Piehota, P., Schneider, T.R., Pizarro, J., Mowad, L. and Salovey, P. (2004) Matching health messages to health locus of control beliefs for promoting mammography utilization, *Psychology and Health*, 19(4): 407–423.

Witte, K. and Allen, M. (2000) A meta-analysis of fear appeals: implications for effective public health campaigns, *Health Eduction and Behaviour*, 27(5): 591–615.

Wolpe, J. (1958) *Psychotherapy by Reciprocal Inhibition*. Stanford, CA: Stanford University Press.

Wortman, C.B. and Silver, R.C. (1989) The myths of coping with loss, *Journal of Consulting and Clinical Psychology*, 57(3): 349–57.

Wright, J.H. (2006) Cognitive behavior therapy: basic principles and recent advances, *Focus*, 4: 173.

Zigmond, A.S. and Snaith, R.P. (1983) The Hospital Anxiety and Depression Scale, *Acta Psychiatrica Scandinavica*, 67: 361–70.

Zwakhalen, S.M.G. Hamers, J.P.H., Abu-Saad, H.H., Martijn, P.F. and Berger, M.P.F. (2006) Pain in elderly people with severe dementia: a systematic review of behavioural pain assessment tools, *BMC Geriatric*, 6(3): 1–15.

INDEX

g indicates glossary

a priori prediction, 14, 246*g*
action planning, stages of change model,
    195, 196
active vs passive coping, 162, 246*g*
acupuncture, 236
acute pain *see* pain, acute
adaptation, 28–9, 246*g*
    assimilation and accommodation,
        developmental stages, 43–4
adherence/compliance, 246*g*
    by health professionals, 203–4
    and concordance, 202–3
    and negative affectivity, 38
    and self-esteem, 140–1
adolescence, development in, 55–7
adulthood, development in, 57–9
adverse reactions to treatment, 233–4
age differences, social cognition models,
    194
ageing, 59–61
    successful, 60, 178
agreeableness, 36
Alzheimer's disease *see* dementia
ambivalent attachment, 52
amnesia, 78, 246*g*
analgesia
    adverse reactions, 233
    patient-controlled (PCA), 228–9, 230
    types, 232–3
analgesic ladder, 230
anticipatory grief, 130–1
anxiety, 6, 34, 88–9, 246*g*
    death, 125
    definition of, 111
    in dementia, 62–3
    and information-giving, 66–7, 228
    management approaches, 111–13,
        114–15
    comparison, 113–14
    as mental disorder, 114
    neuroticism, 36, 37, 100–1, 114
    reduction in hospital settings, 89–90,
        179–80
    separation, 51
    see also avoidance; stress

appraisal, 110, 159, 175–9, 246*g*
    primary, 161, 248*g*
    and reappraisal, 161
    secondary, 161, 249*g*
arousal
    and attention, 66–7
    stress response, 158, 164–6
Asch, S.E., 143–4
assimilation and accommodation,
    developmental stages, 43–4
attachment, 7, 50, 120, 246*g*
    and loss, 125, 128–9
    stress, coping and, 172, 173
    types, 51–3
    see also bonding
attention
    arousal and, 66–7
    selective, 68–9, 135, 140
attitudes, 29–30, 148, 191
attractiveness of information source, 136
attribution error, 34–5
attribution theory, 33–5, 246*g*
authoritarian leadership, 155
authoritarian parents, 54
authoritative parents, 53–4
authority figures, 142
    obedience to, 141–3
avoidance, 115, 246*g*
    of eye contact, 148, 150
    fear-avoidance and management,
        90–1, 234
avoidant attachment, 52

babies
    pain and pain assessment, 216–17, 224
    see also child development
Bandura, A., 23, 102, 103–4, 198, 199,
    208
behaviour modification, 96–8
behavioural symptoms of stress, 157
behaviourism (behavioural psychology),
    5, 6, 85, 246*g*
    anxiety management, 112
    depression management, 102, 119–20
    health education programme, 106–7

self-management, 208
bereavement, 246*g*
  stages, 126–7
  see also loss
biographical approach *see* narrative
    psychology; narrative therapy
biographical disruption, 72–3
biographical memory, 77–8, 123
biospychological model, 3, 246*g*
bipolar dimension of personality, 36,
    246*g*
body ideal, 24–5
body image, 23–7
body movements, 25
body posture and gestures, 25, 148–9,
    150
body reality, 24
bonding, 93, 246*g*
  see also attachment
Bowlby, J., 50, 51, 120, 126, 128, 173
brain injury, 78
breaking bad news, 80–2
burnout, 158, 246*g*
  organisational stress and, 181–2
bystander apathy, 147–8

cancer, chronic pain in, 226, 229–31
caregivers' stress-related illness, 77,
    170–1
catastrophizing in chronic pain, 234
catharsis, 7, 246*g*
child development, 42–54
chronic illness, 204–11
  aim of management, 205
  assessing outcomes, 205–7
  self-management, 207–11
chronic pain
  cancer, 226, 229–31
  case study, 237–42
  global assessment, 223–4
  persistent/benign, 226–7, 231–2
  quality of life improvement, 232–5
  transition from acute to, 232
classical conditioning, 86–91, 246*g*
clinical psychologists, 15
cognition, definition of, 5, 246*g*
cognitive appraisal *see* appraisal
cognitive behavioural therapists, 16
cognitive (behavioural) therapy (CBT),
    121–2, 208, 246*g*
  anxiety, 112, 113
  chronic pain, 237
  depression, 118–19
  systematic desensitization, 90–1, 124
cognitive development theories, 42–6

cognitive dissonance, 74, 137–8, 246*g*
cognitive science, 5, 6
cognitive symptoms of stress, 157
communication
  conflict management, 151–3
  effective, 78–80, 119–20, 149–53
  impairment, and pain assessment,
    224–5
  non-verbal, 25, 148–9, 150, 248*g*
complexity of information, 138–9
compliance *see* adherence/compliance
concordance, 202–3
conditioning, 85–6, 246*g*
  classical, 86–91, 246*g*
  emotional responses, 88–9
  operant, 50, 86, 91–5, 248*g*
conflict management, 151–3
conformity, 29, 143–6, 247*g*
conscientiousness, 36, 38
contemplation, stages of change model,
    195, 196
context-specific memory, 74
control, 100
  gaining and promoting, 171
  locus of (LOC), 33–4, 104–5, 178, 248*g*
  perceived, 101, 102, 167, 168–70,
    191–2
  and perceived uncontrollability,
    100–2, 119, 167, 168, 170–1, 216
  stimulus, 95, 250*g*
coping/coping strategies, 6, 58, 162–3,
    247*g*
  in dementia, 62–3
  health-related behaviours, 194
  mediators, 175–9
  in pain, 217–18, 223
  see also stress
counselling psychologists, 15
counselloring/counsellors, 15–16, 183
  person-centred/Rogerian, 121, 249*g*
credibility of information source, 135
cues, 94–5
cultural differences, 20, 25, 125

daily hassles, 181, 247*g*
daily living help, 235
death
  anxiety, 125
  approaching, 61–3
  children's understanding of, 48–9
defence mechanisms, 125–6, 247*g*
dementia, 62–3, 76–8
  caregivers' stress-related illness, 77,
    170–1
  pain assessment, 224

democratic leadership, 155
demographic influences on stress response, 175–6
denial, 7, 82, 247g
depersonalization, 62–3, 247g
depression, 6, 247g
  in adolescence, 56
  definition of, 116
  diagnosis, 117
  learned helplessness model, 100–2, 119
  maintaining factors, 117
  in older people, 61
  theories and management approaches, 102, 117–21
  triggers, 117
  vulnerability, 117
Diagnostic and Statistical Manual (DSM IV), 114, 117, 122
disengagement theory of ageing, 60
'dual process' model of grief, 127
dualism, 3–4, 247g

eclecticism, 16, 247g
educational attainment and stress response, 176
'effort-reward imbalance', 182
ego, 7, 247g
ego defence, 125–6
emergency, taking responsibility in, 147–8
emotion
  definition of, 109–11
  vs reason, in information-giving, 136–7
emotion-focused coping, 247g
  vs problem-focused coping, 162–3
emotional responses
  conditioned, 88–9
  and perceived control, 168–70
  to stress, 157
emotional support, 172, 247g
empiricism, 85, 247g
Erickson, E.H., 42, 60, 61
ethnography, 13
evidence-based advice/therapies for pain, 233–4, 235–42
experimental methods, 11
experimental neurosis, 100–1
Expert Patient Programme, 209–11, 231
external locus of control (LOC), 105, 106
extroversion, 36, 38
eye contact, 148, 150

facial disfigurement, 26

facial expression, 150
facts vs theory in psychology, 9–10
false memory, 73–4
fear-avoidance and management, 90–1, 234
fight or flight response, 164–5, 247g
focus groups, 13, 247g
Folkman, S. and Lazarus, R.S., 162, 163, 164
forgetting, 74–5
  bad news, 81–2
Freud, S., 7, 41–2, 55, 81–2, 120, 126
fundamental attribution error, 34, 247g

gender differences in stress response, 175–6
goal orientated behaviour, 198
Goffman, E., 9, 26, 27, 28, 113
grief, 125, 247g
  anticipatory, 130–1
  'dual process' model, 127
  see also loss
grief therapy, 128
grief work, 126, 128
grounded theory, 13
group interaction, 153–4
groupthink, 153–4, 247g

habits, 193–4, 247g
hardy personality, 177
health behaviour, 2, 143, 247g
health belief model (HBM), 189–91, 193, 195, 202
health education/promotion programme, 106–7, 187–8
  see also information
health professionals, 15–16
  adherence, 203–4
  motivation of, 146–8
health promotion, 187–8
health psychologists, 15
health, WHO definition of, 2, 186
helping
  as motivation, 146–8
  see also learned helplessness
homeostasis, 165, 247g
hope, 131–2
hospital settings
  anxiety reduction, 89–90, 179–80
  chronic pain, 233
hostility, 178
humanistic psychology, 5, 7–9
  anxiety management, 112–13
  depression management, 121
hypothesis, 10, 247g

ICD 10, 114, 117
identity, 21–3
  see also personality; self
illness behaviours, 32–3, 99–100, 247*g*
illness, definitions of, 186–7
illness management, 201–4
Illness Perception questionnaire (IPQ),
    204–5
immune function in stress, 165–6,
    170–1, 172–3
implementation, stages of change
    model, 195, 196
individual differences in stress-related
    illness (psychoneuroimmunology),
    176–9
inductive methods, 13, 247*g*
information-giving, 69–70, 78–80
  and anxiety, 66–7, 228
  bad news, 80–2
  individualized, 82
  see also memory; persuasion
informational support, 146–7, 172
instrumental support, 146–7, 172, 174,
    247*g*
internal locus of control (LOC), 105, 106
*International Classification of Diseases
    (ICD 10)*, 114, 117
interpersonal/social skills, 119–20,
    149–53
interprofessional/interagency working,
    3–4, 154
intervention, 2, 248*g*
introspection, 20, 248*g*

Kitwood, T., 62–3
Klein, M., 7, 120
Kohlberg, L., 47–8
Kulber-Ross, E., 126

labelling/stereotyping, 20, 30, 32, 33, 39
lay understandings of medicine, 71
Lazarus, R.S., 159–61
  Folkman, S. and, 162, 163, 164
leadership styles, 155
learned helplessness, 248*g*
  perceived uncontrollability, 100–2,
    119, 167, 168, 170–1, 216
  undoing, 102
learning
  in pain, 216–19, 225
  social learning theory, 102–3, 208
  theory development, 85–9
  types, 84–5
life events, 9, 180–1, 248*g*
life review therapy, 61–2, 129

life 'stages', 41–2
lifestyle and behaviour, 95–6
Likert scale, 11, 248*g*
listening, 115, 183
locus of control (LOC), 33–4, 104–5, 178,
    248*g*
long-term memory, 70–1
looking-glass self, 20
loss, 2, 124–31, 248*g*
  of memory, 75–8
  social support and health outcomes,
    172–3
  traditional models, 125–7
    challenges to, 127–9

McGill Pain Questionnaire (MPQ), 221,
    222
maintenance, stages of change model,
    195, 196
Maslow, A., 8
medical errors, 35
medical help-seeking, 200–1
memory, 65–7
  context-specific, 74
  false, 73–4
  and forgetting, 74–5
  long-term, 70–1
  loss of, 75–8
  schemas and scripts, 71–3
  short-term, 67–70
  see also information-giving
meta-analysis, 49, 248*g*
Milgram, S., 141–2, 155
mindfulness mediation, 236
mnemonics, 68, 248*g*
modelling, 27, 103, 248*g*
moral reasoning, development of,
    47–8
motivation, of health professionals,
    146–8
motivational interviewing, 200
mourning, 125, 248*g*
MYMOP (Measure Yourself Medical
    Outcomes Profile), 207

narrative psychology, 5, 9, 13, 22–3,
    248*g*
narrative therapy, 61–2, 129–30, 200,
    248*g*
nativism, 85, 248*g*
nature–nurture debate, 35–6
needs
  in chronic pain, 232
  hierarchy of, 8
negative affectivity, 38, 177–8

negative aspects
  of social support, 173–4
  of stress, 166
neuropathic pain, 226–7
neuroticism, 36, 37, 100–1, 114
nocebo response, 218
non-verbal communication, 25, 148–9,
    150, 248g
NSAIDs, 232–3
numerical rating scale (NRS) of pain, 221

obedience, 141–3
observational learning, 102, 103
older people
  depression in, 61
  development in, 59–61
  see also death; dementia
operant conditioning, 50, 86, 91–5, 248g
opioid analgesia, 232–3
optimism vs pessimism, 177
organisational/work-based stress, 181–3

pain
  acute, 226, 227–8
    transition to chronic pain, 232
  aim of management, 225–6
  anxiety and information, 228
  coping strategies, 217–18, 223
  gate control theory, 214–16
  nocebo response, 218
  perceiving and expressing, 213–14,
    216–19
  placebo response, 218–19
  post-operative and post-trauma,
    227–8
  sensory description, 222
  as stressor, 216, 235
  temporal pattern, 222
  triggers and contextual factors, 223
  types of, 226–7
pain assessment
  location, 220
  measuring and recording, 220
  pain relief, 222
  principles, 219–25
  severity/intensity, 220–1
parenting styles, influence on
    development, 53–4, 56, 57
Parkes, C.M., 126
partnership, 203
patient-controlled analgesia (PCA),
    228–9, 230
peer pressure, 199–200
  see also conformity
peer teaching, 209–11

perceptions
  of information source, 135–6
  pain, 213–14, 216–19
  of punishment and reinforcement,
    92–3
  see also under control
permissive parents, 54
person-centred approaches, 39, 121,
    249g
personal space, 150
personality
  and change, 36–7
  and health, 35–9
    outcomes, 37–9
  measurement, 36, 37
  stress and stress-related illness, 176–9
  traits, 35–6
  see also identity; self
persuasion, 134–9
  audience factors, 140–1
  conformity, 143–5
  message factors, 136–9
  obedience, 141–3
  source factors, 135–6
  see also information-giving
pessimism vs optimism, 177
phenomenology, 7–8, 13, 248g
phobias and management, 90–1
Piaget, J., 42–5, 48, 55
pectoral scale of pain, 222
placebo/placebo response, 11, 248g
play, importance of, 49
'pop psychology' see pseudoscience
positive psychology, 132
positivism, 4, 248g
post hoc explanations, 7, 248g
post-traumatic stress disorder (PTSD),
    89, 122–4, 181
  in chronic pain, 235
  management, 124
pre-contemplation, stages of change
    model, 195, 196
preventative approaches, 187–8
  primary, 186, 187–8, 248g
  secondary, 186, 187, 188, 249g
  tertiary, 186, 187, 188, 201–4, 250g
primacy effect, 69, 137, 248g
primary appraisal, 161, 248g
primary prevention, 186, 187–8, 248g
primary reinforcement, 91
problem-focused coping, 171, 248g
  vs emotion-focused coping, 162–3
progressive muscular relaxation (PMR),
    235–6
pseudoscience, 7, 14, 248g

psychiatrists, 16
psychoanalysis, 5, 248*g*
psychoanalysts, 16
psychodynamic psychology, 5, 7, 248*g*
  anxiety management, 112, 113
  depression management, 120
psychodynamic psychotherapists, 16
psychoeugenic illness, 7, 249*g*
psychological measures, 11
psychology
  current schools of thought, 4–9
  definition of, 1–2
  facts vs theory, 9–10
  importance in health and social care,
    2–3
  practice, 16–17
  research methods, 10–14, 249*g*
psychoneuroimmunology, 2–3, 164–6,
  249*g*
psychosocial processes, 6, 249*g*
psychosomatic disorders, 7, 249*g*
punishment, 42, 91, 249*g*
  consequences of, 93–4
  schedule of, 92
  subjective perception, 92–3

qualitative research, 10, 11–12, 14, 249*g*
quality of life, 205–6, 232–5
quantitative research, 10, 13–14, 249*g*

randomized controlled trial, 11, 12, 249*g*
reappraisal, 161
reason vs emotions, information-giving,
  136–7
recall, 73–4
recency effect, 69, 137, 249*g*
reciprocal altruism, 146
reciprocity in communication, 150
reductionism, 3–4, 249*g*
reference group, 21–2, 249*g*
reinforcement, 50, 91–2, 249*g*
  consequences, 93–4
  depression management, 119–20
  schedule of, 92, 249*g*
  secondary, 91–2
  subjective perception, 92–3
  vs control, 100
relaxation and imagery, 235–6
reliability, 11, 249*g*
religion, 174–5
repertory grid, *22*, 249*g*
repression, 7, 81–2, 120, 249*g*
research methods, 10–14, 249*g*
risk behaviours in adolescence, 56–7
rituals, 125

Rogerian/person-centred counselling,
  121, 249*g*
Rogers, C., 8–9
role play in conflict management, 152–3

'scaffolding', 45
schedule of punishment, 92
schedule of reinforcement, 92, 249*g*
schemas, 30, 42–3, 71–3, 129, 249*g*
schools of thought in psychology, 4–9
scripts and schemas, 71–3
secondary appraisal, 161, 249*g*
secondary prevention, 186, 187, 188,
  249*g*
secondary reinforcement, 91–2
secure attachment, 52
selective attention, 68–9, 135, 140
'selective optimization with
  compensation' (SOC), 57–8
self, 8, 249*g*
  defined by social comparison, 21
  looking-glass, 20
  see also identity; personality
self-actualization, 8, 249*g*
self-concept, 19–23, 28–9
self-efficacy, 11, 102, 103–4, 180, 249*g*
self-esteem, 21, 23, 25, 103–4, 249*g*
  and compliance, 140–1
  and perceived control, 168
self-fulfilling prophecy, 32–3
self-help/support groups, 173, 174, 210,
  231
self-management, 33, 180, 207–11, 231,
  249*g*
self-modification, 98–100
self-regulation/theory, 104, 198–200,
  208, 249*g*
  critique, 199–200
Seligman, M.E.P., 100–1, 119, 132
sense of belonging, 172
sense of coherence, 178, 249*g*
sensory description of pain, 222
separation anxiety, 51
severe learning difficulties, pain
  assessment in, 225
short-term memory, 67–70
Skinner, B.F., 92, 96
social affiliation/networks, 172, 176
social cognition, 5, 102, 164, 249*g*
  models, 189–93
  critique, 193–5
social comparison, 21
social desirability, 145–6
social development, 49–54
social learning theory, 102–3, 208

social norms, 23, 143, 249*g*
social psychology, 5, 9
    anxiety management, 113
Social Readjustment Rating Scale (SRRS), 180
social roles, 27–9
social rules, 28
social space, 150
social support, 4, 164, 168–70, 171–4, 249*g*
    at work, 182
    and health outcomes, 172–3
    negative aspects, 173–4
social/interpersonal skills, 119–20, 149–53
socialization, 250*g*
    pain, 217–18
sociocultural theory of cognitive development, 45–6
space, personal and social, 150
spiritual support, 174–5
stages of change (transtheoretical) model, 195–8
    critique, 196–8
'stages' of life model, 41–2
stereotyping/labelling, 20, 30, 32, 33, 39
stigma, 26–7, 250*g*
stigmatization, 30–2
stimulus, 89, 250*g*
stimulus control, 95, 250*g*
stimulus-response theory, 85
stress
    in caregivers, 77, 170–1
    definitions of, 158–9
    in different contexts, 179–82
    individual differences, 176–9
    mediators, 167–79
    physiological response, 164–6
    positive vs negative effects, 166
    reduction and management, 182–4
    symptoms, 157–8
    transactional model, 159, 163–4
    see also anxiety; coping/coping strategies
stressor
    definition of, 159, 250*g*
    pain as, 216, 235
subjective norm, 191
successful ageing, 60, 178

support
    emotional, 172, 247*g*
    informational, 146–7, 172
    instrumental, 146–7, 172, 174, 247*g*
    self-help groups, 173, 174, 210, 231
    spiritual, 174–5
    see also social support
survey methods, 12
systematic desensitization, 90–1, 124
systematic review, 81, 250*g*

temporal pattern of pain, 222
tertiary prevention, 186, 187, 188, 201–4, 250*g*
theory of planned behaviour (TPB), 191–3, 194, 204
threats, 56–7, 250*g*
transactional model of stress, 159, 163–4
transcutaneous electrical nerve stimulation (TENS), 215, 235
transtheoretical model *see* stages of change (transtheoretical) model
traumatic events *see* post-traumatic stress disorder (PTSD)
trustworthiness of information source, 135
twin studies, 36

uncertainty/unpredictability, 168, 216
unconditional positive regard, 9, 121, 250*g*
uncontrollability, perceived, 100–2, 119, 167, 168, 170–1, 216
uninvolved parents, 54
unpredictability, perceived, 168, 216

validity, 11, 250*g*
verbal rating scale (VRS), 221
visual analogue scale (VAS), 221
volunteers, 146
Vygotsky, L., 45–6, 56, 209–10

whistleblowers, 145
work-based stress, 181–3
World Health Organization (WHO)
    definition of health, 2, 186
    quality of life measure (WHOQOL), 205–6

SAFEGUARDING CHILDREN AND YOUNG PEOPLE
A GUIDE FOR NURSES AND MIDWIVES

Catherine Powell

While many nurses and midwives are in an ideal position to prevent, identify and respond to child maltreatment, they may not currently have a clear understanding of the theory, policy and practice of safeguarding children. This book, which has been written specifically for a nursing and midwifery audience, provides an accessible text that outlines and explores professional roles and responsibilities in the context of inter-agency working.

Importantly, it has chapters on:

- Child neglect
- Fabricated or induced illness
- Child death and child maltreatment
- Safeguarding vulnerable children

This groundbreaking book provides a much needed education, research, practice and evidence-based evaluation. The book also:

- Includes case examples and points for reflection
- Provides an analysis of children's rights and child protection
- Enables readers to understand and apply theory and policy to practice
- Outlines the roles and responsibilities of other agencies
- Helps readers develop skills to deal with sensitive and traumatic issues
- Addresses the importance of confidentiality and information sharing

Safeguarding Children and Young People is core reading for all nursing and midwifery students and practitioners.

Contents
Introduction: Why a safeguarding children guide for nurses and midwives? – Why every child matters – Child maltreatment – Safeguarding children: Professional roles and responsibilities – Safeguarding vulnerable children – Fabricated or induced illness – Child neglect – Child death and child maltreatment – Conclusion: Knowledge for practice.

July 2007 256pp
ISBN-13: 978 0 335 22028 1 (ISBN-10: 0 335 22028 2) Paperback
ISBN-13: 978 0 335 22029 8 (ISBN-10: 0 335 22029 0) Hardback

AN INTRODUCTION TO PUBLIC HEALTH AND EPIDEMIOLOGY
SECOND EDITION

Susan Carr, Nigel Unwin and Tanja Pless-Mulloli

The contents are not specifically nursing orientated but very neatly balanced to be of relevance to all working in the public health arena...the book is well written, the language is clear, and the concepts clearly and simply explained and easily understood

Journal of Biosocial Science

- What are epidemiology and public health?
- What is the nature of public health evidence and knowledge?
- What strategies can be used to protect and improve health?

The second edition of this bestselling book provides a multi-professional introduction to the key concepts in public health and epidemiology. It presents a broad, interactive account of contemporary public health, placing an emphasis on developing public health skills and stimulating the reader to think through the issues for themselves.

The new edition features additional material on:

- Historical perspectives
- Public health skills for practice
- Evaluation of public health interventions
- The nature of evidence and public health knowledge
- Translating policy and evidence into practice

An Introduction to Public Health and Epidemiology is key reading for students of public health and healthcare professionals, including: nurses, doctors, community development workers and public health workers.

Contents
Introduction – Lessons from the history of public health and epidemiology for the 21st century – Sources and critical use of health information – Measuring the frequency of health problems – Measures of risk – Epidemiological study designs – Weighing up the evidence from epidemiological studies – The determinants of health and disease – Health promotion – Health needs analysis – Principles of screening – Changing public health: What impacts on public health practice?

July 2007   192pp
ISBN-13: 978 0 335 21624 6 (ISBN-10: 0 335 21624 2) Paperback
ISBN-13: 978 0 335 21625 3 (ISBN-10: 0 335 21625 0) Hardback

COUNSELLING SKILL

John McLeod

- Does your job involve working with people?
- Do you know what to do when your clients or colleagues want to talk to you about difficult issues in their lives?
- Would you like to improve your ability to listen and help others?

This book is written for practitioners such as teachers, doctors, community workers, nurses and social workers, whose counselling role is embedded within other work functions. A framework is introduced, that allows the reader to draw on knowledge and competencies from their own personal and professional experience, as well as from a range of approaches to counselling, that will help them to help others.

The majority of people who seek help for personal issues do not consult specialist counsellors or psychotherapists, but instead look for support from people who are close to hand. In many instances, the counselling conversations that they have may last for no more than a few minutes. This book equips readers with methods and strategies for working effectively in such circumstances.

Counselling Skill outlines the abilities needed for counselling others – listening carefully, self-awareness, instillation of hope, being reliable and trustworthy, a capacity to engage with emotion – and suggests how these everyday skills may be used to help others to help themselves. In order to help those new to the ideas in the book, each chapter is supported by examples, as well as evidence from research studies.

This book is key reading for people working in helping, managing or supervisory roles: it provides efficient and ethical strategies that will improve their ability to assist or advise others. It is also of use to counsellors and counselling students who wish to develop a better understanding of their craft.

Contents
Preface – Introduction – Defining counselling – Basic principles of embedded counselling – The counselling menu: Goals, tasks and methods – Setting the scene: Preparation for offering a counselling relationship – Making a space to meet – Working collaboratively: Building a relationship – Having a useful conversation: 'Just talking' – Resolving difficult feelings and emotions – Learning to do something different: Working together to change behaviour – Dealing with difficult situations in counselling – Putting it all together – Doing good work – References – Index.

March 2007   288pp
ISBN-13: 978 0 335 21809 7 (ISBN-10: 0 335 21809 1) Paperback
ISBN-13: 978 0 335 21810 3 (ISBN-10: 0 335 21810 5) Hardback

SOCIAL POLICY FOR NURSES AND THE HELPING PROFESSIONS
SECOND EDITION

Stephen Peckham and Liz Meerabeau

- What is social policy and why is it relevant to nursing and other caring professions?
- How has the welfare state changed in response to new social problems?
- What roles do professionals and lay people play in providing welfare services?

This fully revised text is one of a series of books providing coherent and multi-disciplinary support for all client groups involved in the provision of health and social care. The book examines the relationship between welfare and health and includes discussion of key policy issues such as changes in health care delivery, regulation of professionals, privatisation, welfare pluralism and the tackling of health and social inequalities. The significance of social policy in preventing ill health and disability, as well as supporting the sick and disabled people, is emphasised throughout the book. This new edition is updated throughout and includes new chapters on:

- Health policy in the post-war period
- The role of health and social care professionals
- The future of social policy and health in the 21st century

Social Policy for Nurses and the Helping Professions equips students with a lively, readable and well-illustrated introduction to social policy. The reader is guided through the material with the help of chapter summaries, further reading and a glossary, as well as new examples and case studies to reflect the different client groups within nursing.

Contents
What is social policy? – The development of the welfare state – Health policy in the post war period – Poverty, inequality and social policy – Public health and health inequalities – Welfare pluralism – The mixed economy of community care – The changing role of the voluntary sector in the provision of social welfare – Lay perspectives and the role of informal care – The role of health and social care professionals – Social policy and health in the 21st century.

March 2007   304pp
ISBN-13: 978 0 335 21962 9 (ISBN-10: 0 335 21962 4) Paperback
ISBN-13: 978 0 335 21963 6 (ISBN-10: 0 335 21963 2) Hardback

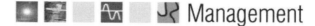
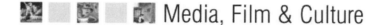
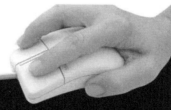
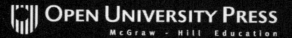